STUTTERING:
RESEARCH
AND
THERAPY

Under the Advisory Editorship of J. Jeffery Auer

STUTTERING: RESEARCH AND THERAPY

JOSEPH G. SHEEHAN

University of California, Los Angeles

Harper & Row, Publishers
New York, Evanston, and London

Stuttering: Research and Therapy

Copyright © 1970 by Joseph G. Sheehan

Printed in the United States of America. All rights reserved. No part of this book may be
used or reproduced in any manner whatsoever without written permission except in the
case of brief quotations embodied in critical articles and reviews. For information address
Harper & Row, Publishers, Inc., 49 East 33rd Street, New York, N.Y. 10016.

Library of Congress Catalog Card Number: 70-108410

CONTENTS

PREFACE

Human problems are largely communication problems. We grope for words to express our meanings and are never entirely satisfied with the result. Imperfect though they are, we can at least convert our word choices into speech. In that last sense, speaking is an easy process, and many are glib with nothing to say. But for the child or adult who has developed the problem called stuttering, the production of a spoken word can be fraught with dread and difficulty. The experience of stuttering is like a slice of life—a mixture of comedy and tragedy.

How can such a problem develop? What are its sources? What do we know about it? Why does it sometimes disappear? How can it be treated? These are just a few of the questions sifted in this book, in which we undertake an examination of the scientific contributions of the past and present, with a view toward the future.

Though the problem of stuttering has been the object of extensive research, and even more abundant speculation, many basic features remain mysterious. In an effort to reduce the mystery and to provide a broader base for future exploration, I have included contributions from disciplines most likely to add to our knowledge of stuttering.

In many respects this book is an effort to systematize, to accelerate the inflow of ideas from logically allied disciplines. Four distinguished colleagues have written chapters especially for this book. Reflected in the result, with inevitable overlap and underlap, are insights from clinical psychology, social psychology, anthropology and sociology, developmental psychology, physiology, behavior modification, research methodology, psychotherapy, and personality assessment. Despite the varied backgrounds of the contributors, and occasional differences in interpretation, the clinician seeking to help the stutterer will find scientifically sound information that is essential to success in treatment.

The Bibliography is a compilation by Charles Van Riper of references on stuttering from the years 1950 to 1970, providing a modern bridge to Elliott's earlier comprehensive bibliography. Throughout the book, chapter references that are given fully in the Bibliography appear by author and year only. In my judgment, the slight inconvenience of referring to two lists is more than outweighed by the value of making the Van Riper Bibliography available as a unit in itself.

Similarly, in Chapter 3 may be found extensive tables providing systematic comparisons of personality studies. While the resulting array makes for sometimes difficult reading, the compilation of these studies in one place provides a unique series of comparisons which should light the way for future researchers on the personality assessment of stutterers. While not presented in tabular form, the extensive summarizing of physiological studies in Chapter 5 serves an analogous function.

Many have contributed to the creation of this book in ways too varied to be fully acknowledged here. Special mention should be made of Waldo Coleman, Malcolm Fraser, Wendell Johnson, Margaret Martyn, Theodore Sarbin, Mimi Sheehan, Vivian Sheehan, and Charles Van Riper.

Finally, along with the contributing authors, I am indebted to the stutterers with whom I have worked. At our present level of knowledge, it may be said that in many ways they have taught us more than we have taught them.

This book is dedicated to stutterers of future generations, in the hope that treatment for them may be better than the treatment available to this generation, and that with the dawn of greater understanding there may be fewer of them.

JOSEPH G. SHEEHAN
Los Angeles, California
January, 1970

No man, for any considerable period, can wear one face to himself and another to the multitude, without finally getting bewildered as to which may be true.

Nathaniel Hawthorne

About the Author JOSEPH G. SHEEHAN, Ph.D., is Professor of Psychology, University of California, Los Angeles, and a Fellow of the American Psychological Association and the American Speech and Hearing Association. Diplomate in clinical psychology. Dr. Sheehan is a contributing author of *Psychopathology, A Source Book; Stuttering: A Symposium; Readings on the Exceptional Child: Research and Theory; Speech Therapy; Stuttering: Significant Theories and Therapies; Learning Theory and Stuttering Therapy; Stuttering and the Conditioning Therapies.* Also a series of seven booklets on stuttering co-authored by Dr. Sheehan has been published by the Speech Foundation of America. Dr. Sheehan was associate editor of the *Journal of Speech and Hearing Disorders* from 1958 to 1965, and associate editor of the *Journal* of the American Speech and Hearing Association *(Asha)* from 1963 to 1968. He is a contributor to professional periodicals including the *Journal of Abnormal Psychology,* the *Journal of Speech and Hearing Research,* and the *Journal of Speech and Hearing Disorders.*

About the Chapter Presented here for the first time is a systematic role-theory interpretation of stuttering, a theory of stuttering as a self-role conflict. Beginning with the observation that the stutterer is strikingly different depending on his role and that some can take part in plays when acting in nonself roles, this chapter develops more systematically the role-conflict interpretation of stuttering begun in presentations of the theory of stuttering as an approach-avoidance conflict. The role-conflict-theory interpretation of stuttering is logically harmonious with approach-avoidance conflict theory. The union of the role-theory model with the learning-theory model paves the way for a new integration of psychotherapy with "speech therapy."

The clinical result, as spelled out here and in Chapter 7, is an advanced form of behavior therapy.

1

ROLE-CONFLICT
THEORY

JOSEPH G. SHEEHAN

1

Stuttering is a disorder of the social presentation of the self. Basically, stuttering is not a speech disorder but a conflict revolving around self and role, an identity problem. In formal role-theory terms, stuttering is most clearly seen as a special instance of *self–role conflict*. As a disorder, stuttering appears to be *role-specific*, calling for a role-specific therapy, a role-taking psychotherapy.

The stutterer typically has no difficulty when alone—a striking and significant feature of the disorder. He can speak freely then, for communication with other human beings is not demanded. Even when with others, he is a stutterer only when he talks—an ancient joke that really tells us something important. For stuttering is role-specific behavior. It is specific to the speaker role and to the listener relationship. Just as it takes two to tango, it takes two to stutter. A listener, as well as a speaker, is required.

In roles removed from the self, as taking part in plays, adopting foreign dialects, using fluent asides, or in other false behavior, many stutterers can be dramatically fluent. Some have even become professional actors, able to speak with ease in character roles or as someone else. Yet, upon return to the self, for example, in saying his own name or in using self-referent words such as "I" or "my," the stutterer again becomes blocked.

As a self–role conflict, stuttering varies in accordance with two principal factors: (1) the self-variable—how the stutterer views himself, particularly in the speaker role, how he views his own status in the social situation requiring speech; (2) the role variable—how the "significant other," the listener or audience, is perceived.

Briefly stated, the foregoing is the central thesis of this chapter. What follows will be devoted to developing the theory of stuttering as a self–role conflict and to integrating therapeutic approaches logically derivative from this theory. Recent advances in role theory are here blended with equally significant advances in learning theory and clinical psychology to build a comprehensive theory and treatment of stuttering. The level of analysis is broad, many-faceted, and complex, resembling in these respects the disorder itself. The role-conflict theory of stuttering presented here is not designed to refute other theories of stuttering, or to imply that other approaches and other levels of analysis could not be employed with profit. Actually, within the pages of this book a variety of approaches flowing from other disciplines may be found.

Taking as its central thesis that stuttering is a role-specific conflict, this chapter seeks to explore the outer limits of a role-theory approach to stuttering. Reciprocally, the "goodness of fit" of the role model to a disorder as complex as stuttering may indicate possible gaps or needed revisions in role theory itself. However, the primary purpose is to build from the role model rather than to build upon it.

KEY CONCEPTS IN ROLE THEORY

Long ago, Plato wrote that people should only be permitted to read or to enact certain roles, because they become imprinted on the soul. In *As You Like It*, Shakespeare penned the famous lines that keynote the significance of role:

> All the world's a stage,
> And all the men and women merely players:
> They have their exits and their entrances;
> And one man in his time plays many parts.

Role theory has a sociological genealogy going back to Cooley (1902, 1909), Mead (1934), and Waller (1932, 1938), among others. In recent years, role theory has captured wider attention, especially from psychology and psychiatry. A popularized though primitive approach to role theory is reflected in Eric Berne's *Games People Play* (1964). Far more scholarly is Cameron's relating of certain role concepts to psychopathology in *The Psychology of the Behavior Disorders* (1947).

Among psychologists, the most comprehensive and systematic development of role theory is contained in the writings of Sarbin (1943, 1954, 1964, 1968), whose works provide the role model upon which this chapter is based. Also utilized is recent work by Goffman on identity, role distance, self-presentation, and stigma (1959, 1961, 1964). Noteworthy with reference to the identity concept are the writings of Erikson (1956) and Wheelis (1958).

According to Sarbin, all society is divided into groups, and these groups in turn are structured into positions or statuses or offices. Position is defined as a system of role expectations. "Roles are defined in terms of the actions performed by the person to validate his occupancy of the position."

Sarbin characterizes role theory in these terms:

> *Role theory attempts to conceptualize human conduct at a relatively complex level. In a sense it is an interdisciplinary theory in that its variables are drawn from studies of culture, society, and personality. The broad conceptual units of theory are* role, *the unit of culture;* position, *the unit of society; and* self, *the unit of personality.*

In understanding behavior in a role-theoretical sense, Sarbin proposed three chief variables: (1) the accuracy or validity of role perception—how well the person locates his position vis-à-vis that of the other; (2) skill in role enactment—how effective the person is in carrying out action systems or roles attached to positions; (3) organization of the self—how the person views himself, his self-concept. Sarbin (1954) writes:

> *Coordinate with role is the concept of self. Its origins and dimensions are described in cognitive terms. The ultimate units of the self are inferred qualities, the conceptualization of which is aided by the use of qualifying terms such as adjectives.*

An important dimension in any role enactment is the depth of self-involvement in the role.

The term "role-playing," which had been used by Moreno

(1946, 1961) and others, has acquired so much surplus meaning connoting superficiality that in this chapter it is restricted to role performance with low self-involvement. Role performance and role enactment are the broader generic terms. Role-taking implies an attitudinal stance, taking the role of the other.

Further delineation of role concepts from the point of view of the sociologist may be found in various writings in the Biddle and Thomas collection, *Role Theory: Concepts & Research* (1966). Lemert, in his chapter on stuttering in this book (Chapter 4), has employed various concepts related to role theory.

Though it places primary emphasis upon cognitive or perceptual terms, role theory is sufficiently broad to be compatible with other psychological systems such as learning theory or conflict principles or even certain parts of psychoanalytic theory.

A ROLE-CONFLICT MODEL

FOR STUTTERING

Stuttering runs on alternating current. A cyclic wavelike characteristic has been observed (Quarrington, 1956; Sheehan, 1969; Sitzman, 1968). Most of the words spoken by stutterers are spoken fluently, and it is typical for stutterers to have some situations in which they have little or no difficulty. Mild and moderate stutterers may handle most occasions with ease and have difficulty only in crucial situations.

In role-theory terms, there is a partial segregation of incompatible roles in stuttering. The stutterer is usually at least a part-time normal speaker. More precisely, most stutterers are just part-time occupants of that role. The experience of speaking normally may set up a role expectation for fluency, and actually lead to more stuttering. On the other hand, when the individual stutters and thereby enacts more fully the role of stutterer, the fear-producing role expectations for normal speech are diminished. In this manner enactment of the stutterer role leads to fluency, and vice versa. Combining role theory with the double approach-avoidance conflict model, we may illustrate and understand the alternating character of the stutterer's roles:

Figure 1 shows that there are approach-avoidance tendencies for both the stutterer role and the normal-speaker role. Each becomes a feared goal. The typical behavior in such a double approach-avoidance conflict is a pendulum-like alternation. We

7

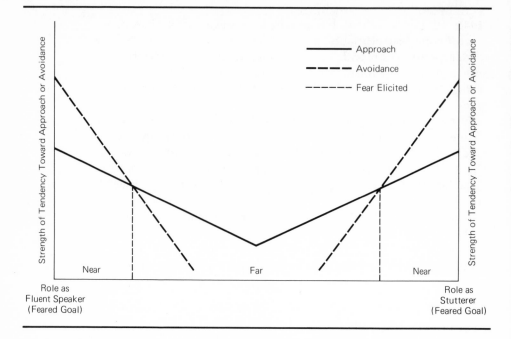

Figure 1   *Role Competition in Double Approach-Avoidance Conflict*

also observe in Figure 1 that most of the difficulty lies in the middle zone where the stutterer role is uncertain. In this region he does not know whether to act like a stutterer or a normal speaker; he does not know what his likely role will be.

We can deduce from the model that there are two apparently opposite ways out of stuttering. One is to be a normal speaker all the way, to wash the stutterer aspect out of the self-concept. Usually this route is available only to young children in whom the development of stuttering has not gone very far. The other way out of stuttering, that which must typically be employed by adolescents and adults, is to become a stutterer all the way, through self-acceptance in this role. Yet even this must be experienced as a mixture of roles, for every stutterer is a part-time normal speaker, and must learn to adjust to himself as a fluent speaker as well (Sheehan, 1954a).

The cyclic variation commonly observed in stuttering (Quarrington, 1956; Sheehan, 1969) may well be understood in relation to the role-conflict model shown in Figure 1 as an alternation of roles following a conflict principle.

THE ROLE OF ROLE IN STUTTERING

Stuttering behavior changes with role change, in turn a self–other change, as noted in earlier writing:

> . . . the occurrence of stuttering is in part a
> function of the relationship between the stut-
> terer and his listener. Some stutterers experi-
> ence no fear when they play a dominant role.
> One may give a fluent public address but stut-
> ter to individuals in the audience before and
> afterward. A child may block severely before
> one parent but speak easily to the other. An
> army enlisted man could never say "sergeant"
> until he became one but he still stuttered on
> "lieutenant," on "sir," and on the titles of all
> the higher ranks. The fact that many stutterers
> can act in plays seems to show the effect of
> changed role.

STUTTERING AS
ROLE-SPECIFIC BEHAVIOR

In many respects, stuttering is role-specific behavior (Shee-han, 1968). It is specific to the speaker role and the listener role. Here are instances to illustrate role-specificity of stuttering.

First, there is the story about the stutterer who read in a magazine about a commercial school that promised a cure. After attending this school and coming back, his friends asked him to say something. He said triumphantly, "Peter Piper picked a peck of pickled peppers." His friends said, "That's great! We never heard you speak like that." He replied, "Y-y-y-yes, b-b-b-b-but it s-s-s-sure is hard to w-w-w-w-w-work that into the c-c-c-c-conversation!" This familiar story does illustrate something significant about the problem. Both stuttering and fluency may be quite role-specific, so that experience in speaking fluently in one role does not automatically beget fluency in another.

To cite another example, one stutterer reported that he had always spoken fluently with his landlady whom he knew quite well in the landlady role. She was unaware that he stuttered and had no conception of the magnitude of his difficulty in some situations. The revelation came when she took a tempo-

9

rary position as a registrar of voters, and he had to give his name, address, and vital statistics about himself to her as she occupied that new status. He reported that she was astonished and so embarrassed that it was a most difficult situation for him. After she relinquished the registrar role, he again saw her in the landlady role. He was able to explain to her, again quite fluently, what had happened. There was no evident transfer of difficulty from the registrar-listener role back to the landlady-listener role.

You stutter to the role, not to the person temporarily occupying the role. And roles are attached to positions, to statuses, not to the person momentarily enacting the role. Stuttering varies both with the role of the speaker and with the role of the listener. Perhaps stuttering is a role disorder primarily, and an interpersonal relations disorder only secondarily. Difficulty with certain classes of persons branches out from the positions they occupy and the roles they perform, not necessarily from their individual personal characteristics.

To illustrate the high degree of role-specificity of stuttering, we may even cite Kinsey:

> *During sexual arousal, inhibitions and psycho-logical blockages are relieved or completely eliminated. A considerable series of histories indicates that stutterers are not likely to stutter when they are with a companion to whom they are sexually responsive."* (Kinsey et al., 1953)

This intriguing observation may point the way to a really exciting new kind of role-taking therapy, but to our knowledge it has never been attempted except on a rather unsystematic basis.

Speech is one of the principal means of social self-presentation, and stuttering is a role-specific self-presentation disorder. Sexual arousal and responsiveness entail presentation of self to a very involved and intimate degree. Sexual self-presentation may also be quite role-specific and, as we know, does not always require expertise in the speaker role. In a situation where the speaker role is subordinated and the self is brought forward more positively, stuttering is likely to decrease. With respect to the sexual role, the stutterer does not always have to speak for himself, like John Alden, in order to gain acceptance.

Three other illustrations highlight the importance of self-regard and body-image along with role-specificity. A girl with a plain face but an attractive figure reported complete relief from her stuttering when she joined a nudist colony. Her new speech freedom persisted after she returned to the world of the clothed. She stated that she now felt differently about herself. For many females, stuttering appears as a stigma preventing fulfillment of the feminine role. Change can of course come about in a variety of ways; this girl's recipe for success might not be appropriate to most female stutterers!

A veteran with whom we worked, a tall, handsome fellow with a somewhat dapper moustache, was proud of his exploits with the opposite sex, with whom he was a very smooth talker. He could pick up girls in bars or elsewhere without the slightest trace of hesitant speech. Yet in the role of job-seeker attempting interviews with prospective employers or personnel men he was unable to give his name and had to resort to paper and pencil to answer questions. He was one kind of speaker with girls and quite another kind with male authority figures. Never did the twain meet—a vivid example of role specificity.

Two telephones sat on the desk of a physician who stuttered severely on one but spoke fluently on the other. How could such a situation come about? The explanation was simple, though it involved different roles, a self-esteem threat, and an identity problem. The phone he found difficult had been on the desk when he had taken over the practice of a physician who had cheated him in the process. Whenever he answered the old phone he felt a blend of resentment at having been cheated and envy of his predecessor's smooth speech. He had installed the second phone himself in the hope that it would be easier, and it was. Even though he knew why the old phone bothered him he continued to have trouble on it. Finally he resolved the problem by taking out the old phone entirely and replacing it with a second new phone.

Role-specificity is a master key to the understanding of stuttering. When stuttering is seen as role-specific behavior, as behavior conditioned to the speaker role, then prevention and treatment should focus on the speaker role. The concept of stuttering as a nonunitary disorder accords well with role-specificity in treatment. If stuttering is role-specific, then stutterers should not have to differ in personality structure or on some physiological basis—as indeed they do not (see Sheehan, Chapter 3, and Perkins, Chapter 5).

Treatment may be problem-specific, a specialized role-taking therapy for stutterers rather than a general psychotherapy. The changes to be made by stutterers are role changes, specifically in terms of the speaker role and the listener relationship.

Both feeling and motor aspects of the needed role-change

11

in stuttering have to be handled in therapy. The stutterer has to change how he feels and what he does, yet not necessarily in that order. If anything, the order is usually reversed—the stutterer is changed by what he does, by successive experiences.

THE RELATIONSHIP
OF SELF AND ROLE IN STUTTERING

We have observed that stutterers can take part in plays as a result of changed role and changed position of the self. These cases may be cited:

One severe stutterer became a professional actor, taking various roles on the stage and on television. He even developed children's puppet shows, taking the voices of each puppet. As he explained it, the characters had nothing to do with his own voice, they had nothing to do with himself. He could step into these nonself roles, as Sarbin calls them, and meet the role demands quite easily. However, even in the midst of these activities he would still stutter when speaking as himself. The actor got along well in such detached-from-self roles until he fell under what proved to be the subversive influence of the Stanislavsky school of acting. Instead of the old acting from "without," he began acting from "within," bringing himself into his stage roles (Stanislavsky, 1938). His stage fluency fell apart on a certain dramatic occasion when he had to enact the role of an anxious expectant father who had a defect— color-blindness. When called upon to say, "Doctor, I have a defect," he thought of his own defect, lost his fluency, and stuttered severely on the word "defect," which, of course, so significantly referred to himself and his feelings about his stuttering.

The involvement of stuttering with the self is shown dramatically in the fact that most stutterers have difficulty with their names, their addresses, their occupations, the names of their families, the significant personal pronoun "I," and other self-referent terms. Some stutterers even use aliases. One stutterer spent most of his army career on K.P. because he could not answer at roll call. Whenever called upon to introduce himself, he would choose among a variety of aliases. He could always be "someone else" and be fluent, so long as he wasn't identifying himself.

Non-self roles used as devices in stuttering may at this point be summarized as follows: (1) taking part in a play; (2) becoming a professional entertainer; (3) adopting foreign dialects; (4) assuming false confidence; (5) "hamming" a social situation; (6) drinking to feel "high"; (7) using props or bystander; (8) murmuring unnecessary asides; and (9) using mannerisms to distract listener and disguise stuttering.

A STATUS-GAP HYPOTHESIS

The role-specific nature of the conflict in stuttering—a conditioned speaker-listener disorder—may be further illustrated by means of a "status-gap" hypothesis.

When alone, that is, when not in social interaction with "significant others" (Mead, 1934), stuttering is either markedly reduced or completely absent (Adler, 1929). When the interpersonal relationships are markedly changed, then the behavior called stuttering changes with them.

As behavior, stuttering is predictable to a high degree from the relative status of speaker and listener. When the perceived status of the speaker is low relative to that of the audience, stuttering tends to be severe. When the stutterer speaks to a peer figure, as to another stutterer or a close friend, stuttering tends to be moderate. And when the stutterer feels high in self-esteem, as by the intoxicating effects of love, or of alcohol, or of observable success, and feels no awe of the listener, he speaks with comparative fluency. What Sarbin calls "role demand" appears to operate at these three levels.

Therapy with stutterers, as all psychotherapy, should aim at enhancing the individual's self-esteem, self-respect, or self-concept, while reducing the awesomeness or fear-eliciting properties of the audience, to use Goffman's term (1959, 1961, 1964), or of significant others, to use Mead's (1934).

THE ICEBERG OF SHAME AND GUILT

Shame is the public failure of a role expectation. The private equivalent is called guilt. When the stutterer attempts to deny his stuttering behavior and to represent himself as a fluent speaker (which he is part of the time), he then creates tensions relating to fear of failure of the role expectation.

Stuttering may be likened to an iceberg, with the major portion below the surface. What people see and hear is the smaller portion; much greater is that which lies below the surface, experienced as fear, guilt, and anticipation of shame. For an adult or an adolescent mature enough to tolerate it, public presentation of the self as a stutterer has major therapeutic effects. The portion of the iceberg exposed to the sunlight of public view melts away more quickly. In Figure 2 we have presented a schema of the relationship between covert and overt aspects of stuttering.

To a large extent, stuttering is a false-role disorder. Without the tricks, crutches, and other false-role behaviors, very little stuttering would remain.

Stuttering appears to involve a certain amount of resistance to self-disclosure (cf. Jourard, 1964). In attempting to hide his identity as a stutterer, the person resorts to false-role or "crutch" behaviors which are intermittently successful and therefore periodically reinforced. Whether successful or not, the stutterer's crutches and other false-role behaviors lead to guilt. Misrepresentation of self to others is always productive of guilt, and the stutterer is no exception.

At least three sources of guilt may be identified: (1) originating guilt, stemming from the origins of each individual's particular case of stuttering, that is, from his route to becoming a stutterer; (2) false-role guilt, resulting from crutches and avoidance devices used to fool listeners; and (3) audience-reaction guilt, a byproduct of the stutterer's knowledge that his speech is distressing to his listeners.

Figure 2 illustrates schematically both the primarily covert character of stuttering and the effect on the total handicap of avoiding by covering up and hiding of self. The stutterer may reduce the guilt portion by working on the shame portion—the open display of oneself in the stutterer role. Among adult therapy techniques directed toward this goal are discussion of stuttering, maintaining eye contact, introduction of oneself as a stutterer, freely given references to receiving therapy, stuttering easily and openly, and building safety margin or showing more disfluency publicly than necessary.

The occurrence of stuttering translates guilt into shame. The stutterer who has been trying to cover up is now forced by his effort to speak to emerge into the open to a certain extent. But shame is more hopeful than guilt; it is a more public, interpersonal event. By experiencing his stuttering, a stutterer can get over his shame. By getting more of the stuttering behavior above the surface, the total amount of fear and handicap may be reduced.

To summarize, the stutterer needs to convert his guilt experiences into shame experiences, for shame reactions can be reconditioned or extinguished but private guilt goes on forever

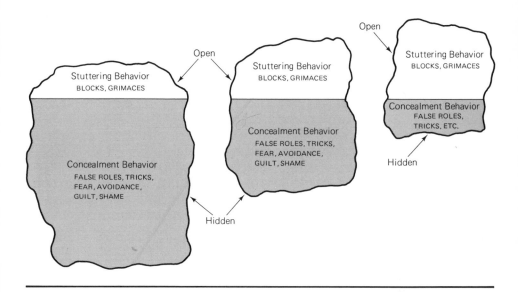

Figure 2 *The Iceberg of Stuttering*

(Mowrer, 1968). The shame above must come to equal the guilt below, so that both may ultimately vanish.

CONCEALMENT

OF STUTTERING FROM THE SELF

An interesting and significant byproduct of the stutterer's concealment of the problem from himself is a narrowing of the cognitive and perceptual field—characteristic behavior of all organisms when high on the avoidance gradient. Under increased motivation, the fine discriminations required in speech may break down. This may be one reason the stutterer so frequently is found stuttering on the wrong sound or continuing to stutter on sounds and words he has already spoken successfully (Sheehan, 1946).

Every time the stutterer has a block, he is reliving one of his most significant experiences—that of finding himself blocked and unable to express himself through speech. He falls victim to many reactions typical of persons undergoing severe emotional stress. During the block, he may come to have a kind of tunnel vision. A professional man with a gift of verbal expression describes this stress-induced egocentricity. **15**

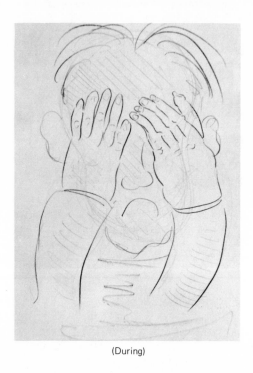

(During)

Figure 3   *Graphic Projection of Stuttering*

When I'm in the situation, I lose all contact with the world around me. I'm completely riveted on this one thing—on my struggles with the stammering. Along with that, there is a real feeling of anxiety and a feeling of real tension. Following it, there is a reduction in the tension, a feeling of embarrassment and shame—almost a feeling of relief that the act is over. Coming up to the stammering, there is an increasing anxiety and tension, which I try to escape from and avoid. And when it occurs, I've gotten myself into a trap that I can't avoid, and must plow through. That probably is fairly typical of my stammering pattern. The stammering itself is interesting in that I'm not aware of anything that is going on around me—surrounding peo-

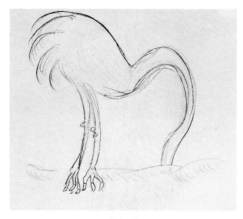

(After)

Figure 4 *Graphic Projection of Stuttering*

> ple, or their expressions or reactions; I'm only
> concentrating on my own struggles . . . . The
> same kind of oblivion that comes during a block
> also comes during moments of anger or great
> fear.

The detachment of stuttering from the self is even more
richly illustrated in the accompanying figures, taken from drawings representing behavior before, during and after the moment
of stuttering (Sheehan, Cortese, & Hadley, 1962).

Another drawing from the same study reflects perception of
self as cast in the role of clown when stuttering.

STUTTERING AND

COGNITIVE DISSONANCE

Why should the stutterer alter his perceptions during the
moment of stuttering? Why should he cover up stuttering from
himself? The theory of cognitive dissonance (Festinger, 1957)
may give us new understanding of the stutterer's self-imposed
blindness.

According to dissonance theory, the person attempts to maintain a balance in his perceptions, including, in the case just
cited, self-perceptions. Discordant perceptions are reduced by

17

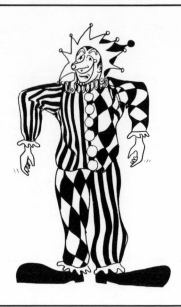

Figure 5   *A Stutterer's Self-Perception*

cognitive shift. The attempt to deny the stutterer role is highly discrepant with the actual occurrence of stuttering behaviors, that is, the blocks and the experiencing of stuttering. Therefore stuttering tends not to be experienced as other things might be experienced, with perceptual clarity. As a result, he loses the kind of perceptual feedback that he needs to regulate his speaking behavior effectively. He develops an incapacity to observe his stuttering behavior. He shields himself from the stutterer role in a fashion that is truly ostrichlike (see Figure 5). In therapy it is important to stress, as a part of self-acceptance in the stutterer role, the need to "experience" the moment of stuttering as fully as possible—to see, hear and feel the stuttering vividly. This process we call "monitoring."

A SELF-PRESENTATION DISORDER

If stuttering is a self–role conflict, a disorder of the social presentation of the self, then in what respects is it a speech disorder? To be sure, speech is involved, in fact so much involved that, except when functioning as himself in the speaker role, the stutterer is not different from anyone else. Personality comparisons and other comparisons of stutterers and normal speakers consistently yield no differences except on the level of aspiration measure. However, level of aspiration is very much a function of the self; in fact, it may be regarded as one of the measures of self-esteem and self-perception (Sheehan & Zelen, 1955; Zelen, Sheehan, & Bugental, 1954; Sheehan, Chapter 3 in this book).

To the puzzle of whether stuttering is a speech disorder should be added this—that most stutterers speak fluently most of the time. Stuttering is unlike other speech disorders in that the stutterer speaks wih complete normality on occasion and, in fact, on most words he utters. Contrast this with cleft-palate speech or speech associated with hearing loss or severe articulatory disorders. To be sure, those with psychogenic voice disorders do sometimes produce normal speech—typically, with some significant shift in their life situation. So, perhaps some voice disorders are not truly speech disorders, either, though the shift to completely normal speaking is much rarer than in stuttering. Stuttering is dramatically more intermittent than any other speech disorder. The stutterer does not have to be taught how to speak, or anything whatever about speech per se.

ROLE-SPECIFICITY IN STUTTERING THERAPY

Just as stuttering is a problem that occurs in a social milieu, so it is to be treated in a social context. It is striking that nearly all modern therapies devised for stuttering—even among authorities who insist on a constitutional factor or a predisposition to stuttering, e.g., West (1958) or Eisenson (1958)—have been socially oriented therapies. Whatever the belief held by any authority concerning the cause of stuttering, the therapy tends to have a social, interpersonal character.

Speech therapy for stutterers is so unique among speech therapies that in many respects it is not speech therapy at all. Among the most commonly utilized and widely accepted techniques of working with adult and adolescent stutterers are: (1) keeping eye contact with the listener; (2) accepting openly the role of stutterer; (3) advertising oneself as a stutterer; (4) discussing stuttering; (5) entering feared situations; (6) changing attitudes to effect a reduction of shame, hatred, embarrassment, guilt; (7) resisting time pressure; (8) stuttering on pur-

19

pose; (9) developing a new style or pattern of stuttering; and (10) learning to stutter smoothly, easily, and even fluently. Only in a very limited sense do these techniques involve speech. Basically they are social interaction methods. Along with all these techniques must be a high amount of social reinforcement from the therapist and significant others if the therapy is to progress. Krasner's notion of the therapist as a social-reinforcement machine seems to apply here (Krasner, 1965).

A ROLE-TAKING PSYCHOTHERAPY

Most of what we call speech therapy for stutterers is, in reality, a role-taking psychotherapy. The logical models are those of role theory, learning theory, and behavior-modification therapy. It is noteworthy that Eysenck (1960), a famous skeptic as to the effects of psychotherapy, has suggested that the field of psychotherapy could learn much from what is done with stutterers. The journal edited by Eysenck and Rachman (1965), *Behaviour Research and Therapy,* has given substantial attention to the problem of stuttering. Moreover, what London (1964) has inaccurately called "action therapy" bears a striking resemblance to "speech therapy" for stutterers. The role-specificity of treatment in stuttering is better captured in the preferable term "stuttering therapy," despite its clumsiness— that is, it can be misread "the therapy stutters." Why not? Sometimes it does!

In working with stutterers, the author has long offered this challenge:

> *You are changed by what you do. Not by what*
> *you think about, read about, or talk about, but*
> *by what you actually do.*

Though the foregoing motto was empirically devised, as a result of experience working clinically, it is interesting that the concept is similar to that to be found in the writings of existentialists:

> *Feeling is formed by the deeds that one does. . . .*

> *Man . . . exists only in so far as he realizes*
> *himself, he is therefore nothing else but the sum*
> *of his actions." (Sartre, 1956)*

It is also striking that role-taking therapy for stutterers has anticipated to a high degree two of the prevailing influences on current psychotherapy, *viz.*, existentialist philosophy and behavior-modification therapy.

"STUTTERING THERAPY" AS A SPECIALIZED PSYCHOTHERAPY

The field of psychotherapy has moved increasingly toward emphasis on experiencing, toward the here and now, and toward action orientation. This trend is evident, in sharply different forms, both from growing emphasis on values and existential concerns, and from the population explosion of behavior modification techniques.

How do we change? The insight model which issued from the work of Freud and Breuer on the kind of hysterics that abounded in turn-of-the-century Vienna is much more difficult to apply to today's problems and today's therapy procedures. In our view, psychotherapy may be seen as a process of role-taking, just as disordered behavior may be seen in terms of role-taking deficiencies. Our thesis is that role change precedes insight and brings about changes in the perception of the self as a by-product. What has come to be called "stuttering therapy" may exemplify this point.

When stuttering therapy is seen as a specialized psychotherapy, some of the haunting concerns of the speech clinician about offering symptomatic treatment are abated. Particularly, our theory of stuttering as an approach-avoidance conflict permits integration of psychotherapy with speech therapy, since reduction of avoidance is an essential feature of each.

To this view, we now add that stuttering is a false-role disorder which is to be treated by the recognition and elimination of false roles, and by the process of experiencing through a role-taking therapy, with a consequent feedback upon the self (Sheehan, 1968; Sarbin, 1964). In these respects what we call stuttering therapy lies at the very heart of psychotherapeutic experience.

What do we mean by "stuttering therapy"? The operations and techniques as applied to adult therapy have been reasonably well spelled out, with numerous examples and some accompanying rationale, in the booklet, *On Stuttering and Its Treatment* (Speech Foundation of America, 1960). Some of the special problems dealing with adolescents and children, with further examples of stuttering therapy techniques, are given in another booklet, *Treatment of the Young Stutterer in the Schools*

21

(Speech Foundation of America, 1964). These publications emphasize practical aspects of therapy, and represent clinical agreement among a fairly diverse group of specialists on the problem of stuttering. They illustrate well the principle that divergence in theory tends to exceed that in therapy, despite a number of differences of importance.

To summarize this section: In the treatment of stuttering, psychotherapy and speech therapy may be combined in varying degrees. In a broad sense, there is some psychotherapy in every clinical interaction. Speech therapists are psychotherapists of a special kind. That word does not belong to the bearded analysts or to the individuals who practice therapy privately in the cloister of the couch. What we have called speech therapy with stutterers is really a behavior therapy, a social relations therapy, a psychotherapy through action—in short, a role therapy.

THERAPY DIRECTIONS
FROM ROLE THEORY

When stuttering is viewed as a self–role conflict, twin aspects of therapy are brought into focus. The needed changes in the self include attitude work, change in the feeling of the stutterer. Role changes required include ease in entering feared situations, modification of the stuttering pattern, elimination of false-role devices or crutches, and acquisition of a new role as a self-accepting, fluent stutterer. Success in therapy then depends upon improved perception of self development of skill in role enactment, and positive growth in self-concept resulting from feedback of role enactment upon the self.

In the case of adult therapy, the result is a person who accepts himself and adjusts freely to either the stutterer role or the alternating normal-speaker role, who struggles minimally against himself when he stutterers and who feels freedom and comfort in the speaker role whether he stutters or not. Combination of self-acceptance with role acceptance leads to freedom and ease in the speaker role, with prevalent fluency as the ultimate product.

FEEDBACK OF PROLONGED
ROLE-ENACTMENT ON THE SELF

How is it that enacting roles can change anyone? After all, we all carry out roles all the time. Some people "go through the motions" or indulge in role-playing in the most limited sense of the term. Such behaviors typically are detached from any central concept of the self, and have little or no permanent impact. Yet prolonged role enactment with self-involvement does result in changes in self-concept (Sarbin, 1964).

Role-taking and role-enactment are not to be confused with role-playing, a more superficial term typically connoting non-involvement of the self. Whether role-taking therapy with stutterers, inappropriately called "speech assignments" is effective hinges largely on the degree of self-involvement in the enactment of the assigned role.

If a person enacts new roles consistently over a period of time with high self-involvement, he is thereby changed, and his self-concept changes. Evidence for the effect of prolonged role enactment on the self has been cogently presented by Sarbin (1954).

Again, this is consistent with the motto that you are changed by what you do, changed by experience. And what is experience, except the assumption of ever-changing and new roles in interaction with significant others with consequent feedback upon the self? It is striking that modern psychotherapists such as Rogers (1961) and Gendlin (1968) increasingly emphasize "becoming," "experiencing," and the realization of the potentialities of the self.

That self, role, and identity factors so dramatically influence the behavior known as stuttering should not really be too astonishing when the reciprocal roles of speaker and listener are considered. In his formulation on ego identity, Erikson (1956) writes:

> *Take for example a child who is learning to speak; he is acquiring one of the prime functions supporting a sense of individual autonomy and one of the prime techniques for expanding the radius of give-and-take. . . . Speech not only commits him to the kind of voice he has and to the mode of speech he develops; it also defines him as one responded to by those around him with changed diction and attention. . . . Thus the child may come to develop, in the use of voice and word, a particular combination of whining or singing, judging or arguing, as part of a new element of the future identity, namely, the element 'one who speaks and is spoken to in such-and-such a way.'*

23

In the stutterer we have a person who knows how to speak, who has uttered normally most words he has spoken in his life, and who has available to him at any moment the capacity for speaking as fluently as anyone else. When alone, or when not himself due to role assumption or inebriation, he exercises his normal speech capacity easily. But under the impact of a decline in self-esteem, an increase in the emotional loading of the utterance, or an increase in the authority and awesomeness of the listener (Sheehan, Hadley, & Gould, 1967), he becomes a different person. Not multiple personality, but rather role-conflict specificity is the central process here.

ROLE ACCEPTANCE VERSUS "FAKING"

Since stuttering is so largely a false-role disorder, it is remarkable that one of the most widely recommended techniques has been called "faking" or pretending to stutter. Is there not too much pretense in the stutterer already? Why increase it by teaching him to fake still more? The trouble with the faking of stutterers is that it is just too fake.

The concept of role-taking with varying levels of self-involvement is useful here. Semantically, the unhappy term "faking" should be supplanted by "voluntary stuttering," which does not have to be fake at all. "Going through the motions" or role-playing the stuttering behavior without self-involvement is illusory and essentially useless, as many of our stutterers and our own common sense tell us. The crucial issue is the genuineness of the role enactment. Nearly the same outward behavior may be accompanied by either high or low self-involvement. Many stutterers show resistance by refusing to perform assigned roles; others by going through the motions in the most superficial, false, and contemptuous way possible. When the stutterer is told to fake stuttering, he may do just that, and the results are as fleeting as the performance.

How can you get a stutterer to stutter with acceptance of the role? *Experiencing* is the key. The stutterer needs to feel his stuttering, to monitor avidly, to experience vividly. In this way he may undo the repression with which he has concealed his stuttering from himself. If he monitors faithfully and experiences fully everything he does when he stutters, with appreciation that *he is doing the doing*, that it is his behavior and not just something that is happening to him, then he will begin to drop the false mannerisms automatically.

ROLE ACCEPTANCE VERSUS "CONTROL"

The acquisition of fluency in stuttering should come about indirectly, through the reduction of avoidance, through being open, through accepting the role of a stutterer. Anything that the stutterer has to do in a special or direct way to "achieve fluency" is probably wrong.

It is a salient feature of stuttering that the stutterer is forever trying to "control" his speech. This is one of the chief ways in which he differs from the normal speaker. The efforts at control used by stutterers are typically suppressive, taking the form of covering up, putting more of the iceberg under the surface, and using tricks, crutches, and false-role behaviors. The control problem probably goes back to the origins of stuttering. Initially unaware of hesitancies, the stutterer is corrected by parents and others. The awareness in and of itself does not produce harmful effects, except that it frequently leads to efforts to control, a major fallacy underlying both development and continuation of the disorder.

Let us consider a parallel to walking, which is, like speech, another acquired skill, and typically operates under what the neurologists call automatic associated function. If we tried to control walking in the same way the stutterer tries to control his talking, a very awkward gait would result. In England over a hundred years ago, James Hunt propounded a theory of stuttering as a conscious interference with an unconscious process. He taught the stutterer to speak consciously, without dodge or trick, as he would ordinarily speak unconsciously (Hunt, 1863). It is interesting that stutterers are able to utter asides and other pat phrases quite fluently. Offhand remarks typically do not involve any special effort to speak and do not involve any "control of stuttering." One stutterer, in trying to read a passage beginning with "I," was unable to get started at all. After several struggling, abortive half-attempts, she looked up in mock futility and said, "I can't say that," uttering in the process the very word that she had been unable to use in a different context. She was astonished when told that she had said in her aside the same word, "I," that she was trying to control. For her, the "I" which began the fluent aside posed no challenge. She made no special effort to say it. The set that the stutterer has toward the act of speaking does much to perpetuate his stuttering. Once the girl gave up the special set and the efforts to control, to keep from stuttering when saying "I," she was able to say it quite fluently.

25

To give up efforts at control, the stutterer can oversatisfy the fear. He can create a safety margin, therefore enjoying periods of fluency as a by-product. But fluency does not beget fluency; it does not lead anywhere. The stutterer may enjoy it, may wallow in it, but it is not productive for the future.

The effort to exert conscious control is a root cause of stuttering. If a child stutters very early, usually there is a conscious effort to control. How do you get away from it? To return to the example of walking as a parallel, suppose people begin to laugh and stare at the way you walk? You begin to exert conscious efforts to control your gait, to put one foot in front of the other, etc. Can you resist the audience pressure and go ahead and walk along naturally, go about your other business? That is what a stutterer needs to do about his talking. Can a stutterer give up conscious efforts at directing the mechanics of speech? A stutterer often has to force himself, to make a conscious effort to go ahead, because he is overmotivated to avoid any appearance of disfluency.

SAFETY MARGIN
AND NATURAL FLUENCY

One way a person can become comfortable about his stuttering, and define himself operationally and vividly as a stutterer, is to use a voluntary stuttering technique such as a bounce or a slide. There are, however, some problems in connection with these techniques in ordinary clinical use. In a study comparing use of the bounce and slide and the imitation of true pattern, Sheehan and Voas (1957) found that imitating the true stuttering pattern reinforces stuttering and increases frequency of blocks. However, using a slide on nonfeared words just before the feared word seems to bring about faster adaptation, to bring about improvement. This result offers experimental support for the concept of the "safety margin." Most important, the slide should be used on nonfeared words rather than on feared words. When used primarily on feared words, the slide can be misused as a kind of control technique. Then the slide becomes a crutch, a way to keep from touching the moment of stuttering, a way to avoid the basic self-confrontation that the stutterer needs. Far better for the stutterer to open up, to monitor, and to let the monitoring process lead naturally to the corrections that follow automatically from monitoring. The stutterer should not have to try to change his pattern too much. He merely needs to develop awareness of it to end the covering up of his stuttering from himself. The most important cover-up in stuttering is not the covering up from others but the concealment from self.

One of the difficulties of the control concept is that without the effort to control his speech the stutterer would probably be able to speak quite naturally and normally. Stuttering is something the stutterer does because he tries very hard not to. The end result of therapy should not be a form of controlled speaking but a form of natural speaking. The end goal is not watching himself all the time but getting beyond that point. It is important to teach the stutterer that speech therapy does not have to be something interminable. He does not want to spend he rest of his life controlling something that really is not there (Williams, 1957).

A DISORDER OF
STARTING AND STOPPING

Stuttering is not just a difficulty of starting; for many stutterers it is a difficulty of terminating. The more severe the stutterer, the more trouble he has getting started, and the more trouble he has getting stopped. An aspect of listening to a severe stutterer that exasperates many people is that he never seems to know when to stop, as hope sags that each next word will be the stutterer's last. Why should this be? Why should one who struggles so hard for each word go on endlessly, because he rations his efforts so poorly? Three hypotheses are offered for this clinically observed phenomenon:

First, since most trouble is experienced at the beginning, the stutterer becomes conditioned to fear silence. Avoidance of silence, or a kind of filibustering is a prominent behavior in stuttering. The stutterer spends much of his time stuttering on crutch words or phrases not needed at all. Silence is avoided as well as speech—this is the other side of the double approach-avoidance conflict (Sheehan, 1958a).

Second, the stutterer keeps on keeping on because previous experience in situational adaptation leads him to be optimistic, to hope that he may get better if he will just keep going. From the studies of adaptation effect it is easy to make this inference. Direct evidence for this interpretation is contained in a study of level of aspiration for fluency (Sheehan, 1963). Severe stutterers were found to show the greatest discrepancies between their performance and their subsequent predictions of degree of fluency, while mild stutterers set more realistic fluency goals and predicted more modest performances. The severe stutterer keeps trying the long shot. His efforts show the triumph of faith over experience.

Third, in severe cases a syntactical disorganization becomes part of the problem. Because the severe stutterer is forever gambling that some phrases may be easier than others, he is constantly shifting, until his sentences become elaborate, stilted, pedantic, or Germanic. His word choices form a Markov chain —a pattern of dependent probability. From word substitution and phrase revision emerges a constant rearrangement of the syntax.

In role theory terms, the severe stutterer shows a compulsion to continue because he has experienced the role of stutterer and is trying to deny it. From Figure 1, depicting the alternating roles of stutterer and normal speaker, it may be seen that enactment of the stutterer role, or absorption in it, leads to an avoidance of that role and an inclination toward the normal speaker role. From the cyclic variation principle, as well as from previous experience in situational adaptation, he may anticipate that he will get better as he goes along. At least, in the gambling psychology of stuttering, stepping back into the normal speaker role is an attractive possibility. Hence, he continues, using filibustering devices such as "uh," or "well," to hold the floor against any interruption threat. To the audience, it always seems as though he is making agonizing decisions to continue beyond necessity.

What are the implications for therapy? The stutterer needs to learn to stutter forward. He needs to go ahead on every originally selected word, without regard to anticipated difficulty. Damn the torpedoes—full speed ahead! This could be every stutterer's motto. Successful avoidance, either word substitution or phrase revision, reinforces the instrumental acts leading to further avoidance, and increases the reservoir of fear. The eventual confrontation with feared words and situations is rendered more difficult. We have never known a stutterer in the clinic who successfully overcame the problem while persisting in word avoidances.

The filibustering behavior of stutterers leads to a failure of normal phrasing, to dead stops before each feared word, and to a robot-like pattern in the speech of many severe stutterers. As a therapy measure, it is often necessary to teach the stutterer that English words are not spoken one at a time with spaces in between as in writing, but are spoken as integrated portions of phrase units. By this we do not mean "phrasing" and "blending" as these have typically been used in speech therapy, merely as devices to avoid stuttering.

Rather, the stutterer can be taught to risk and to court the fear of silence, by permitting pauses in his speech. Pauses to built up fear, not to avoid possible blocks. Pauses to permit the stutterer sufficient breath so that he is not trying to force out words on residual air. When this is accompanied by "safety margin" through exercise of voluntary stuttering or tolerated disfluency, the change in the stutterer's phrasing can result in striking improvement. Moreover, pausing helps the stutterer resist pressure from the audience and to reject the self-imposed time pressure set (Sheehan, 1958; Stunden, 1965).

The time pressure set is one important source of the inability to terminate, for it is related to the syntactical disorganization, the fear of silence, and the fluency optimism. The stutterer can develop a tolerance of silence, of disfluency, can reject every invitation to substitute, can phrase reasonably, and learn to quit when he should. Since an important source of the filibustering is an effort to deny the stuttering he has just done, the therapy steps just outlined will be catalyzed by open stuttering and matter-of-fact acceptance of the stutterer role.[1]

FEATURES OF ROLE-TAKING THERAPY

Every stutterer has to select from the smorgasbord that we offer him in therapy those things which are most pertinent to him. After he leaves the clinic he begins to lose some of the

---

[1]As we have stressed throughout this book, stuttering is not a condition, but a style of behavior. Dean Williams (1968) has recently criticized the acceptance-of-stuttering approach on the grounds that it grew historically out of an organic predisposition, or dysphemia concept of stuttering. We agree with Williams that dysphemia is a discredited concept; however, our own advocacy of acceptance-of-stuttering has a different source. From approach-avoidance conflict theory, the "holding back" behavior is basic to stuttering. Why does the stutterer struggle, grimace, and develop the "walking museum"? Because he does not accept stuttering as something he does, as his own learned behavior. We have never believed in the organic causation of stuttering even though we cut our academic teeth on the early writings of Travis and West. We accept stuttering not because we believe it to be organic but because such acceptance is a social and clinical necessity, following logically from our view of stuttering as a false-role disorder based on approach-avoidance conflict.

guilt that is produced by the doing kind of therapy, by the performance kind of therapy.

One of the disadvantages of role-taking therapy is that if the stutterer is not really enacting the roles he feels guilty. As indicated earlier, guilt may be viewed as the private experiencing of failure of role-enactment in accordance with conception of self. Shame is the public equivalent of guilt. Shame and guilt are basically important in stuttering. Tension often results from the person's effort to resist exposing himself, that is, his effort to keep the guilt part below the surface from coming up to equal the shame part above.

To a stutterer, the term "working on your speech" is so vague as to be treacherous. Often it means any old effort to get the word out. It is much harder to teach by-product fluency, but it is vastly more important. To get by-product fluency, we must tell the stutterer: First, eliminate all islands of avoidance, every last reservation. Keep the initiative, go into every situation that offers challenge. Second, monitoring. Third, open up and stutter smoothly and easily. Let the other person know what you are doing—that is the basic principle of open stuttering. Fourth, the idea of Karma can become important. What you are doing today is important to what you were doing yesterday and what you are going to be doing tomorrow is a product of what you are doing today. Build for the future: oversatisfy the fear in the present, and the next time you enter a situation you will have less fear and you will be able to speak better in it. (This was one of my own personal mottoes and it had a profound effect on my improvement.) Fifth, you should try to do more stuttering in any situation than you have to. If you keep oversatisfying the fear instead of short-changing it as nearly every naive stutterer tries to do, you produce a profound reduction of the tendency toward avoidance.

Why is it that professional stutterers—those who have gone into speech pathology—tend to get better? It is not just the vague magic of the clinic atmosphere. Rather, it is the fact that we are constantly presenting ourselves as stutterers. We are curious about it, we are fascinated by it. And this is all very important. It is not just being in a clinic: it is a complete role acceptance.

For adults, a paradoxical feature of the problem is that role acceptance as a stutterer leads to being able to perform the role of a normal speaker, and the attempt to become a completely normal speaker leads back again to the role of a stutterer.

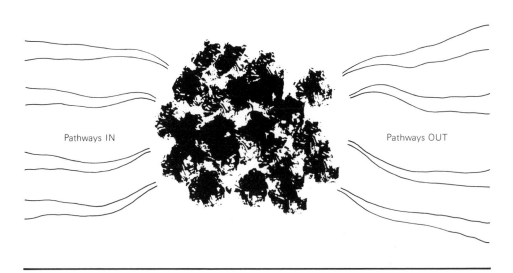

Pathways IN   Pathways OUT

Figure 6 *The Jungle of Stuttering*

THE JUNGLE OF STUTTERING

How does one acquire the role of a stutterer, and how does he emerge from the role? How is it that those with stuttering in common have so little else in common? To throw some light on this question, we have to summarize much of what has been said here. The schematic diagram called "The Jungle of Stuttering" is presented in Figure 6. Following first the arrow on the left, many pathways lead into the central portion, the jungle called stuttering. Many roads lead to Rome and to stuttering. Once inside, the path of entry is less important than the ongoing conditions—the struggle for survival of the ability to communicate.

From looking at a denizen of the jungle, we cannot always tell how he got in, or which of many routes may provide him the best exist. The routes of exit, shown on the right, all lead from the interior of the jungle but do not bear any necessary relation to point of entry. Similarly, the processes of recovery, with or without therapy, may not correlate highly with the origin and onset factors.

However, we can make some statements about recovery as a role-learning process. First, it is gradual. No one gets a cata-

31

pult ride from the jungle. Second, four out of five will find their own way out. Those coming into the clinics as adults are an unlucky one-fifth (Sheehan & Martyn, 1966, 1970; Martyn & Sheehan, 1968). Third, ages crucial in role change also offer best hope of spontaneous recovery. The years of transition from childhood to puberty, 11 to 14, and from adolescence to adulthood, 19 to 22, seem especially propitious for recovery. Inferentially, these should be years of optimum readiness for assimilation of the role changes involved in therapy. These might be the best years to guide the stutterer toward a pathway out, toward the full recovery which we now know to be not only possible but highly attainable.

References

References that are listed here only by author and year of publication appear in complete form in the Bibliography.

Adler, A.   (1929)   *Problems of neurosis.* London: Kegan Paul, Trench, Trubner.

Berne, E.   (1964)   *Games people play.* New York: Grove Press.

Biddle, B. J., and Thomas, E. J., eds.   (1966)   *Role theory: Concepts and research.* New York: Wiley.

Cameron, N.   (1947)   Language, thought and role-taking. In *The psychology of the behavior disorders.* Cambridge, Mass.: Riverside Press, 4, 89–102.

Cooley, C. H.   (1902)   *Human nature and the social order.* New York: Scribner.

Cooley, C. H.   (1909)   *Social organization.* New York: Scribner.

Eisenson, J.   (1958)

Erikson, E.   (1956)   The problem of ego identity. *Journal of the American Psychoanalytic Association,* 4, 56–121.

Eysenck, H. J., ed.   (1960)   *Behaviour therapy and the neuroses.* New York: Pergamon.

Eysenck, H. J., and Rachman, S.   (1965)   *The causes and cures of neurosis.* San Diego, California: Robert R. Knapp.

Festinger, L.   (1957)   *A theory of cognitive dissonance.* New York: Harper & Row.

Gendlin, E. T.   (1968)   Focusing ability in psychotherapy, personality, and creativity. In J. Schlein, ed., *Research in psychotherapy. Vol. III.* Washington, D.C.: American Psychological Association, pp. 217–241.

Goffman, E.   (1959)   *The presentation of the self in everyday life.* New York: Doubleday.

Goffman, E. (1961) *Asylums.* New York: Anchor, Double-day.

Goffman, E. (1964) *Stigma: Notes on the management of spoiled identity.* Englewood Cliffs, N. J.: Prentice-Hall.

Hunt, J. (1863) *Stammering and stuttering, their nature and treatment.* London: Longmans, Green.

Jourard, S. R. (1964) *The transparent self.* New York: American Book, Van Nostrand.

Kinsey, A. C., Pomeroy, W. B., Martin, E. C., and Gebhard, P. H. (1953) *Sexual behavior in the human female.* Philadelphia: Saunders.

Krasner, L. (1965) Verbal conditioning and psychotherapy. In L. Krasner and L. Ullmann, eds., *Research in behavior modification.* New York: Holt, Rinehart and Winston.

London, P. (1964) *The modes and morals of psychotherapy.* New York: Holt, Rinehart and Winston.

Martyn, M. M., and Sheehan, J. G. (1968)

Mead, G. H. (1934) *Mind, self and society from the standpoint of a social behaviorist.* Chicago: University of Chicago Press.

Moreno, J. L. (1946) *Psychodrama.* New York: Beacon House.

Moreno, J. L. (1961) The role concept, a bridge between psychiatry and sociology. *American Journal of Psychiatry, 118,* 518–523.

Mowrer, O. H., in Gregory, H. H. (1968)

Quarrington, B. (1956)

Rogers, C. (1961) *On becoming a person: A client's view of psychotherapy.* Boston: Houghton Mifflin.

Sarbin, T. R. (1943) The concept of role-taking. *Sociometry, 6,* 273–285.

Sarbin, T. R. (1954) Role theory. In G. Lindzey, ed., *Handbook of social psychology.* Reading, Mass.: Addison-Wesley.

Sarbin, T. R. (1964) Role theoretical interpretation of psychological change. In P. Worchel and D. Byrne, eds., *Personality change.* New York: Wiley.

Sarbin, T. R., and Allen, V. L. (1968) Role theory. In G. Lindzey and E. Aronson, eds., *Handbook of social psychology.* Reading, Mass.: Addison-Wesley.

Sartre, J. (1956) *Being and nothingness.* New York: Philosophical Library. (Translated by Hazel Barnes.)

Sheehan, J. G. (1946) *A study of the phenomena of stut-*

33

tering. M. A. thesis, University of Michigan, Ann Arbor.

Sheehan, J. G.   (1953)

Sheehan, J. G.   (1954a)

Sheehan, J. G.   (1968)   Stuttering as a self-role conflict. In H. H. Gregory, ed., *Learning theory and stuttering therapy*. Evanston: Northwestern University Press.

Sheehan, J. G.   (1969b)

Sheehan, J. G., Cortese, P. A., and Hadley, R. G.   (1962)

Sheehan, J. G., Hadley, R. G., and Gould, E.   (1967)

Sheehan, J. G., and Martyn, M. M.   (1966)

Sheehan, J. G., and Martyn, M. M.   (1970)   Stuttering and its disappearance. *Journal of Speech and Hearing Research, 13,* (in press) Reprinted in E. P. Trapp and P. Himelstein, eds., *Readings on the exceptional child: Research and theory*. (Revised). New York: Appleton, 1970.

Sheehan, J. G., and Voas, R. B.   (1957)

Sheehan, J. G., and Zelen, S. L.   (1955)

Sitzman, R. B.   (1968)   *Stuttering as a function of word predictability*. Ph.D. Dissertation, University of California, Los Angeles.

Stanislavsky, C.   (1938)   *My life in art*. Boston: Little, Brown.

Waller, W.   (1932)   *The sociology of teaching*. New York: Liveright.

Waller, W.   (1938)   *The family: A dynamic interpretation*. New York: Cordon Company.

West, R.   (1958)

Wheelis, A.   (1958)   *The quest for identity*. New York: Norton.

Williams, D. E.   (1957)

Zelen, S. L., Sheehan, J. G., and Bugental, J. F. T.   (1954)

About the Author CHARLES VAN RIPER, Ph.D., is Distinguished Professor in the Department of Speech Pathology and Audiology, Western Michigan University and a Fellow of the American Speech and Hearing Association. Dr. Van Riper is the author of *Speech Correction: Principles and Methods, Speech Therapy, Speech in the Elementary Classroom, Teaching your Child to Talk,* and *Casebook in Speech Therapy;* he is coauthor of *Casebook in Stuttering* (with Leslie Gruber), *Introduction to General American Phonetics* (with Dorothy E. Smith), and *Articulation and Voice: Abnormal and Normal* (with John V. Irwin). Professional periodicals to which Van Riper has contributed articles include the *Quarterly Journal of Speech* and the *Journal of Speech and Hearing Disorders.*

About the Chapter The history of the treatment of stuttering is as fascinating as the disorder itself. In this chapter Dr. Van Riper traces with admirable conciseness the evolution of therapeutic approaches from ancient and medieval philosophers, through ensuing centuries of misconception, ignorance, and malpractice, to the present. Along with Demosthenes of the famous pebbles we find such personages as Avicenna, an Arabian philosopher of the 10th century who advocated that the stutterer take a deep breath before speaking—a method still widely recommended though it has failed for a thousand years. Van Riper concludes with a brief consideration of major modern therapists and their contributions.

2

HISTORICAL
APPROACHES

CHARLES VAN RIPER

2

When we find a disease or disorder in which multiple or unknown causes seem to be present, in which the symptoms are widely varying from case to case and intermittent in the same case, we always find a wide variety of remedial measures being advocated. Asthma, to cite but one of many such disorders, has plagued the human race for as long as stuttering, and we find in it the same multiple or mysterious etiology, the same intermittency, and similarly wide variations and contradictions in the treatment used. Many widely differing theories explain its nature and govern its treatment. Claims are made for psychotherapy, for regimentation of the environment, for various medications. Even breathing exercises, hypnosis, and relaxation training have been employed. Desensitization therapy is widely used. Symptomatic relief seems to be the criterion of success, but relapse is common. Often the victim seems to "outgrow" his asthma. Emotional stresses seem to precipitate attacks, but not predictably. (According to reports in the literature, the incidence of asthmatic attacks in London decreased markedly during the bombing raids of World War II.) Treatment that is successful with one patient fails abjectly with another. Some cases are "cured," many others are improved, but asthma presents much the same difficulty to the physician that stuttering does to the speech therapist. The great difference is that the speech therapist, newly become professional, becomes upset, whereas the physician merely does his best and goes on to his next patient.

In reviewing the various kinds of treatment used for stuttering, it is interesting that, from the very first, theory has determined therapy. What evidently happens in the therapeutic mind, whether it be that of the Oracle of Delphi, a surgeon of the eighteenth century, or a Salish Indian of the present day, is that the therapist looks at the disorder, makes a guess at its nature, and then devises a treatment in terms of the guess. Thus, the Oracle of Delphi, observing that one Battos stuttered more in his familiar surroundings than in any other place, recommended that he banish himself forever, a prescription many a modern speech therapist would occasionally like to use. And Dieffenbach (1795–1847), noting (1841) that in stuttering the tongue "clave to the roof of the mouth," treated it by cutting out a triangular wedge from the base of the tongue, which certainly prevented the tongue from taking this abnormal action even if the stutterer had to learn to stutter in a different way, which he doubtless did. Dieffenbach devised his therapy to fit his theory, which was that stuttering was a lingual cramp. Quite as logical were the Tlahoose Indians, who, according to Lemert (1953), required the stutterer to find a board with a knothole in it and every morning upon rising to recite to it, "I give my stuttering to you," and then to spit or blow through the hole to get the stuttering devil out of his throat. These Indians, too, had a theory concerning the nature of stuttering and a therapy based upon it.

In each of these three instances we see a therapist scrutinizing the disorder, seizing upon one little facet of the problem as significant of the whole, and then developing a theory concerning the nature of stuttering in terms of the therapist's own culture and knowledge and, finally, prescribing a treatment based upon that theory and that culture. The sources of error in such a *modus operandi* are apparent, and doubtless they continue to operate, at least to some degree, in contemporary speech therapy. Perhaps by reviewing the different types of therapy used with stutterers, in terms of this frame of reference, we may be less likely to go as far astray, though stray we shall.

The history of the treatment of stuttering is interesting but not particularly illuminating. Satyrus treated Demosthenes by requiring him to declaim with pebbles in his mouth and lead plates upon his chest while climbing hills. In Roman times, stutterers were viewed as being possessed by evil spirits and various types of exorcism were employed. In the Middle Ages, the tongue was viewed as the seat of the trouble and hot irons, spices, and noxious substances were applied to that organ to drive away the evil. Francis Bacon, noting that the tongue seemed to be stiff and frozen in the act of stuttering, recommended that the tongue be thawed with hot wine, a procedure which undoubtedly produced more fluency. Stuttering was also treated by purging and bloodletting. Even as late as 1830, Bostock, an English physician, cites the cure of a case of stammering by the prolonged use of powerful cathartics. The poor devils were either afraid to stutter lest an accident occur or too weak to do so. In the late seventeenth century, Amman, a Swiss physician, believed "hesitantia" to be merely a vicious tongue habit, and recommended tongue exercises and gymnastics, procedures still being used today by a few uninformed therapists. Itard, a French doctor, felt that stuttering was due to muscular weakness, and invented a little fork made of gold or ivory, which the stutterer had to wear inside his mouth to support the tongue during speech. We could continue to cite some of the more bizarre teatments used by early practitioners, but we doubt the value of such an account. We go, therefore, to the direct antecedents of modern stuttering therapy.

Early in the last century some serious investigators and observers began to appear, and the European literature that developed on the subject of stuttering is still fascinating. In contrast to the prescientific remedies we have been describing, we find in this literature instances of keen observation and a vigorous attempt to make stuttering and stuttering therapy make sense (see, for example, Hagemann [1845], and H. Gutzmann [1887]).

In 1832, Otto described stuttering as a transitional phenomenon, an inability to shift from one sound to another. "By stuttering is meant the utterance of a sound unit, syllable or word, made faulty by severance, extension or repetition of the initial sound." He differentiates between normal nonfluency or the nonfluency of stage fright and that of stuttering by saying that in the former, the difficulty is with the whole word or phrase and not with the syllable. He recommends phonetic drills, and conscious utterance to integrate the faulty transitions. These are still being used today.

In the same year, Colombat (1830) popularized the time-beat method originally conceived by Dupuytren in 1817, in which the stutterer was asked to speak in a singing or chanting tone, marking the intervals with a foot tap or a finger movement. Colombat felt that stuttering was a disorder of rhythm and of tone, hence his time-beat method. Rate control and rhythmic timing are still in use. As recently as 1964, Andrews and Harris report dramatic results especially in young stutterers by using syllable tapping, a procedure also recommended by Van Dantzig in 1940.

In 1836, Bell called attention to the *"involuntary* action of the organs, which are not obedient to the will. In stuttering, the articulating organs—the lips and tongue—rebound again and again before the subsequent vowel can find egress." Bell's therapy was largely phonetic drill, done in a highly conscious manner, so as to bring the articulators under control of the will. Therapies today still reflect the need to get voluntary control of stuttering behavior.

In 1841, Braid, who did some of the early experiments with hypnosis, explored the use of suggestion in the treatment of *begaiement* (stuttering). He was not the last. Suggestion seems to play a vital part in much of modern speech therapy.

Also in 1841, Malebouche defended his secret "American Method" for treatment of stuttering, which he made "scientific" and sold to the Belgian and Prussian governments. This cure consisted of curling the tongue tip and keeping it in firm contact with the palate during all speaking. Hagemann (1845) describes it thus: "The one forceful remedy in its simple but superb entirety is as follows: Always keep the tip of the tongue in the upper part of the mouth and when no speaking is taking place, keep the body of the tongue high in the mouth also. Keep it next to the palate so that the tip of the tongue continually rests against the upper incisors or better still against their roots." It takes some doing! This method had been widely though secretly used in England and America for several years before. The originator, possibly a Dr. Yates, felt that stuttering was a spasm of the glottis, and this concept found many believers throughout the next hundred years, although the method for treating the spasm soon fell into disrepute. This idea, that the stutterer is momentarily unable to produce voice, is an item easily demonstrated by direct observation of many stutterers. It is not true of all stutterers. Arnott (1827) seems to have been among the first to state that the stutterer had indeed a transient inability to produce voice, a momentary aphonia. This inability was later felt to be due to a muscular spasm, or as Ssikorski (1891) described it, a muscular cramp. (Makuen [1941], a physician of great influence in the second decade of

41

the present century, and Kenyon [1940] have been modern advocates of this concept.) Three types of treatment were used by believers in the laryngeal spasm theory: relaxation, retraining by phonetic drills, and the positioning of the suprahyoid musculatures in such a way as to prevent laryngeal spasm. Again we see the beginnings of much of the therapy used today.

Skipping the sad era of surgical butchery which we have already referred to in connection with Dieffenbach, we come to Herman Klencke (1862), whose work has had a profound influence on speech therapy. He was among the first to describe the anxieties and personality features of the stutterer. A brief excerpt might be instructive: "Stutterers have certain characteristics which are associated with the inclination toward secrecy, indolence. They show a suspicious, passive opposition against any inconvenience of the treatment which leads them to a sanguine devotion to anything which seems to point to an easier and rapid cure." In a sense, he anticipates the semantic treatment of stutterers, speaking in most vivid terms of their confused thinking. Klencke advocated an all-out attack on the stuttering problem and combined in his therapy many of the older methods. For example, he used the finger-pinching technique to time the moment of speech attempt. He used breathing exercises, the blending of consonants and vowels, the use of measured talking (rate control). He felt that any of the bizarre abnormalities shown by stutterers were secondary symptoms used to avoid or release the stutterer from his transient phonetic inability to utter a syllable. Klencke insisted that his patients plan to spend at least twenty weeks in therapy and warned them of relapse. He also anticipated some of the modern feedback and automatic control theory. In this regard he says, "At this juncture comes another and more important point—placing the speech under the control of the ear and therefore under the judgment and control of the mind . . . His speech must be placed under the direction and control of the ear."

In 1868, Wyneken propounded the theory that stuttering was a neurosis and only a neurosis. He attacked all older workers with an energy equal to advocates of the present day, but he localized the neurotic system in the larynx as his predecessors had done. He stressed that there was no organic pathology or deficiency, and that anything that contributed to the morale of the stutterer would decrease his symptoms. He emphasized the contribution to severity of shame and embarrassment and described the role of both situation and phonetic fears in increasing the moments of stuttering. He correctly described how secondary symptoms arise as the result of avoidance and came close to the modern approach-avoidance explanation of stuttering. Much of Wyneken's clarity no doubt came from self-observation, for he himself was a stutterer. Wyneken's therapy was less advanced than his theory and seems to have been based primarily on that outlined earlier by Klencke. One of his innovations, however, was the prescription of complete silence during the first stage of treatment; another was his insistence that the stutterer be isolated from all but other stutterers during the first part of therapy. Both of these practices are still found in modern therapy in some clinics. He used breathing exercises, phrasing, and phonetic drills, all structured so as to build up the stutterer's confidence that he could talk without stuttering. It is also interesting that Wyneken concludes his paper with a description of how relapse occurs, and hints that it is very likely to happen.

Ssikorski (1891), who, as we mentioned earlier, believed stuttering to be of the nature of a muscular cramp or spasm, gives us some of the clearest descriptions of symptomatology ever written. His main contribution seems to be that of showing that these spasms may exist not only in the larynx but in the breathing and articulatory apparatus as well. He also showed that stuttering symptoms vary according to the course of the disorder. He felt that treatment should be specific to the localization of the muscle spasm. In general, he follows Klencke in his therapeutic regime.

Denhardt (1890), like Wyneken, emphasized psychological factors. His description of the conflict aspect is vivid: "If we examine the mental processes during stuttering, we see that the disturbance typifies the struggle between two opposing forces. The volition which tries to convert the thought into speech is pitted against the belief that we are unable to accomplish what we intend. One drives, the other restrains." Denhardt's therapy consisted of exercises and speech drills intended to convince the stutterer that he could talk without stuttering and to increase the urge to move forward in utterance. Besides the inevitable breathing exercises, he taught his patients to slur or slight the initial consonant of the word that was feared, to ease the voice into the succeeding vowel, and to link and blend each new word with the last part of the preceding word. He also

43

recommended training in timing the speech attempt at the beginning of exhalation. These techniques are still being used in many clinics today.

Wyllie (1894) was an English physician whose book, *The Disorders of Speech*, became a medical classic and dominated the thinking on stuttering in England and America for many years. He described the development of symptom formation and gives us a clear picture of the disorder in its advanced stages. His major contribution concerns the role of tension in stuttering. He feels that most of the involuntary movements and spasms are produced by this tension. For example, he says, "From the nerve centers of oral articulation thus surcharged, an overflow in many cases occurs; so that spasmodic movements thus produced may be enumerated: trembling movements and spasmodic twitchings of the lips and cheek, working of the jaw, forcible winking of the eyes, twitching or tonic contradictions of the sterno-mastoid on one or both sides, and sometimes spasmodic working of the arms." Wyllie felt that many of the symptoms of stuttering were first practiced voluntarily and then became involuntary as they became habitual. He recommended that intelligent stutterers should not have a therapist but should solve their own problems by learning to speak without the extreme tension and abnormal movements and to keep their speech on as voluntary a level as possible.

In the same year, 1894, Leopold Treitel divided the spasm of stuttering into tonic and clonic blockings and describes the vicious circle of stuttering begetting fear and fear begetting stuttering. He felt that stuttering was nervous illness arising early in childhood from these causal factors: (1) the child speaks faster than his immature and awkward organs can move (dysphemia?); (2) the child stutterers are usually delayed in the ability to form and articulate certain difficult sounds; (3) the child may have experienced some illness or shock which set off the stuttering; (4) the child may have learned his stuttering by imitation. Treitel gives some interesting accounts of the development of the disorder in specific cases.

Sandow (1898) was one of the first to protest against the use of breathing exercises and phonetic drills. Ascribing the difficulty to excessive nervous tension, he treated the stutterer primarily by relaxation. He says, "Away with these dangerous speech exercises! The only way of dealing with overexcited nerves is with a type of intermittent rest between natural and unforced movements, and accompanied by much dream-free sleep." In modern speech therapy there is little stress on dream-free sleep, except that which can be provided by psychotherapy, but relaxation techniques are widely used, and phonetic drills are fast disappearing.

Liebmann (1895) prescribed unison reading, whispering, repeating, and drawling in order to convince the stutterer that he can speak without his interruptions. He also described the development of stuttering as being gradual, with the secondary symptoms and facial contortions coming later. Changes in the personality of the stutterer are recommended, since most are hypersensitive, morose, and nervous.

It has long been known that stutterers speak more fluently when reading aloud or speaking in unison with a normal speaker. This has been experimentally corroborated by Barber (1939) and others, and it has been explained as being due to the distraction or lack of propositionality involved. Nevertheless, the technique has been used for many years. In 1956, Cherry and Sayers proposed a modification of unison-speaking, termed "shadowing," in which the stutterer repeats echoically the words uttered by another speaker. They report an almost total inhibition of stuttering under these conditions.

There were three Gutzmanns who wrote on stuttering. In 1898 Henry, the elder, published *Das Stottern*, which became a classic and influenced many later writers. He felt that in stuttering there was some central deficiency in the cerebral apparatus responsible for syllable coordination. He was greatly interested in the stuttering of aphasics, who he felt demonstrated the validity of his thesis. He, like Ssikorski, described the interruptions in fluency as spasms, and his description of the symptoms of stuttering is accurate. He was convinced that the emotional and personality abnormalities shown by adult stutterers were the result rather than the cause of stuttering. Much of his therapy consisted of phonetic drills, but when aspirated vowels were feared he advocated their use also.

In this country, Scripture (1912) published his book *Stuttering and Lisping*, in which will be found some excellent descriptions of stuttering together with case reports. He believed that stuttering was largely a learned response which had become habitual, maintained by anxiety, and precipitated as muscle spasms by excessive tension. He describes the role of anxiety and how *starters* and avoidance devices can become involuntary accompaniments of the utterance. He speaks of the substitution of synonyms as contributing to the severity by increasing the mental confusion. He speaks of inner stuttering, of stuttering during thinking. He felt that stutterers speak too rapidly. Much

45

of his therapy was traditional: slow speech, relaxation, phonetic drill, and breathing exercises, but he also introduced the so-called octave-twist, in which the stutterer, when he feels himself in a spasm, immediately shifts his intonation to a full octave above the normal starting point. This is one of the first instances of the use of a different type of stuttering response, albeit a most unpleasant one.

In the first and second decades of this century, therapy for stutterers in this country consisted chiefly of relaxation, breathing exercises, phonetic drills, and rate control or timing devices. Strong suggestion, the use of abnormal speech patterns such as the prolongation of the vowels, chanting and inflected speech, all designed to prevent the patient from stuttering, served as the core of therapy. Much of the treatment was in the hands of commercial schools and quacks with secret cures. These schools provided a safe and highly regimented environment, in which a period of mandatory silence served as the penalty for not following "the method," that is, for stuttering. Stuttering was generally considered a bad habit, like thumb sucking, which must be broken. Most of the techniques used were those developed on the continent of Europe during the preceding century, though a few variations appeared, such as the distracting visualization of words prior to utterance (Swift, 1915), the use of an arm-swinging figure-eight to time the moment of speech attempt (Lewis, 1903). The Martin School in Rhode Island probably presented the therapy of the time at its best, and the Lewis and Bogue Schools at its worst.

There developed a rising protest against these methods during the 1920s. Tomkins, as early as 1915, protested against the drilling, pointing out that normal speech is highly automatic and that the stutterer's chief problem was that words and sounds were receiving too much attention, that the stutterer was reacting to his reactions. In many ways, Tomkins anticipated much of the thinking of the semanticists. He insisted that the stutterer should merely try to talk without stuttering, and he advocated the use of distraction devices, strong clinical suggestion, and demand for fluency.

Bluemel (1913) made a strong protest against the practices of the "stammering schools," and his books were some of the first in America to acquaint the public with German literature. Influenced perhaps by Gutzmann, he developed first the transient auditory aphasia theory of stuttering and later (1935) his view of stuttering as phenomena due to conditioned inhibition. He gives a clear picture of the development of stuttering and uses the terms "primary and secondary symptoms." In his earlier work he advocated strong reauditorization of speech as had Klencke long before. In his later work he advised using highly conscious speech and the elimination of secondary symptoms through training. He says, "I feel that the stammerer's first task in speech correction is to learn to stop the physical struggle with which he has formerly met his speech block. . . . When he has checked the struggle, the stammerer is admonished to give his whole attention to mental speech. He is taught to regard the act of speaking as the process of thinking aloud, and when speaking he is urged to listen quietly to his thoughts. He is told to make no attempt to control the organs of speech but to let the mind broadcast to the mouth and to permit the speech to produce itself." Bluemel also stressed the need for building confidence and morale.

With the Blantons (1919), who established one of the first university speech clinics in this country and helped to bring therapy into the public schools (as had Martin), we find the transition from speech drills to psychotherapy. The Blantons used both, but their chief emphasis was on improving the mental hygiene and emotional control of their patients. The study of the self was emphasized. The family environment was subjected to change. Physical hygiene was also stressed. The individual rather than the stuttering became the focus of therapy.

Beginning in 1911 and continuing to the present day, Froeschels (1914, 1935, 1943), formerly of Vienna but now in this country, has written prolifically on the subject of stuttering and has made many contributions to our knowledge of the disorder. His views concerning stuttering and its treatment have been widely adopted in Europe, with the exception of England and France, and his recent publications in English have found interest if not acceptance in the United States. Froeschels is a keen observer with a wide experience in stuttering. Probably his major contribution to our understanding of stuttering is his description of how it develops. He feels that stuttering begins in the child's search for words and thoughts, a search which creates syllable and word repetitions. These early repetitions are of normal tempo and without tension. He terms these the primary clonus. Frustration and the need to make his wants known evoke tension, which alters the tempo of the repetitions and gradually causes them to turn into tensed prolongations of an articulatory posture (tonus). As he becomes aware of these repetitions and prolongations, he begins to struggle and then to

47

avoid, with the distortion of the personality and anxiety following later. This view is achieving wide acceptance as describing the manner in which the majority (but not all) of stuttering develops.

Froeschels rebelled against the drills and exercises current at the time he began to practice. He doubted that broken speech could be integrated by practicing any of the parts of speech whether they be breathing or the utterance of vowels or syllables. He felt that, since the stutterer could talk normally part of the time, any concentration on the stuttering itself was unwise, since it was this which caused the abnormality in the first place. Accordingly, he used ventriloquism and other distractive techniques in his therapy, along with strong suggestion and clinical demand for fluency. He is probably best known as the author of the chewing method, in which the stutterer is required to chew his breath and to synthesize his broken speech by associating it with a highly organized integrated biological function. He and his students feel that this chewing-speaking is useful and effective with all speech disorders. It has not found wide adoption or acceptance in this country or in England.

The third decade of our century showed a great upsurge of interest in stuttering, especially in the United States. Much experimentation was done, especially at the University of Iowa, where Travis (1940) and his students investigated many phases of the disorder. Travis's theory of cerebral dominance, which had its origins in the thinking of Orton and before him in several German and English workers, had a strong impact on the thinking at that time. In essence, the theory held that stutterers possessed a different type of neural organization than did normal speakers, that they lacked a dominant controlling and integrating mechanism in the cerebral cortex sufficient to withstand the disintegrating effects of emotional stress. Travis originally felt that this lack of a margin of dominance could be produced by a shift of handedness as well as by other factors. The stuttering was seen as a breakdown in the integration of speech due to the fact that the paired musculatures did not receive their proper innervation at the proper moment to permit fluency to flow unimpaired. Stuttering was conceived as consisting of blockings, neurological in nature, which could be precipitated by psychological factors.

At about the same time, West (1936), at the University of Wisconsin, introduced the concept of dysphemia to explain the sex ratio, the heredity factor in stuttering, the biochemical differences, poor diadochokinesis, and other so-called character-istics of the person who stutters. The influence of Travis and West was widespread. A great amount of research was done to support or deny the validity of cerebral dominance and dysphemia. Unfortunately, neither concept was sufficiently precise to permit adequate testing, and the belief in a constitutional factor (in certain stutterers at least) is still commonly held. Greene (1935), a physician who specialized in speech disorders, likewise held to a belief in a constitutional predisposition to stuttering. He felt, however, that the predisposition was in terms of personality structure, a thesis which is also untestable. In Germany, Seemann (1936) and others also became interested in establishing a constitutional difference as basic to stuttering.

Since we are here primarily interested in therapy and not in the validity of theory, let us consider some of the changes that occurred as the result of the widespread interest thus engendered. At first there was a shifting of the handedness of stutterers and the use of simultaneous talking and writing so as to help to build up the margin of dominance of the presumed unilateral speech-integrating apparatus. Also, since stuttering was conceived as a breakdown in normal functioning, various measures were taken to increase the threshold of breakdown and to maintain speech on a highly voluntary and conscious level, especially under conditions of stress. It was in the latter connection that Bryngelson (1943) used voluntary stuttering to replace the involuntary variety. By deliberately stuttering in a highly conscious and controlled fashion and with slow repetitions, the stutterer was freed from the upheaval of involuntary abnormality. The stutterer was urged and trained to control his behavior under stress, to control the form of the abnormality so that breakdown would not occur, so that his dysphemia or low margin of dominance would not produce disintegration. Dunlap (1917), from the logic of his beta hypothesis, had urged the voluntary practice of ticlike behavior, and his application of negative practice technique specifically to stuttering has undoubtedly influenced the genesis of voluntary stuttering as a technique. Voluntary stuttering as a therapy is quite logically related to the theory Dunlap developed.

Accompanying the cerebral dominance and dysphemic theories was the therapeutic concept of the "objective attitude," which insisted that the stutterer accept his stuttering as a part of the self, refusing to hide or avoid its occurrence, common practices among most advanced stutterers who use many devices to deny their problem as a problem. Since stuttering was thought to have a constitutional basis, this acceptance logically followed. We see here also the influence of the Blantons, whose insistence on the mental hygiene concept of knowing one's self and self-acceptance has won widespread adoption. Since the cerebral dominance and dysphemic theories permitted the constitutional predisposition to stuttering to be thwarted by the efforts of the stutterer to keep his speech under voluntary control or by reducing the vulnerability to stress or by reducing the stress itself, they offered a wide field for various therapeutic measures. Perhaps the greatest value of these theories was that they freed the therapist to experiment and to explore new types of treatment. Therapists could experiment with group therapy, with self-confrontation, with the modification of the stuttering behavior, with environmental manipulation, with psychotherapy of all types. It freed the therapist from the search for the secret method, the talismanic trick or training which would erase and eliminate the stuttering devil from the mouths of men. These theories, in their emphasis upon the individual's responsibility for his own behavior (that is, whether he would permit dysphemia or breakdown to produce speech abnormality), set the stage for the application of learning theory and semantic reorientation to the stuttering problem.

In 1932, Van Riper, a student of Bryngelson and Travis, challenged the thesis that stuttering was a form of behavioral disintegration and the product of a breakdown of fluency. He showed that on the contrary the abnormality of stuttering was a highly integrated act, and the result of a learning process. He viewed the symptoms as learned responses to the expectation or experience of some momentary interruption in the flow of speech. Espousing the principle of multiple causation, he held that stuttering could originate in emotional conflict affecting speech, in dysphemia or a poorly coordinated speech apparatus, or in the stresses of speech acquisition in infancy where fluency interruptors were especially frequent or potent. He showed that stuttering symptoms could be modified, unlearned, or replaced. Much of his effort was spent in experimental therapy in an attempt to find a type of fluent stuttering which could be used as a replacement for the abnormal symptoms presented by the stutterer. He held that avoidance and frustration responses conditioned to situational and phonetic cues can be weakened by the application of learning principles and that new responses to these cues can be taught. In his later work he equated the presence of tremor with what he had earlier considered to be a neurological block, and felt that this too could be modified and prevented. He structured his therapy so that the patient, by working with the stuttering, became acquainted with the self and learned to accept the responsibility for his own behavior and for modifying it in the direction of normality. His major contribution seems to be his evidence that the form of stuttering can be modified to produce fluency within the normal limits.

Johnson (1956a), in 1934 one of Travis's students at the University of Iowa, rebelled against the implication that stutterers were constitutionally different from normal speakers, as he had previously rebelled against the thesis that stutterers were primarily neurotics. A series of researches by his students challenged the dysphemic hypotheses. Influenced by Korzybski, he began to apply the principles of general semantics to stuttering, developing a therapy which sought to modify the stuttering symptoms in the direction of normal nonfluency through perceptual retraining. It is interesting that in his therapy many of the techniques evolved earlier were kept with some modification. Voluntary stuttering, for example, was transformed into "the bounce," a form of easy, automatic, rhythmic repetition which the stutterer was to substitute for the more bizarre symptoms when he felt he had "to hesitate to hesitate." All avoidance behavior was rejected, and stuttering was seen as the product of a learning process, originating in the incorrect labeling of childish nonfluency as pathological by the parents or associates of the stutterer. Self-confrontation, training in realistic evaluation of the symptomology, "semantic relaxation," the "bounce," the acceptance of stuttering as a problem (objective attitude), and the prescription of much speaking under stress comprise the core of his therapeutic program. In later years he discontinued his advocacy of the bounce, insisting that the stutterer use any form of normal disfluency instead of his struggle or avoidance. Johnson's influence has been very potent in modern speech therapy, both in the stimulation of research and in theoretical formulation.

Modern speech therapy, in its evolutionary course, still shows many of the old practices. Practitioners still advocate relaxation, the sigh technique, suggestion, and phonetic drills. Rate control is still to be found in many clinics, as are unison speech, rhythmic time beating, and chanting. Therapists still use phrasing, relaxation, exaggerated inflections, and blending. Distraction techniques are in current use in many places.

The psychoanalysts and psychiatrists have not neglected the

51

stutterer. Stein, in England, and Coriat (1915), Cooper, (1942), Solomon (1938), Despert (1946), and Barbara (1946) in the United States, have continued to view stuttering as a neurosis and to insist on deep psychotherapy as the only legitimate treatment. Unfortunately, as Fenichel (1945) himself admits, speech, the healing tool of psychotherapy, is itself affected in stuttering, and the results of psychoanalysis have not been impressive. Despite this, there seems to be a growing conviction on the part of some speech therapists (one which has been fostered by clinical psychologists as well) that stuttering treatment could well be surrendered to the psychotherapists. This alternative would certainly decrease the professional burden on the speech therapist, but we do not feel that it would be wise either for the stutterer or for the professional speech therapist. Our record for helping the stutterer can well stand comparison with that of the other professions.

The current trend in speech therapy for the stutterer, if we can discern it with any degree of clarity, seems to be that of a growing emphasis on viewing stuttering as learned behavior, susceptible to unlearning if proper training procedures can be devised. Influenced by Johnson and Spence, Wischner (1950) has proposed a systematic attack on stuttering in terms of conditioning and learning theories, especially those of Clark L. Hull of Yale. Skinnerian psychology has also had its effect. Viewing stuttering as operant behavior, various conditioning schedules have been used experimentally to bring it under control, as demonstrated in the studies of Shames and Sherrick (1965), Goldiamond (1960a), and Flanagan, Goldiamond, and Azrin (1958).

The approach-avoidance conflict theory advanced by Sheehan (1951, 1953, 1958a) has produced wide interest, especially since through analysis of conflict levels Sheehan has shown that psychotherapy and speech therapy can be brought under the same concept. Sheehan suggested that speech therapy be offered first and that the stutterer's response be used as an index of his need for more extensive psychotherapy. Sheehan advocated a behavioral approach involving the modification of stuttering through nonreinforcement (1951). Psychotherapy and speech therapy were seen as twin routes to the common goal of reducing the fear and avoidance tendency responsible for the stutterer's conflict.

Brutten and Shoemaker (1967) ingeniously applied Mowrer's two-factor learning theory to the modification of stuttering, covering both conditioned negative emotionality and instrumental behaviors.

Training in frustration tolerance, in desensitization to stress, in self-confrontation, in semantic reorientation, in conditioning new responses to stuttering cues will improve as soon as more workers experiment with therapy. Tranquilizing drugs show some promise. Van Riper's efforts (1957) to devise a speech therapy that is also a nonverbal psychotherapy show promise. Various techniques based on feedback controls are being tested. Continuous and intermittent masking noise usually creates a marked reduction in stuttering frequency and severity, and this has been employed recently by Cherry, Sayers, and Marland (1955) and Van Riper (1963a). Experimentation with the control, modification, and prevention of the stuttering tremor creates hope that we are on the threshold of a new and effective therapy for the confirmed stutterer. Treatment of the beginning stutterer is already quite standardized and effective. Public education and the development of public school speech therapy have reduced the number of severe cases. Prevention, in terms of better home policies and methods for teaching speech to infants, is growing in effectiveness. There remains much to be done, incredibly much, but we can now feel that we are on our way.

Contemporary speech therapy for the stutterer seems to aim at several major goals: (1) to improve the general security and morale of the patient; (2) to reduce the situational and phonetic anxiety; (3) to weaken the strength of the stereotyped stuttering responses; (4) to increase the threshold of discharge; (5) to reduce the reinforcement the stuttering responses acquire by avoidance, repression, and escape-reward (anxiety reduction and frustration release); (6) to give the existing fluency some stimulus value. Therapy is conceived as a process of learning and unlearning, and the stutterer is envisaged as being trainable to an extent that the frequency and severity of his stutterings can be reduced to a position within the limits of normal nonfluency. The trend seems to be away from the use of techniques used to prevent the occurrence of stuttering (which dominated speech therapy of the past) and toward techniques aimed at modifying the stuttering when it does occur so that the stutterer may stutter and still be fluent. Some experimental therapy indicates that a synthesis of both points of view may be emerging, with the preventive techniques being used in terminal therapy once the stuttering reactions have been weakened and modified.

Unfortunately for the stutterer, no unified program of experimental therapy exists. Communication between training centers, so far as therapy is concerned, is practically nil. Indeed, the state of stuttering therapy in this country generally is inadequate, largely in the hands of untrained graduate students, superficial and confused in goals and methods. Therapy time is woefully inadequate. Follow-up is almost nonexistent. Criteria for evaluating therapeutic progress are unsystematized. Protocols are missing. A few isolated workers are experimenting with therapy, but their accomplishments are seldom written up or available. Most of the research on stuttering has been descriptive, and, for therapy, rather sterile. With more than a million and a half victims of the disorder in this country alone, some integrated attack on the problem is sorely needed. No single person or training center can hope to make more than a minimal contribution to its solution. What is needed is a strongly sponsored team approach to the problem similar to that now being employed with polio and cancer and other human ills. Most of the groundwork has been laid, the time is ripe, and we are ready.

References

References that are listed here only by author and year of publication appear in complete form in the Bibliography.

Andrews, G., and Harris, M. (1964)

Barbara, D. A. (1946) A psychosomatic approach to the problem of stuttering in psychotics. *American Journal of Psychiatry, 103,* 188–195.

Barber, V. (1939) Studies in the psychology of stuttering: XV chorus reading as a distraction in stuttering. *Journal of Speech Disorders, 4,* 371–383.

Bell, A. (1836) *Stammering and other impediments of speech.* London: Sherwood, Gilbert, and Piper.

Bender, J. F., and Kleinfeld, V. M. (1938) *Principles and practices of speech correction.* New York: Pitman.

Blanton, M. G., and Blanton, S. (1919) What is the problem of stuttering? *Quarterly Journal of Speech Education, 5,* 340–350.

Bluemel, C. (1930) *Mental aspects of stammering.* Baltimore: Williams & Wilkins.

Boome, E. J., and Richardson, M. A. (1932) *The nature and treatment of stuttering.* New York: E. P. Dutton.

Brutten, E. J., and Shoemaker, D. J. (1967)

Bryngelson, B. (1943) The stuttering personality and development. *Nervous Child, 2,* 162–171.

Cherry, C., and Sayers, B. M. (1956)

Cherry, E. C., Sayers, B. M., and Marland P. (1955) Some experiments upon the total suppression of stuttering. *Nature, 176,* 874.

Colombat, M. (1830) Du begaiement et de tous les autres vices de la parole. Paris: Mansut Fils.

Cooper, C. A. (1942) Discussion on the relationship between speech disorders and personality defects in children, and how stuttering may unfavorably affect children's personality development. *Journal of Pediatrics, 21,* 418–421.

Coriat, I. H. (1915) Stammering—A psychoanalytic interpretation. *Journal of Abnormal Psychology, 9,* 417–430.

Denhardt, R. (1890) *Das Stottern, Eine Psychose.* Leipzig; Ernest Keil's Nachfolger.

Despert, J. L. (1946) A psychosomatic study of fifty stuttering children. *American Journal of Orthopsychiatry, 16,* 100–116.

Dieffenbach, J. F. (1841) Die heilung des stotterns durch eine neue chirugishche operation; ein sendschreiben an das Institut von Frankrech. Berlin: A. Forstner.

Dunlap, K. (1917) The stuttering boy. *Journal of Abnormal Psychology, 12,* 44–49.

Fenichel, O. (1945) Stuttering. In *Psychoanalytic theory of neurosis.* New York: Norton, 311–317.

Flanagan, B., Goldiamond, I., and Azrin, N. (1958)

Froeschels, E. (1914) Ueber das Wesen des stotterns. *Wien med. Woch, 64.*

Froeschels, E. (1935) Speech defects in children. *Wien Klin Wchnschr, 48,* 874–875.

Froeschels, E. (1943) Survey of the early literature on stuttering; chiefly European. *Nervous Child, 2,* 86–95.

Goldiamond, I. (1960a)

Greene, J. S. (1935) Treatment of the stutter type personality in a medical-social clinic. *Journal of the American Medical Association, 104,* 2230–2242.

Gutzmann, A. (1890) *Das Stottern und Seine Grundliche Beseitigung Durch Ein Methodisch Geordnetes und Praktisch Erporbtes Verfahren.* Berlin: E. Staude.

Gutzmann, H. (1887) *Euber das Stottern.* Berlin.

Hagemann, H. (1845) *Die Untrugliche Heilung des Stotter-und stammeluebels Nachesechszehn-jahringer Behandlung Desselben Largest-ellt. Breslau Trewendt.*

Johnson, W. (1956a)

Jones, M. V. (1948) Leopold Treitel on stuttering. *Journal of Speech Disorders, 13,* 19–22.

Kenyon, E. L. (1940) A critical examination of the foundations of 'the recoil of the vowel' theory of the cause of the impediment of the speech in stammering. *Journal of Speech Disorders, 5*, 97–112.

Klencke, H. (1860) *Heilung des Stotterns.* Leipzig.

Klingbeil, G. M. (1939) Stuttering and stammering. *Journal of Speech Disorders, 4*, 115–32.

Larson, M. (1949) Representative 19th century stuttering therapists. M.A. thesis, University of Denver, Colo.

Lemert, E. M. (1953)

Lewis, G. A. and Hyson, G. B. (1902) *Methods of attack, a textbook for students of the Lewis Phono-metric Institute and School for Stammerers.* Revised ed. Detroit: Phono-meter Press.

Liebmann, A. (1895) *Stottern und Stammeln.* Berlin: Steinnitz.

Makuen, G. H. (1841) Psychology of stammering. *Journal of Nervous and Mental Disorders, 43*, 68–72.

Malebouche, F. (1841) *Precis sur les causes du begaiement et sur les moyens de guerin.* Paris: Fortin, Masson.

Sandow, I. (1898) *Mechauik des Stotterns, Grundliche, Selbatheilung Ohne Akem-Artikulations-, Stimmbildungs- und Sprechubungen.* Norhausen: E. Edler.

Scripture, E. W. (1931) Stuttering, lisping, and correction of the deaf. Macmillan. 399–404.

Seemann, M. (1936) Contribution to the pathogenesis of stuttering. *Rev. Neurol. Psychiat., 33*, 399–404.

Shames, G. H. and Sherrick, C. E. (1965)

Sheehan, J. G. (1951)

Sheehan, J. G. (1953)

Sheehan, J. G. (1958a)

Solomon, M. (1938) The psychology of stuttering. *Journal of Abnormal Psychology, 3*, 59–61.

Ssikorski, J. A. (1891) *Ueber das Stottern.* Berlin.

Swift, W. B. (October–November 1915) A psychological analysis of stuttering. *Journal of Abnormal Psychology.*

Tompkins, E. (1916) Stammering and its extirpation. *Pedagog. Seminary, 23*, 151–174.

Travis, L. W. (1940) The need for stuttering. *Journal of Speech Disorders, 5*, 193–202.

Van Dantzig, M. (1940) Syllable-tapping, a new method for the help of stammerers. *Journal of Speech Disorders, 5*, 127–31.

Van Riper, C. (1957) Symptomatic therapy for stuttering.

In Travis, L. E., ed., *Handbook of speech pathology*. New York: Appleton, 818–896.

Van Riper, C.   (1963a)

Van Riper, C.,   (1965)   What next? *WMU Journal of Speech Therapy, 2,* 1–2.

West, R.   (1936)   Is stuttering abnormal? *Journal of Abnormal Psychology, 31,* 76–86.

Wilton, G.   (1950)

Wischner, J. W.   (1950)   A preliminary theoretical formulation of stuttering behavior and learning. *Journal of Speech Disorders, 15,* 324–335.

Wyllie, J.   (1894)   *The disorders of speech.* Edinburgh: Oliver and Boyd.

Wyneken, C.   (1868)   Ueber das Stottern und dessen heilung. *Zeitschrift fur Rationelle Medicin, 31.*

About the Author (Dr. Sheehan is identified at the beginning of Chapter 1.) Dr. Sheehan teaches graduate courses at UCLA in clinical psychological methods, psychological testing, projective techniques, and psychotherapy.

About the Chapter From at least the time of Aristotle, in numerous attempts to understand stuttering, people have pondered over the personality of the stutterer. What must he be like, to speak so haltingly in this glib world of ours? Is there a personality type in stuttering? Do stutterers differ from nonstutterers? If there are differences, are they causes of stuttering or results? What personality changes need to be made in treatment? These are some of the questions sifted in this chapter.

3

PERSONALITY
APPROACHES

JOSEPH G. SHEEHAN

3

The inner workings of the person who speaks with a stutter has always puzzled and intrigued those who come in contact with him. In the midst of a glib world, what must go on in an individual to produce halting speech or blocked and grimacing speech? The mystery deepens as the stutterer is observed to have less difficulty speaking to one person than to another, or to speak fluently on occasion. It is therefore not too surprising that much of the vast research on stuttering has focused on personality assay of the stutterer. What is surprising is that so little systematic effort has gone into combining, systematizing, and reconciling the myriad of assertions, speculations, clinical studies, and occasional objective studies of personality factors in stuttering.

1. Are there systematic personality differences between stutterers and nonstutterers?
2. Is stuttering a unitary disorder with common personality types, or is it a conflict that can be found with many different personality patterns?
3. Are there, psychologically speaking, several different kinds of stutterers? What subtypes exist within the group known as stutterers?

4. What psychological factors lead to the development of stuttering in one child and not in another?
5. How does the child who stutters differ from the child who does not?
6. How does the adult who stutters differ from the adult who does not?
7. How does the stuttering child differ from the stuttering adult?
8. How does the female stutterer differ in psychology from the male stutterer?
9. Do those who stutter and seek therapy differ in personality from those who stutter and do not?
10. In what respects, if any, do the parents of stutterers differ from the parents of nonstutterers?
11. If differences between stutterers and nonstutterers, or between different types of stutterers, can be found, are they to be regarded primarily as causes or as effects?
12. If stuttering is to be regarded as an anxiety condition, how are we to account for the absence of stuttering in many anxious children?
13. How are we to account for the relatively good adjustment of many stuttering children and their parents?
14. If stuttering is to be regarded as a form of neurosis, or merely as "persistent maladaptive behavior," what are the paths of symptom formation?
15. If no systematic personality differences emerge, then for what does a stutterer need psychotherapy?
16. What personality changes pave the way for accomplishing behavioral change?
17. What behavioral changes bring about personality change?
18. What personality changes accompany recovery from stuttering in the absence of treatment?
19. What personality changes occur during successful treatment?
20. How do stutterers with a good prognosis differ in personality from stutterers with a poor prognosis?
21. What is the role of the therapist's personality in determining the outcome of treatment?
22. What is the influence of therapy on the therapist's own personality?
23. What personality factors in the therapist make for success or failure in working with stutterers?

24. What is the range of personality diagnosis in stuttering (normal, neurotic, psychotic, psychopathic, etc.)?
25. What can personality-assessment approaches offer future investigators of stuttering, both in basic research and in therapy?

Interest in the personality characteristics of stutterers is as old as the history of the disorder. Aristotle was perhaps the first to advance the theory that stuttering was due to thinking faster than one spoke, and he attributed the disorder to the inability of the tongue to keep up.

From a variety of observations of what today should be called the social psychology of stuttering, Moses Mendelssohn (1729–1786) concluded that stuttering was psychological in origin and not due to any kind of physical difficulty. Comments on personality aspects of the stutterer have been offered by nearly every writer in the history of stuttering, especially the Germans. James Hunt, writing in Great Britain over a century ago, thought stuttering to be due to a conscious interference with what should be basically an automatic process. Wyneken, at about the same time, called a stutterer a *sprachsweifler*, a "speech doubter." Attributing stuttering to a fear of failure, Wyneken compared the fear and doubt in the stutterer to that involved in leaping across a chasm or to a fear of sexual impotence. The fear in these instances was held to aggravate the problem. Nearly all other writers of the last century offered some assertions or implicit hypotheses concerning the personality of stutterers.

As a clear modern landmark, the investigation by Wendell Johnson in 1930 and 1931 deserves first mention. Whereas nearly all previous writers had confined themselves to assertions that stuttering was the result of various personality factors, Johnson explored comprehensively the influence of the experience of stuttering on the personality. Those few personality differences which did appear were held to be the result of the stuttering rather than its cause. Mostly, however, stutterers were seen by Johnson as essentially normal, a view he not only held but strengthened as he continued his long scientific career.

During the 1930s, at the universities of Iowa and Wisconsin and at a few other places, numerous investigators—led by Travis, Johnson, Bryngelson, West, and Van Riper—explored a vast range of possible differences between stutterers and nonstutterers. Comparisons included physiological, neurological, biochemical, electroencephalographic, electromyographic, and diadochokinetic measures. For reasons spelled out by the author in Chapter 8, a vast array of false positive differences were reported on these dimensions. As methodology improved, the evidence turned negative and the search for physiological differences "slowed from a swift scurry into a slow meander" (Johnson, 1955).

With the growth in clinical psychology and the more promising techniques (especially projective methods) in the psychological test battery that grew out of World War II, the exploration of the personality of stutterers resumed in earnest, though it had never entirely ceased.

In an accumulating array of personality researches, stutterers have been studied by means of the Rorschach, the Thematic Apperception Test, the Minnesota Multiphasic Personality Inventory, the Picture-Frustration Test, level-of-aspiration measures, self-concept measures, paper-and-pencil personality inventories, IQ test comparisons, graphic techniques, various other projective techniques, and clinical interviews. By far the most frequent technique, especially in the earlier literature, has been the argument from authority, the bearded pronouncement.

Free-flowing speculation and armchair psychology may serve a highly useful function in the investigation of stuttering or any other phenomenon, provided that they are not mistaken for evidence. In this chapter, following an extensive survey of the literature on stuttering and personality, the focus will be on those contributions which can truly be regarded as studies, i.e., which are based on some publicly identifiable evidence.

The literature search undertaken for this chapter turned up innumerable purely descriptive papers and case studies, some of which presented so little in the way of contribution to the psychology of stuttering that they were not accorded space in this review. Since the better and more recent descriptive papers may be found in the Bibliography prepared by Charles Van Riper, they are not cited here.

Tables have been prepared to facilitate reader comparison of the findings of published studies, their methodology, the interpretations offered by the original investigators, and their relationship to one another.

When the studies are laid end to end, a striking result is that so many seem to have been carried out with little or no regard for other highly relevant studies using the same instrument. Virtually no attempts have been made to relate the find-

TABLE 1	RORSCHACH STUDIES
Investigator	Ingebregtsen, 1936
Subjects	40 stutterers. Ages: 8–26
Controls	None.
Significant Findings	One fourth gave a mediocre number of total answers. 21 gave no answers of motion, 18 gave no color responses. 10 gave "Hell-dunkel" answers. 60% of subjects had "unanswered plates."
Interpretation	On the basis of this and other tests given, the stutterer presents the following characteristic pictures of symptoms: reduced attention, great suggestibility, reduced language memory, logical displacement, motorial amusi, tendency to perseveration, indolence, derangements of motility, signs of depression, repressions and restrictions.

ings of one study to those of another, except for separately published reviews (Sheehan, 1958b; Goodstein, 1958). The investigators themselves, remarkably incurious, have frequently exhibited *la belle indifference* toward the central findings of others, even on such supposedly basic dimensions as anxiety, hostility, dependency, or degree of contact with reality. Personality studies of stuttering have thus grown and flourished in a kind of grand academic schizophrenia.

RORSCHACH STUDIES

Possibly the most prestigious and certainly the most famous of the widely used measures of personality is the Rorschach test. The Rorschach investigation of the stutterer began early and has not really abated, although the findings have not been overly exciting. However, the comparison of the Rorschach studies on stuttering is especially important as a beginning point, because so many of the methodological pitfalls in the

Meltzer, 1944	Richardson, 1944
50 stutterers. Ages: 8–17. Mean age: 12.46. IQ: 97.20.	30 stutterers.
50 matched controls. Age 8–17. Mean: 12.67. IQ: 97.20.	30 controls, matched for age, sex, mental ability, and education.
a) Lower F+ %. b) Higher Z. c) Higher W.	No significant differences.
Galaxy of interpretation of nonsignificant differences. Stuttering children more productive and more responsive but less well-balanced than control group.	Stutterers more detailed in their approach to problems. Average amount of inner living, more constricted than average, and tendency not to respond impulsively to outside stimuli.

personality assessment of stuttering have been illuminated by researchers using and misusing this instrument.

Though the Rorschach is an enormously rich and sensitive technique in clinical usage by experienced clinicians, it carries with it some inherent drawbacks as a research instrument. Productivity varies widely among individuals in a way that complicates statistical analysis; ratios such as M:C,W:M are less reliable in records with low productivity than in records with high productivity. Determinant variables and the personality dimensions that they tap are not normally distributed. Validation studies have turned up negative or positive results predictable from the bias of the experimenter, and highly questionable choices have been made on the crucial issue of criterion validity.

In the history of projective testing, the principal failures have not been those of the instrument but those of the investigator. Rorschach research on stuttering has been no different. With few exceptions, each researcher has operated as

TABLE 1	(continued)
Investigator	Krugman, 1946
Subjects	50 stutterers. Ages: 6½–15.
Controls	50 problem children, matched case by case for age, IQ, and sex.
Significant Findings	a) F − higher. b) More refusals. c) Low productivity.
Interpretation	Stutterers showed wide range of personality traits. Stuttering closely associated with emotional and personal maladjustment frequently manifested by obsessive compulsive traits of obsessional neurosis.

though in solitary confinement, with little reference to previous Rorschach research, either in planning the study or upon publishing it.

Table 1 presents, in chronological order, findings of the major Rorschach studies on stuttering. In Table 1, subjects, controls, significant findings, and interpretations have been

Pitrelli, 1948	Haney, 1951
311 hospitalized patients; Psychotics, nonpsychotic stutterers, psychotic stutterers, psychotics who had been stutterers (Exact numbers not reported).	6 stutterers.
None.	None.
Stuttering far less prevalent among psychotics than among the general population.	Primary findings derived from an experimental projective technique in which subject was asked to visualize an imaginary white card and then to project upon it. Each subject carried out this experimental procedure for 90 (sic) hours. Results were "submitted to test-retest appraisal by the Rorschach Ink Blots and Thematic Apperception Test."
Stuttering is symptomatic of a character neurosis. It is a defense against the coming into awareness of repressed instinctual urges.	Subjects began to project themselves. The speech mechanism "was perceived as spatially disoriented, structurally confused, and functionally self-contradicted." The stutterer's "perceptual distortions were (seen as) motives implied by the speech maladjustment termed stuttering."

summarized for each study. Only the better, more objective studies that can justifiably be called research have been included. Purely speculative papers, case reports, and reports based loosely on clinical impression have been omitted.

The findings are not particularly consistent with one another, and some studies are not consistent internally. Even when

TABLE 1	(continued)
Investigator	Wilson, 1951
Subjects	30 stutterers.
Controls	Parents of 30 stutterers; 30 nonstuttering siblings.
Significant Findings	Stutterers had a high S response. Mothers and stutterers showed similarity with regard to emotional immaturity as judged by the high percentage of CF over FC. Mothers showed strong anxiety tendencies. No such marked similarity between fathers and stutterers, although they both showed lack of positive identification with either sex, indicating considerable ambivalence.
Interpretation	Findings point up indications of a mother-stutterer relationship, with possibility of stutterers having introjected characteristics of mother. Findings do not suggests a pattern of parent-child relationship.

investigators agree on basic findings, their interpretations often differ considerably.

For example, Meltzer found that stutterers had a lower F+ percent compared with a clinical control group. Krugman, on the other hand, found that stutterers had a higher F—, which he attributed to alleged obsessive-compulsive tendencies (Fenichel, 1945). Though a higher F— might indicate other kinds of disturbance, it undermines rather than supports the notion that stutterers are obsessive-compulsive.

When Krugman and Meltzer's actual findings are compared, they are not too far apart. But they arrived at opposite conclusions from essentially similar data. Thus, in one of the few instances when the findings are in agreement, the interpretations are not. This situation seems to illustrate a tendency noted earlier:

> *For many researchers, the Rorschach has seemed to offer an amorphous flux from which any*

Christensen, 1952	Shames, 1953
30 stutterers. Ages: 4½–12½.	27 stutterers; 10 others with speech problems.
30 siblings. Ages: 5–14.	Stutterers compared before and after treatment.
a) Significantly more Hd and At responses to card VI. b) Significantly faster reaction to achromatic cards. c) Projected significantly more additional space and additional CF. d) No significant differences in F responses.	None better than .05 level. Factors related to improvement at 10% level of confidence: Sum C > Fc + c + C'; P, 4 or more; F%, 50% or less; M, 3 or more).
	These factors tentatively related to improvement although statistics inconclusive.

> *desired interpretation could be pulled, independently of the statistically defensible data.*
> *(Sheehan, 1958b)*

Though Krugman noted that stutterers varied in their personality traits, the observation did not seem to prevent him from agreeing with Fenichel's assertion that stutterers were basically obsessive-compulsive.

Upon examination and comparison of the Rorschach studies since Ingebregtsen's in 1936, it is disappointing that so little systematic effort has been made to cross-validate findings. For example, Ingebregsten reported suggestibility and reduced attention among stutterers, with signs of depression. But references to these possible factors are lacking in subsequent studies. Pitrelli reported stuttering to be less prevalent among psychotics, a logical finding in terms of the postulated relationship between anxiety and stuttering. Haney noted perceptual distortions, while Wilson noted a Rorschach similarity between stut-

TABLE 1	(continued)
Investigator	Sheehan, 1954
Subjects	35 stutterers.
Controls	Dropped patients compared to continued; most improved to least improved.
Significant Findings	Those with more movement responses M, FM, m, more likely to remain in therapy and to improve (P < .02).
Interpretation	Stutterers relatively good treatment prospects—high unused ego strength shown on Klopfer's RPRS scale.

terers and their mothers. Christensen's atomistic report of "significantly more Hd and At responses on Card VI," bears all the stigmata of having emerged from a long search through the sample for chance differences. It is puzzling that Santostefano, using the Rorschach Content Test, found in his sample more anxiety and hostility, when these factors had not shown in the samples of previous investigators. However, Rosenberg's conclusions agreed partially with those of Santostefano in emphasizing passivity-aggressivity. In finding no "stutterer personality" among 100 child and adolescent stutterers, Speidel appears to have reached a conclusion in congruence with those of reviewers (Sheehan, 1958b; Goodstein, 1958; Johnson, 1961d; Johnson *et al.*, 1967).

What have the Rorschach studies comparing stutterers with nonstutterers shown? For a considerable amount of effort, the

Santostefano, 1960	Rosenberg, 1961
26 stutterers. Mean age: 20. Mean IQ: 121.	16 male stutterers.
26 nonstutterers, matched for sex, age, IQ.	Subjects were own controls in before and after treatment paradigm.
Stutterers projected more content indicative of anxiety and hostility than did nonstutterers. In the laboratory situation, stutterers showed a significantly greater decrement in performance under stress than did nonstutterers. (Rorschach Content Test anxiety and hostility scores higher. P < .01).	None.
By adulthood a stutterer develops an enduring emotional disposition characterized by anxiety and hostility, a product of continual stress, which interferes with personal adjustment and efficiency.	Qualitative analysis indicated common psychological influences related to passivity-aggressivity.

return has been pitifully meager. While some possibilities remain for using the Rorschach in investigation of change during therapy or prediction of response to therapy, further expenditure of effort merely comparing stutterers with nonstutterers on this projective instrument is unwarranted.

The use of the Rorschach in investigating response to therapy has shown promise. Shames (1953) concluded that some Rorschach factors could be tentatively related to improvement, though his statistics were inconclusive. Sheehan (1954b) found that Klopfer's movement variables, M, FM, and m, could discriminate those who dropped out of therapy and those who continued, as well as those who showed most improvement on psychotherapeutic dimensions. The Rorschach Prognostic Rating Scale accomplished the same result, though more laboriously. Sheehan suggested that though the Rorschach might

TABLE 1	(continued)
Investigator	Speidel, 1963
Subjects	100 child and adolescent stutterers of normal intelligence.
Controls	36 nonstutterers.
Significant Findings	No "stutterer-personality" found.
Interpretation	Some significant differences seen in stutterer's attitudes: they "gave more" in the inquiry part of test; behaved more indifferently; were, in some respects, more inhibited.

aid in prognosis, the task might well be accomplished by simpler means. Sheehan has recently cross-validated successfully his earlier positive result on the prognostic value of the Rorschach with stutterers (Sheehan, 1970).

In the tables presented in this chapter, it is inevitable that some authors' contributions or conclusions will have been lost or slighted in the condensation necessary for systematic comparison of results. It is always difficult to summarize the results of the research findings of another, particularly if he has not summarized his own findings very ably. Therefore, where possible, the original references should be pursued.

Even with the above limitation, it is amply clear that no consistent finding has emerged across the board on the Rorschach studies. Virtually no agreements appear except by a fairly generous inference process on the part of the reader.

TAT STUDIES

Since stuttering occurs primarily in a social context, the widely used (second to the Rorschach) Thematic Apperception Test (TAT) should be an investigative instrument of choice. The TAT yields much of the content of social rela-

Sheehan, 1970
50 college stutterers.
Served as own controls.
Found M, FM, m distinguished between Improved Most and Improved Least, as well as between Continued and Dropped.
Rorschach can be used to predict psychotherapeutic improvement, but not speech improvement. Rorschach usable for prognosis, but other methods may be less costly.

tionships and frequently sheds light on family interaction patterns. The TAT protocol may be viewed clinically as latent autobiography.

Since stuttering begins typically in early childhood, the TAT should be able to tap not only initial personality differences between stutterers and nonstutterers, but also to reflect the influence of stuttering on the personality. On either count, differences ought to appear if they exist.

What are the findings? Table 2 summarizes the results of major investigations of the TATs of stutterers. Again, no unique pattern emerges, and no systematic differences appear from one study to another. Few TAT investigators show that they have examined previous findings and used them as prior hypotheses, or even considered other findings in interpreting their results. Again, we are faced with the puzzling lack of significant dimensions. Even if personality dynamics were not a factor in onset, the experience of growing up a stutterer might logically be expected to produce differences.

Either stutterers differ in dimensions which are not reflected in their TAT (or Rorschach) protocols, or the experience of growing up a stutterer somehow has an offsetting effect.

Most TAT investigators, beginning with Richardson, have

TABLE 2	TAT STUDIES
Investigator	Richardson, 1944
Subjects	30 stutterers.
Controls	30 controls, matched for age, sex, and college experience. Decile rating for mental ability.
Significant Findings	
Interpretation	Stutterers showed greatest needs for achievement and affection. (Controls showed higher proportion.)

concerned themselves with such factors as the needs for achievement and for affection, with dependency, and with mechanisms for handling feelings of hostility. Richardson found stutterers somewhat lower in achievement orientation, a finding indirectly corroborated in Sheehan and Zelen's later study of level of aspiration (Sheehan & Zelen, 1955). However, TAT investigators either did not follow Richardson's lead or found no significant differences in achievement motivation.

The lack of consistently appearing differences in comparisons of stutterers and normals on the TAT is primarily due to a

Haney, 1951	Wilson, 1951
6 stutterers.	30 stutterers.
None.	30 nonstuttering siblings. Parents of 30 stutterers.
Primary findings derived from an experimental projective technique in which subject was asked to visualize an imaginary white card and then to project upon it. Each subject carried out this experimental procedure for 90 (sic) hours. Results thus obtained were "submitted to test-retest appraisal by the Rorschach Ink Blots and Thematic Apperception Test."	Stutterers were extremely aggressive (.01 level) and displayed a significant amount of inverted hostility (.05 level).
Subjects began to project themselves. The speech mechanism "was perceived as spatially disoriented, structurally confused, and functionally self-contradicted." The stutterer's "perceptual distortions were [seen as] motives implied by the speech maladjustment termed stuttering."	Stutterers and mothers of stutterers showed significant similarity in areas of aggression and hostility, suggesting some introjection by the stutterers of maternal characteristics.

simple reality: Stutterers are normal. At least, they cannot be said to differ from normal controls on those dimensions tapped by the TAT.

Possibly the more sophisticated techniques developed by Atkinson (1958, 1967) to measure need for achievement and need for affiliation will eventually yield more precise data on the achievement motivations of stutterers. Since this factor relates to self-esteem and level of aspiration, it is one of the more promising leads for research on personality factors in stuttering.

75

TABLE 2	(continued)
Investigator	Christensen, 1952
Subjects	30 stutterers. Ages: 4 1/2–12 1/2.
Controls	30 siblings. Ages: 5–14.
Significant Findings	Projected significantly more in situation involving nursing at breast. Identified significantly more with male figure in pictures that furnished opportunity for aggression. Projected significantly more sadness and choking.
Interpretation	More unfavorable outcomes in pictures that furnished opportunity to express attitudes of aggression.

ROSENZWEIG PICTURE-FRUSTRATION STUDIES

An aspect of the personality of stutterers frequently alleged in the literature is hostility, or its behavioral representative, aggression. Psychoanalytic writers have been especially prone to attribute hostility to stutterers. Logically, from the frustration-aggression hypothesis (Dollard *et al.*, 1939), the experience of stuttering should be sufficiently frustrating to lead to aggression. Van Riper (1963b) has emphasized the frustration

Lowinger, 1952	Silverman, 1952
29 nondelinquent neglected and orphaned stuttering children. Ages: 8–15.	10 male Negro stutterers.
29 controls, matched for age and WISC IQ (70 or better).	10 male Negro nonstutterers.
Stutterers do not differ significantly in degree of aggression. Stuttering girls significantly less aggressive than stuttering boys (.05 level). Stutterers more guilt burdened, but not significantly. Correlation between aggression and guilt, .63–.84, significant for both groups. No difference between groups on orality. Girls of both groups manifest significantly more orality. No significant relation between TAT and Rosenzweig P-F aggression and guilt or overt aggressive behavior for either group.	Stutterers had more dominant mothers than nonstutterers.
Findings on aggression and orality did not reveal a dynamic pattern specific for stutterers.	

aspects of stuttering in his acronym PFAGH, and in other writings.

Against this backdrop, four investigators have used the Rosenzweig Picture-Frustration Test (P-F) to study the personality of stutterers. Madison and Norman (1952) reported compulsive, anal-sadistic tendencies. It should be noted that they did not gather a control group but compared their experimental group of 25 stutterers against Rosenzweig's P-F normative group. These findings were not confirmed by Quarrington, whose methodological criticisms of the Madison-Norman study

TABLE 2	(continued)
Investigator	Goodstein, Martire, and Spielberger, 1955
Subjects	30 male stutterers.
Controls	30 male nonstutterers.
Significant Findings	No significant differences found between stutterers and nonstutterers on achievement imagery responses to card 10.
Interpretation	Findings do not support hypothesis of difference between stutterers and nonstutterers in achievement imagery.

included the charge of failure to control experimenter bias. When Quarrington did contol experimenter bias, no significant differences were obtained. In another study bearing on the handling of hostility, Murphy (1953) found significantly more extrapunitiveness and significantly more intrapunitiveness, exactly opposite to the Madison and Norman findings. Obviously, Quarrington's results failed to confirm the differences reported

Bloodstein and Schreiber, 1957	Solomon, 1963
15 adult stutterers; 15 adult non-stutterers.	35 stutterers. Ages: 14–35.
30 parents.	35 with normal speech; 35 with speech defects other than stuttering.
Analysis of variance yielded non-significant F on checklist for obsessive-compulsive characteristics.	When a particular kind of intense aggression is considered (i.e., murder or intent to kill), stutterers appeared to respond with significantly less aggression. In the face of an intense aggressive stimulus, stutterers in contrast to nonstutterers seemed to express significantly less aggressive stories where a hero in the story must assume full reponsibility for the aggression. Stutterers in contrast to nonstutterers appeared to indicate significantly more physical aggression of a certain kind—e.g., fighting, hitting.
Stutterers no different from non-stutterers in obsessive-compulsive tendency.	Stutterers in contrast to nonstutterers appeared to express significantly more subtle aggression (natural death themes) and defensive aggression (verbal aggression in a story without a definite hero).

by Murphy. The study by Lowinger (1952), using 29 child stutterers with 29 controls matched for age and IQ, found no difference in aggressive responses and no specific dynamic pattern characteristic of stutterers. This negative result is in agreement with Quarrington's on adults and supportive of the generalization that stutterers do not differ from controls on most personality measures.

TABLE 3	ROSENZWEIG P-F COMPARISONS
Investigator	Madison and Norman, 1952
Subjects	25 stutterers. Ages: 14–59. Mean age: 23.3.
Controls	Rosenzweig's norm group.
Significant Findings	Significantly higher intropunitiveness and need-persistence. Significantly lower on obstacle dominance and extrapunitiveness.
Interpretation	Findings seem to correspond to psychoanalytic contention that stuttering is compulsive in nature, with anal-sadistic tendencies resulting in turning-in of aggression.

SELF-CONCEPT STUDIES

The self-perceptions and self-concepts of stutterers were investigated in studies by Fiedler and Wepman (1951) and by Zelen, Sheehan, and Bugental (1954), with essentially negative findings. Zelen, Sheehan, and Bugental reported that stutterers tended to make more positive-toned statements about themselves and that those for whom therapy was successful made fewer negative statements initially.

Though the role of self-concept in stuttering has been stressed by Sheehan (1953; 1954a; 1958a), Murphy and Fitzsimons (1960), and Rieber (1963), surprisingly few studies have provided data on this potentially important variable.

Redwine (1958) used an adjective check list on 30 stuttering children and 30 controls, found no significant differences, and rejected the idea that a distinct stuttering personality

Quarrington, 1953	Murphy, 1953
30 stutterers. Mean age: 30.4	30 adult stutterers.
Rosenzweig's norm group.	30 adult nonstutterers.
No significant differences.	Stutterers showed higher percentage of ego defensiveness, at .05. Stutterers showed less intrapunitiveness (.01), less group conformity (.01), more extrapunitiveness (.05).
Study failed to confirm Madison and Norman findings. Their findings may be due to bias in sampling or in method employed. Efforts to eliminate hypothetical expectations from scoring not set forth. In this study, two psychologists scored tests independently; they were unaware of purpose or opinions of research group.	

existed. Fitzpatrick (1959) concluded that the speech disorder becomes a vital element in the personality of the stutterer. Using a variety of projectives with no controls, Broida (1962) reported that boys who stutter differ from the "normal population" and concluded that stuttering was a result of neurotic conflict related to identification. Using the Sarbin-Hardyck stick-figure test, Buscaglia (1962) reported stutterers to be inferior in role perception and empathy. Gildston (1964) reported less self-acceptance.

Recently, Sheehan and Martyn (1966, 1970) and Martyn and Sheehan (1968) have reported that those who develop self-concepts as stutterers are less likely to experience a spontaneous recovery. The experiment by Bardrick and Sheehan (1956) showing that a self-esteem threat increases the frequency of stuttering has been cited as supportive of a self-other, status-gap factor in stuttering (Sheehan, 1968).

TABLE 3	(continued)
Investigator	Lowinger, 1952
Subjects	29 stutterers. Nondelinquent neglected and orphaned children (children's form). Ages: 8–15
Controls	29 nonstutterers, matched for age and WISC IQ (children's form, 70 or better).
Significant Findings	No difference in frequency and intensity of guilt or aggressive responses. Inverse relation between manifested aggression and guilt, but not statistically significant.
Interpretation	No specific pattern characteristic of stutterers.

LEVEL-OF-ASPIRATION STUDIES

Level-of-aspiration behavior (LOA), which is related to self-concept and self-esteem, is the one dimension that has shown some promise in distinguishing the personalities of stutterers from those of nonstutterers. Sheehan and Zelen (1951; 1955) found that stutterers were significantly lower in level of aspiration, that they stayed in the success area of goal-setting, predicted more modest performances for themselves, and tried to avoid the possibility of failure. Mast's results (1952), using a different level of aspiration measure, agreed with these findings. Using other measures, Trombly (1958) found LOA scores unrelated to severity of stuttering.

Sheehan (1963) studied level of aspiration for fluency in a role-theory framework, finding:

1. Severe stutterers differed from mild stutterers in that they bid more ambitiously for fluency.
2. When severe stutterers set more modest fluency goals, they stuttered less.
3. The highest role-commitment to fluency, as reflected in the level of aspiration D-scores, was associated with the most severe stuttering.
4. The mild stutterers were more likely to underestimate their performance, whereas severe stutterers were more likely to overestimate their performance.

Using Rotter board and a speech task, Goldman and Shames (1964a, 1964b) studied 24 family units of stutterers and 24 control units, consisting of mother, father, and child. The stutterers' fathers set higher goals on speech tasks. They concluded that stutterers' parents set higher goals for their children. For a more complete discussion of the Goldman-Shames, Sheehan-Zelen, and other LOA studies, see Table 5 and the original articles.

VARIED PROJECTIVE STUDIES

Not all projective studies of stuttering have employed the more common instruments such as the Rorschach and TAT. In Table 6, various other projective studies are summarized. Here the same situation applies as noted previously, that is, the studies do not report on common dimensions and their authors make few efforts to relate findings to one another.

In general, the earlier and more poorly controlled studies report differences and the more recent and methodologically refined researches do not. Using a modified Blacky test, Boland (1952) came up with the interesting and possibly very significant finding that speech anxiety and general anxiety may be relatively independent of one another. Boland found that stutterers had a higher level of anxiety associated with the speaking situation, but not a general higher anxiety level. Kurshev (1961) noted differences between mild and severe stutterers in reactions to drawings and words. Using the Blacky pictures, Carp (1962) failed to confirm previous Blacky results by Merchant (1952) and Bernhardt (1954). Reference here should be made to Carp's discussion and to that of Boland, who used a modification of the Blacky pictures.

PARENT-CHILD RELATIONSHIP STUDIES

Since stuttering has its onset early in childhood, and personality develops in interaction with parental figures, it was natural and inevitable that investigators should turn to parent-child relationships in stuttering. A number of these efforts, along with studies of the children themselves, are summarized in Table 7.

Johnson (1942) was more impressed by the similarities than the differences between 46 stuttering children and 46 control-group children. Rotter (1939) stressed pampering, while Despert (1946) cited pressure by the compulsive mother. Glasner (1949),

83

TABLE 4	SELF-CONCEPT STUDIES
Instrument	Q-technique
Investigator	Fiedler and Wepman, 1951
Subjects	10 stutterers.
Controls	6 nonstutterers, matched for sex, age, education, socioeconomic status.
Significant Findings	On composite scales for group of clinical psychologists and mental hygiene patients, stutterers looked on themselves more like psychologists than patients.
Interpretation	No trends between stutterers and nonstutterers.

in a study of 70 young stutterers without a control group, reported other associated emotional disturbance, and, like Rotter, stressed overprotection. Bloodstein, Jaeger, and Tureen (1952) found that parents of stuttering children evinced a higher fluency standard and were quicker to diagnose stuttering. However, both these results could be interpreted as secondary or as results of experience with a stuttering child.

Moncur (1952) emphasized parental domination in mothers of stuttering children. Darley (1955) found families with one stuttering child markedly similar to families with one matched control child, with further investigation indicated into areas of parental standards and sensitivity to speech deviations. Glasner and Rosenthal (1957) reported a relationship between active parental correction of disfluency and perpetuation of stuttering.

W-A-Y technique	Q-Sort of 100 self-referent statements structured into 6 personality-trait categories
Zelen, Sheehan, and Bugental, 1954	Wallen, 1959
30 stutterers in group therapy.	30 adolescent male stutterers.
160 nonstutterers.	30 nonstutterers, matched for age, IQ, socioeconomic status, school locale.
Stutterers made more positively toned statements about themselves. Normals mentioned age and sex more frequently. Stutterers for whom therapy was successful made fewer negative statements initially.	Stutterers exhibited significantly less similarity between actual-self concept and ideal-self concept.
Stutterers who have decided to go into therapy may have resolved a conflict in the self, hence feel more positive about themselves.	Contrary to several previous studies, stutterers exhibit significant differences in terms of specific self-concept relationships and specific personality traits in comparison with nonstutterers.

But Holliday found that parents of stutterers were not more dominating than parents of nonstutterers, and stressed the interaction of parent and child. A further illustration of contradictory results is Abbott's finding (1957) that mothers of stutterers displayed more empathy and affection toward their children than mothers of nonstutterers. Wyatt (1958) confirmed her previous writings in reporting higher "distance" anxiety in stutterers.

In a large and carefully controlled study, Johnson *et al.* (1959) compared 150 parents of child stutterers with matched controls. In the large majority of interview items, the two parental groups did not differ significantly. However, parents of stutterers did operate with somewhat more demanding expectations and were more striving and perfectionistic. Berlin (1960) found that par-

TABLE 4	(continued)
Instrument	Projective Drawings
Investigator	Fitzpatrick, 1959
Subjects	32 secondary stutterers. Ages: 8–14.
Controls	None.
Significant Findings	Significant statistical difference found between 8 of 11 categories evaluated in drawings. The "self" drawings depicted a lesser degree of speech proficiency than did drawings of the "ideal" self.
Interpretation	Regardless of etiology, speech disorder becomes a vital element in the personalities of stutterers.

Experimenter-designed self-concept inventory (check-list of adjectives)	It Scale for Children, Draw-A-Person Test, Structured Story Completion Test, Structured Puppet Play Test, questionnaires for parents and teachers to rate subjects' sex-typed behavior
Redwine, 1958	Broida, 1962
15 4th-grade stutterers; 15 8th-grade stutterers.	45 male stutterers, Caucasian, middle socioeconomic status. Ages: 5–10. Parents and teachers of subjects.
15 4th-grade nonstutterers; 15 8th-grade nonstutterers.	None.
No significant differences found between self-acceptance of stutterers and nonstutterers. There are self-descriptions significantly unique both to particular groups of boys who stutter and to particular groups of boys who do not.	Subjects had strong preference for the masculine role at every age past 5. Ambivalence in sex-role identification increased with age. Fathers preferred to mothers, particularly at ages 5 and 6. After age 5, parents perceived to be far more punishing than nurturing ($p < .001$).
Findings reject the concept that a distinct "stuttering personality" exists.	Boys who stutter have a higher preference for masculine role earlier, more frequently and with less variance than normals; they are more ambivalent in sex-role identification; they differ in their development course of parental preference; they perceive their fathers as more punishing than nurturing. Findings support theory that stuttering is result of neurotic conflict developing from disturbances in the identification process in early childhood.

TABLE 4	(continued)
Instrument	Sarbin-Hardyck Stick Figure Test (modified form)
Investigator	Buscaglia, 1962
Subjects	30 male stutterers.
Controls	56 male nonstutterers; 26 psychotic male adolescents (demonstrating total role disintegration).
Significant Findings	Comparison of scores for stuttering group compared to nonstutterers significant beyond .05 level; scores for nonstutterers versus psychotics significant, $P < .001$; stutterers versus psychotic population, no significance, $P > .10$.
Interpretation	Compared to nonstutterers, stutterers are less able to perceive their own and others' life roles. Assuming correlation between role inadequacy and social behavior, stutterer is socially more inadequate. Assuming correlation between role perception and empathy, stutterer has less empathic ability and his future role-learning will be negatively affected.

ents of stutterers were not unusually intolerant of nonfluency, thus differing from Johnson, from Darley, and from Bloodstein, Jaeger, and Tureen.

Attempting to tap possible covert rejection in the mothers of stutterers, Kinstler (1959) compared mothers with prodigiously matched controls on the University of Southern California Maternal Attitude Scale. Although it tackles a dimension of possible importance, the method of analysis suggests a possible capitalization on chance differences in the sample. An interesting finding was that the mothers of normal-speaking children were more overtly rejecting than the mothers of stutterers. If this result could be verified it would have vast implications for learning-theory conceptions of the origins of stuttering.

Hilden Q-Sort
Gildston, 1964
55 junior-high-school stutterers.
55 nonstutterers, matched for age, sex, IQ, grade, school, socio-economic level.
Stutterers were less self-accepting than nonstutterers and they perceived their parents to be less accepting of them. No significant difference found between maternal and paternal acceptance for either group.

MMPI STUDIES OF STUTTERERS

Probably the best standardized and certainly the most widely used paper-and-pencil personality test today is the Minnesota Multiphasic Personality Inventory (MMPI). It is an empirically derived test that reveals the similarity of the response pattern of the subject to those of established clinical categories. The clinical scales of the MMPI contain both a "neurotic" and a "psychotic" side. In addition, four validity scales provide built-in safeguards by yielding information on the subject's comprehension of the items, degree of defensiveness, and test-taking attitude.

The MMPI does discriminate successfully among clinical

TABLE 5	LEVEL-OF-ASPIRATION STUDIES
Instrument	Rotter Board
Investigator	Sheehan and Zelen, 1951
Subjects	20 stutterers.
Controls	20 nonstutterers.
Significant Findings	No significant differences; stutterers somewhat lower than controls.
Interpretation	Statistical "Zone of Uncertainty."

categories, indicated by score elevations on clinical scales. These categories include hypochondriasis (Hs), anxiety-depression (D), psychasthenia, obsessive-compulsive tendencies, (Pt), hysteria (Hy), nonconformity, psychopathic deviation (Pd), cultural interests, liberalism, masculinity or femininity (Mf), paranoid tendency (Pa), hypomanic, acting-out tendency (Ma), reality contact, schizophrenia (Sc), and social introversion (Si). Moreover, a vast number of special scales have been derived from the MMPI—Barron's ego-strength (Es) scale, Navran's dependency scale, and many others. Taylor's manifest anxiety scale was developed largely as a modification of the MMPI "D" scale. Entire handbooks have been developed giving MMPI profiles relating to a wide range of personality types (Dahlstrom & Welsh, 1960).

In other words, the MMPI should be an excellent instrument for detecting personality differences between stutterers and nonstutterers or between their parents, if such differences actually exist. What are the findings?

The pattern of nonrelatedness among results already noted on the Rorschach, the TAT, and other projective tests is found on the MMPI. Pizzat (1949) reported a slightly elevated mean profile for stutterers compared with test norms. Thomas (1951) found a slight elevation within the range of normal adjust-

Carl Hollow Square	Rotter Board
Mast, 1952	Sheehan and Zelen, 1955
Stutterers.	40 stutterers.
Discrepancy scores.	60 matched controls.
Significantly lower discrepancy scores.	Stutterers show lower discrepancy score (P= .05), more range (P= .05), and greater frequency of success (P= .02).
Indicates that stuttering group was overly cautious in defenses against failure—in the defeatist category.	Stutterers signicantly lower in level of aspiration: they stay in success area, avoid threat of failure.

ment. Boland, using a variety of MMPI-derived measures, did not find "neuroticism" more prevalent in stutterers. It should be noted that whereas Thomas merely referred to test norms, Boland actually obtained a control group. One of Boland's findings, which we feel to be quite significant, is that speech anxiety and general anxiety may be relatively independent. This finding fits well with the role-specificity concept in stuttering (see Sheehan, Chapter 1).

Dahlstrom and Craven (1952) found much heterogeneity, but no significant differences between stutterers and university counselees. They also reported no relationship between MMPI scores and stuttering severity. The college-student stutterers resembled general college students rather than general psychiatric cases. Walnut (1954) found that stutterers do not differ from controls except in their reaction to speaking situations. Frederick (1955) found that stutterers do not necessarily have common psychodynamics despite apparent commonality in presenting symptom. More recently, Lanyon (1966) found that ego strength was positively related to improvement in therapy.

From the foregoing, it may be seen that MMPI comparisons of stutterers and nonstutterers have failed to turn up differences, even on this well-standardized instrument.

TABLE 5	(continued)
Instrument	Graphomotor Test; Oral Reading Test; Knower Speech Attitude Test
Investigator	Trombly, 1958
Subjects	30 stutterers, Ages: 13–54. Mean age: 21.5. 26 male, 4 female.
Controls	None.
Significant Findings	Severity of stuttering not significantly related to any of LOA scores. Attitude toward speech was significantly and negatively related to 3 speech scores and positively related to 1 of graphomotor scores.
Interpretation	Significantly more stuttering in speaking following success than in speaking following failure.

Rotter Board; Speech Task	Level of Aspiration for Fluency
Goldman and Shames, 1964	Sheehan, (1963)
24 family units of stutterers (mother, father, child 8–12).	60 adult stutterers. Mean age: 27.3
24 units of nonstutterers (mother, father, child 8–12).	Subjects served as own controls.
Differences between 2 groups of mothers on Rotter Board not statistically significant. On speech tasks, nonstutterers' mothers set goals lower than stutterers' mothers. Fathers of stutters differed significantly from fathers of nonstutterers on both tasks in 2 ways: (1) they predicted fewer speech difficulties for their children, and (2) they didn't lower their estimates of performance following failure on Rotter Board as frequently as nonstutterer' fathers.	Highest role commitment, as reflected in level-of-aspiration D-scores for fluency, was associated with the most severe stuttering. Mild stutterers were more likely to underestimate their performance, severe stutterers were more likely to overestimate their performance. Level-of-aspiration-for-fluency D-scores tended to reduce somewhat through successive readings of five 100-word passages, with varying individual patterns relating to the mild-severe dimension.
Results support contentions that stutterers' parents set higher goals for their children generally, and higher speech goals specifically. Stutterers' fathers appear less realistic in their goal-setting behavior for their children's speech under conditions of failure. This lack of readjustment by fathers could possibly be a pressure-producing agent involved in the etiology or perpetuation of stuttering.	The greater the role commitment to fluency, the greater the pressure toward perfect speech and the greater the anxiety regarding the speaker role.

TABLE 6	VARIED PROJECTIVE STUDIES
Instrument	Duss's Fables; Case History and Interview (part of larger study)
Investigator	Despert, 1946
Subjects	50 stutterers. Ages: 6 1/2–15
Controls	None.
Significant Findings	Stutterers showed a greater frequency of deviation from "normal" developmental history, and greater frequency of early neurotic characteristics with obsessive-compulsive traits predominating. Sadistic fantasies commonly brought out in fables.
Interpretation	As a group, stutterers are more intelligent but more rigid than nonstutterers. While there is no specific personality type characteristic of stutterers, specific neurotic trends are found with obsessive-compulsive traits predominating.

MMPI STUDIES OF PARENTS

Perhaps then, differences should be expected between parents of stutterers and parents of nonstutterers. Comparisons of the parents are summarized in Table 9. The MMPI seems to have been first used by Grossman (1952), who reported no differences in pattern analysis, though stutterers' parents seemed to interpret MMPI items more atypically. Goodstein and Dahlstrom (1956) found more defensiveness in control parents, though no significant differences appeared in T scores above 70. They concluded that parental attitudes involved in the etiology of stuttering are problem-specific to the speech situation. In a cross-validation, Goodstein (1956) confirmed his previous conclusion that the etiology of stuttering is not related to severe

Bender Visual Motor Gestalt Test	7-Point Rating Scale for 10 personal and nonpersonal cartoons
Burleson, 1949	Staats, 1955
40 male child stutterers. Grades: 4, 5, 6	26 male stutterers (University speech clinic) and 63 male nonstuttering college students.
40 male child nonstutterers. Grades: 4, 5, 6	57 male nonstuttering college students.
No significant observable differences between the two groups in psychomotor performance nor in perseveration or hesitancy.	No statistically significant differences found between nonstuttering control group and stutterers. Only 1 nonpersonal cartoon showed a significant difference (at 5% level) between nonstutterer controls and nonstutterer experimental group.
Stutterers do not differ from nonstutterers as measured by the Bender.	A difference in sense of humor between stutterers and nonstutterers was not demonstrated.

psychopathology in the parents. More recent studies have been similarly negative.

There appears to be here a discrepancy between what we are able to show through clinical instruments and what most clinicians believe. Stuttering is widely assumed to be the "parent's symptom" as Travis (1946) aptly put it.

We hold to the belief that members of the family are members of the problem and are to be treated as such. Yet it is hard to justify these beliefs with data. Kinstler's study on overt and covert maternal rejection (1961) opened up an area of investigative promise, despite a number of methodological limitations. Even more promising may be the work of Goldman on matriarchal and patriarchal patterns in Negro and white stutterers. Among anthropological approaches, the

TABLE 6	(continued)
Instrument	Travis-Johnston Projective Test
Investigator	Wilson, 1951
Subjects	30 stutterers.
Controls	Parents of 30 stutterers; 30 nonstuttering siblings.
Significant Findings	Mothers of stutterers showed significantly higher level (.01) on aggression-hostility and significantly fewer withdrawal tendencies in face of environmental stimuli.
Interpretation	The possibility that stutterers have introjected approximate characteristics of the mothers is tenable. Pattern of parent-child relationship not suggested by findings.

work of Aron (1962) on stuttering among the Bantu, and Lemert on stuttering in Pacific and Polynesian groups is especially promising. It may be eventually that anthropological approaches will yield more than studies employing psychological test instruments.

CALIFORNIA TEST OF PERSONALITY STUDIES

Five studies have appeared employing the California Test of Personality. These are summarized in Table 10, along with

Blacky Test	Speech Anxiety Projective Test (Modified Blacky Test)
Merchant, 1952	Boland, 1952
20 stutterers, 15 male and 5 female.	24 stutterers.
20 nonstutterers, matched for sex, age, family constellation, aptitude.	24 nonstutterers.
Stutterers differed from controls on 7 out of 14 Blacky dimensions at significant level. More disturbance on Oral Eroticism, Oral Sadism, Castration Anxiety and Penis Envy, Identification Process, Guilt Feeling and Anaclitic Love-Object. On Anal Expulsion stutterers received significantly fewer strong scores.	Level of anxiety associated with speech situation is significantly greater for stutterers.
Suggestion that this is a validation of the Blacky Test because it is sufficiently sensitive to pick up these consistent developmental patterns with only 20 pairs of subjects. Fenichel views appear to be supported.	Speech anxiety and general anxiety may be relatively independent.

Richardson's study using the Guilford inventory, which taps some similar dimensions. Powers's study in 1944 found no significant differences in self-adjustment nor in total adjustment. Though Perkins (1947) and Schultz (1947) reported some differences, negative results appeared in the studies by Elliott (1952) and by Horlick and Miller (1960). Essentially, the findings in this series must be viewed as negative.

VARIED MOTOR STUDIES

Not all personality studies of stuttering can be grouped via comparisons of different investigators using the same instru-

TABLE 6	(continued)
Instrument	Blacky Pictures
Investigator	Bernhardt, 1954
Subjects	44 male stutterers. Ages: 11–22
Controls	None.
Significant Findings	Certain psychosexual dimensions evoked significantly more stuttering. Subjects with highest amount of conflict show highest amount of stuttering.
Interpretation	Stuttering is related to personality difficulties of the stutterer, and certain environmental stimuli related to personality affect his stuttering.

ment. In Table 9 we have grouped a number of varied motor studies involving such instruments as the Tachistoscope (Eisenson & Winslow, 1938; Franks & Rousey, 1958), serial learning tasks (Hill, 1942), tests of motor proficiency, (Kopp, 1946), the Bender (Wilson, 1951), tests of perseveration (King, 1954, 1961; Martin, 1962), EEG (Murphy, 1953), pursuit tasks under stress and Saslow screening test for anxiety (Berlinsky, 1954), palmar sweating (Brutten, 1957), electromaze (Kapos & Standlee, 1958), auditory visual perception (Froeschels & Rieber, 1963), critical flicker frequency (Kamiyama, 1964). Other tests

Sacks Sentence Completion Test	Blacky Pictures Test
Snyder, Henderson, Murphy, and O'Brien, 1958	Eastman, 1960
75 adult stutterers.	Male stutterers, child group and adult group. Ages: 8–13; 16–38
75 parents of stutterers, matched for age, socioeconomic background and education.	None.
Attitudes of stutterers varied significantly from parents of stutterers with respect to family, sex, interpersonal relationships and self-concept.	Hypotheses confirmed at high level of confidence (for both groups): (1) More stutterers will show disturbance on the dimensions of Anal Sadism and Guilt Feeling on Blacky than on any other dimensions. (2) Fewer stutterers will show disturbance on Sibling Rivalry than on any other dimension.
Stutterers as a group present a more disturbed personality structure than parents of stutterers. Many similarities were found between the two groups in the area of emotional dynamics.	

that might have been included under the heading of varied motor tests were omitted from this chapter because they are covered by William Perkins in his review of physiological studies, Chapter 5.

In general, the findings of the varied motor studies are negative. First, as may be seen by the summary of the findings in the tables, most of these studies directly reported no differences between stutterers and nonstutterers. Where differences were noted, they did not emerge in other studies—they appeared to be *ad hoc*, for that case only, conclusions from sample characteristics rather than probable universe characteristics. The

TABLE 6	(continued)
Instrument	Special Aggressive and Non-Aggressive Stimulus Cards
Investigator	Aten, 1961
Subjects	24 stutterers. Ages: 7–14
Controls	24 nonstutterers, matched for age, sex, race, occupational status of parent.
Significant Findings	Significant differences found on response to male peer aggressive stimulus picture.
Interpretation	Theme avoidance or "perceptual defense" of stutterer and possible inhibition of aggressive activity to peers.

Ivanov-Smolenski Method (reactions to drawings and words)	Blacky Pictures
Kurshev, 1961	Carp, 1962
16 stutterers. Ages: 15–39	20 college stutterers, 15 male and 5 female. Ages: 19–39. Median age: 22
Subjects served as own controls.	20 college nonstutterers, matched for sex, age, family constellation, and classification in Ohio college aptitude test.
In forming varied responses (conditioned, differential, inhibitory, disinhibitory), some differences were found between mild and severe stutterers. In severe stutterers there is a predominance of inhibitory and disinhibitory responses with words difficult to pronounce acting as stronger stimuli. In the milder group a summation effect takes place in the sense of an influence exerted by the verbal reaction upon the motor response.	In Anal Retentiveness, stutterers did not differ significantly from nonstutterers in any scoring category. On Anal Expulsiveness, stutterers scored lower (significant at .05% level) than nonstutterers on ODS. On the three scorable secondary components (phallic, oral, erotic, and anal sadistic) stutterers obtained higher scores than nonstutterers. In every case, Spontaneous Story scores supported the psychoanalytic predictions for secondary components.
	Predictions concerning personality characteristics of stutterers derived from psychoanalytic theory were affirmed in regard to secondory components but not in regard to primary impulse. Anal Retentiveness and Anal Expulsiveness scoring artifacts of the test may have caused the discrepancy.

TABLE 7	CASE STUDIES
Instrument	Case History
Investigator	Rotter, 1939
Subjects	522 stutterers, 425 male and 97 female. Ages: 2.5-44. Median age: 14
Controls	Nonstuttering population from White House Conference and Child Health and Protection.
Significant Findings	Statistically significant findings of more only children and fewer middle children among stutterers. Mean number of years between stutterer and next sibling were greater than normal.
Interpretation	Data suggests that "there is a direct relation between development of stuttering in a child and degree to which he becomes dependent on others to do things for him and to solve his own problems successfully." (Rotter uses term "pampering" to describe this evident dependency and loss of self-esteem). Child feels inadequate to solve his own problems successfully.

regularity of directly negative findings and "findings that do not lead anywhere" becomes a monotonous procession.

INTELLIGENCE STUDIES

Nothing we know about the social psychology of stuttering should have been especially predictive of intelligence as a major factor in the disorder. Yet, because articulate speech is so often lacking in the retarded, it was perhaps inevitable that intelligence was one of the first personality dimensions to be explored. Then, too, research is often shaped by the available measuring instruments. At the time systematic studies of stut-

Interview and Case Study	Parental Interview and Case History
Johnson, 1942	Despert, 1946
46 stutterers, 32 male and 14 female. Ages: 2–9	Parents of 50 stutterers. Ages of Children: 6 1/2–15
46 nonstutterers, 33 male and 13 female. Ages: 2–9	None.
Birth conditions, developmental data, age of onset of speech defect essentially the same for both groups. More stutterers in the families of stutterers than nonstutterers.	Majority of the mothers were domineering, overanxious, overprotective and perfectionistic. 31 mothers and 20 fathers were considered neurotic. Fathers played secondary role.
Similarities between the two groups more significant than differences. Parental evaluations of child's speech a determining role in subsequent speech development of child.	Pressure by the often compulsive mother at critical periods of the speech development in "somatically sensitized individuals" is viewed as a catalyzing agent for speech and associated pathology.

tering were begun, IQ tests were well developed and standardized, while techniques for assessing other personality dimensions were relatively crude.

Do stutterers differ from nonstutterers in intelligence? If so, are they more intelligent or less intelligent than nonstutterers? If differences exist, are they among the causes of stuttering or among the results? These and similar questions were the focus of the first investigations of stuttering and personality. Fairly early, there was an impression that although stutterers did not differ from nonstutterers, college stutterers were more intelligent than college nonstutterers, on the ground that a person would not attempt college with the handicap of stuttering unless

TABLE 7	(continued)
Instrument	Case Study
Investigator	Glasner, 1949
Subjects	70 stutterers under age 5. Median age: 3.6
Controls	None.
Significant Findings	All exhibited some degree of emotional manifestation other than stuttering. 54% characterized as "feeding problems," 27% were enuretic, 20% had exaggerated fears and/or nightmares. Over half the children showed 2 or 3 other indications of emotional disturbance.
Interpretation	Stuttering children under the age of 5 can be roughly divided into 3 main types: (1) the healthy child whose stuttering closely follows the introduction of a disturbing element into his environment; (2) the child who in addition to stuttering has a whole constellation of neurotic symptoms and tendencies; (3) the "sensitive" child, standing somewhere between type 1 and type 2. Stutterers generally show a long history of overprotection and pampering and have overanxious, excessively perfectionist parents.

he possessed good intelligence. In *Speech Pathology,* Travis (1931) reported that the average stuttering child was retarded about one and a half years in school. Travis noted:

> *It must also be observed that intelligence tests, especially those which involve speaking, tend to*

Bell Adjustment Inventory (using "home adjustment" section scores only)	Response to 2-minute recorded samples of stuttering and nonstuttering speech
Duncan, 1949	Bloodstein, Jaeger, and Tureen, 1952
62 stutterers, 49 male and 13 female. Ages: 16–27. Median age: 18	24 parents of stutterers. Ages of children: 3.5–8. Median age: 6
62 nonstutterers with varying degrees of articulatory defects. Age: 16–25	24 parents of nonstutterers. Children's ages: 4–10
Responses to 5 of the 35 items were significantly different at the .01 level. The discriminating questions dealt with feelings about lack of parental affection, recognition, acceptance, and understanding.	Parents of stutterers made a significantly larger number of diagnoses of stuttering than parents of nonstutterers.
Significant differences shown point toward an unwholesome situation somewhere in the relations between the stutterer and his parents, or they may indicate a higher incidence of neurotic characteristics among stutterers.	Existence of higher standards of fluency for parents of stuttering children. The extent to which a child's nonfluency is excessive or conspicuous is determined not only by amount of repetition in his speech but by fluency standards of listener.

depreciate the stutterer's ability. It would be interesting to compare I.Q.'s obtained before and after the cure of stuttering. It is reasonable to say that in so far as intelligence involves adaptability and in so far as adaptability involves normal speech, stuttering is certainly a

105

TABLE 7	(continued)
Instrument	Personal Interview Data, revaluated on Dominance Scale
Investigator	Moncur, 1952
Subjects	Mothers of 48 stutterers. Ages of children: 62–98 months
Controls	Mothers of 48 nonstutterers matched for sex, grade, residential area. Children's ages: 65–95 months
Significant Findings	More mothers of stuttering children gave answers indicating parental domination. Difference was statistically significant.
Interpretation	An environmental syndrome of factors precipitating or aggravating stuttering (e.g., oversupervision, overprotection, excessively high standards, adverse parental criticism) may be a variety of dominating parental actions.

deterrent in the stutterer's attempts to exhibit his native intelligence. The stutterers in the University of Iowa have been distinctly superior to the average college student in intelligence. (The selective factor at work operates more completely in the case of the stutterer who hesitates to go to college with two handicaps, stuttering and mental dullness.)

The first systematic survey of intelligence and personality data on stuttering should be credited to Wendell Johnson for his classic monograph, *Influence of Stuttering on the Personality*, in 1931. Basing his conclusions in part on data from McDowell (1928) and others, Johnson noted:

The influence of stuttering on the personalities of these individuals has been chiefly that of

Case Study, Direct Observation	Iowa Scale of Attitude Toward Stuttering
Moncur, 1955	Darley, 1955
48 stutterers. Median age: 79.6 months	50 families, each with stuttering child.
48 nonstutterers, matched for age, sex, school placement. Median age: 80.2 months	50 control families, matched for age and sex of child and socio-economic status.
Stutterers averaged 8.8 symptoms of maladjustment and controls averaged 4.0.	No significant intragroup or inter-group differences were found.
Stuttering children display more symptoms of maladjustment than nonstuttering children. Symptoms of maladjustment most character-istic of stuttering children are nervousness, enuresis, nightmares, aggressions, fussiness in eating, and frequent need for discipline.	

*frustration and discouragement. Stuttering lim-
ited the possibilities for adaptation to social situations.*

*The reactions of the individuals were mainly
of two kinds: Those of rebellion against, and
those of acceptance of and acquiescence to the
stuttering and its implications.*

In the light of Johnson's later formulation of the semantogenic hypothesis, the following passage in *Influence of Stuttering on the Personality* makes fascinating reading today:

*Which appeared first, the stuttering or the fear
of it? In this case the answer is obvious. She
says, "For two weeks I expected each new attempt at speech to be successful and was surprised at the interrupted rhythm. Now, what is*

107

TABLE 7	(continued)
Instrument	Guilford's Inventory of Factors STDCR
Investigator	Darley, 1955
Subjects	50 families, each with a stuttering child.
Controls	50 control families, matched for age and sex of child and socioeconomic status.
Significant Findings	STDCR differences between the two groups of parents are not statistically significant at the 5% level on any of the 5 factors.
Interpretation	Neither the experimental group cases nor their parents present pictures of marked maladjustment or strong family discord. However, areas that appear to warrant closer investigation included parental standards and expectations, early management of observed nonfluencies, parental drive and dominance characteristics.

Interview and Case Study (II)	California Test of Personality; Allport Ascendance-Submission Reaction Study; Psychosomatic Inventory of McFarland and Seitz; Ammons-Johnson Test of Attitude Toward Stuttering; Test constructed by author to measure parental attitudes toward the role of boys and girls
Darley, 1955	LaFollette, 1956
50 families, each with a stuttering child. Ages of children: 2.4–14.4. Mean age: 9.2	85 families of stuttering children.
50 control families, matched for age and sex of child and socioeconomic status.	50 families of nonstuttering children.
On 12 of 15 personality traits the stuttering children were rated significantly less favorably by their parents. 32% of 238 items yielded intergroup differences: Stutterers' parents were somewhat older; they had smaller, better educated families and higher standards of neatness; they were less well satisfied with their children's achievements; mothers were more socially active.	Parents in the experimental group showed a greater tendency toward submissiveness than did control group. Fathers in experimental group showed greater submissive tendencies and less satisfactory mental health when compared with controls. No dependable differences found between the 2 groups of mothers nor between parents of male stutterers and those of female stutterers.
While the two groups are markedly similar on the vast majority of items studied, areas warranting closer investigation include: parental standards and expectations generally and specifically with regard to speech, early management of observed nonfluencies, parental sensitivities with regard to speech deviations, and parental drive and dominance characteristics.	

TABLE 7	(continued)
Instrument	Interview
Investigator	Glasner and Rosenthal, 1957
Subjects	153 parents of stuttering 1st-grade children.
Controls	843 parents of nonstuttering 1st-grade children.
Significant Findings	70% of stutterers' parents actively sought to correct child's speech. Parents attributed cause of disorder to emotional disturbance in 62% of cases. When emotional problems posited as cause, 41% said to have stopped stuttering; when environmental influences thought to be cause, 82% said to have stopped.
Interpretation	Relationship found between active correction of the nonfluency and the perpetuation of the stuttering.

just is—but I'll probably get over it. I must. And each morning I rather expect to be well again." Pointed questions were put to her. There was no sign of fear during the first week or two of stuttering. The stuttering always came as a distinct surprise to her. Then she began inter-

Edwards's PPI; Edwards's Social Desirability Scale; USC Parent Attitude Survey (Shoben's)	Observation Scale of 10 Behavioral Qualities; Structured Interview (228 items); Parental Attitude Research Instrument; Iowa Scale of Attitudes Toward Stuttering
Holliday, 1958	Abbott, 1957
58 pairs of parents of stutterers.	30 stutterers, 30 mothers of stutterers. Ages of children: 4.9–11.11
58 pairs of parents of nonstutterers, matched for age, education, and father's occupation.	30 nonstutterers, 30 mothers of nonstutterers, matched for age, sex, familial socioeconomic status.
Fathers of stutterers tended to be more compulsive, less exhibitionistic, and less aggressive than fathers of nonstutterers. Mothers of stutterers were more abasing in their attitudes toward themselves, but more aggressive than the mothers of nonstutterers. Parents of stutterers were not more dominating than parents of nonstutterers.	Mothers of stutterers displayed more affection and empathy toward their children. Tendency towards overprotection revealed by the PARI and items concerned with Developmental History obtained from interviews. Children in both groups did not display any differences regarding their reactions to their respective mothers.
Not only is the individual personality structure of each parent important in the child's environment, but also the pattern of behavior or interaction between the personalities of the two parents.	

preting certain kinaesthetic strains as being indicative of on-coming stuttering, and she began to regard certain social situations as particularly difficult to manage. Then, since stuttering meant something extremely undesirable to her, a fear of it began to develop.

111

TABLE 7	(continued)
Instrument	Mother-Child Relationship Test (battery of projective tests) measuring distance anxiety, mother devaluation, and fear of disaster
Investigator	Wyatt, 1958
Subjects	20 child stutterers.
Controls	20 nonstuttering children, matched for age, sex, intelligence.
Significant Findings	Higher incidence of "Distance Anxiety" among stutterers significant at .005 level; "Fear of Disaster" approached .05 level. Coincidence of FD with advanced stuttering was significant at .05 level.
Interpretation	Combination of acute "Distance Anxiety" and feelings of devaluation of mother as love object is characteristic of stuttering child, rather than the anxiety or aggressive feelings seen in isolation.

Comparisons among principal studies of stuttering in relation to IQ measurement are summarized in Table 12. Not included are "studies" based loosely on clinical impression, or without verifiable methods of data collection.

Using the Ohio State Psychological Examination, Fruewald (1936) found that college stutterers ranked higher in intelli-

Interview and Case Study (III), Iowa Scale of Attitude Toward Stuttering	Recorded Samples of nonfluent speech
Johnson *et al.*, 1959	Berlin, 1960
Parents of 150 stutterers. Ages of children: 27–96 months. Mean age: 59.9 months	67 parents of stutterers. Mean age of children: 10
Parents of 150 nonstutterers, matched for age, sex, socioeconomic status. Ages of children: 28–103 months. Mean age: 60.2 months	57 parents of children without speech problems. Mean age of children: 11.5. 86 parents of children with misarticulations. Mean age of children: 10.5
Experimental-group parents operated with more demanding expectations regarding the fluency of their children's speech. They were also somewhat more dissatisfied with their children and with each other, had higher standards of child development and were, in general, more discontented, more perfectionistic and striving.	Mean number of diagnoses of stuttering remained approximately the same for all groups of parents.
In their responses to a large majority of the interview items, the two parental groups did not differ to a statistically significant degree.	The parents of stuttering children were not unusually intolerant of nonfluency compared to the other parents; members of all parent groups misdiagnosed some normal nonfluency as stuttering.

gence than the general college population, an agreement with Travis's statement cited above.

While it did not provide a direct IQ measure, Hill's study of perseveration in stutterers and nonstutterers involved a serial-movement learning task, which could probably be related to certain visual-motor subtests on the Wechsler. He reported a

TABLE 7	(continued)
Instrument	Case Study Interview
Investigator	Bloodstein, 1961b
Subjects	5 adopted child stutterers.
Controls	None.
Significant Findings	In 4 of the 5 cases there was no known stuttering in the adoptive families. In the 5th case, the adoptive mother stuttered and described herself as being an excessively demanding parent.
Interpretation	

slower performance speed for stutterers, and found perseveration in both stutterers and controls.

Carlson (1946) compared 50 child stutterers with problem children, and found no direct relationship between stuttering and intelligence.

Projective questionnaire	Rotter Board
Kinstler, 1961	Goldman and Shames, 1964
30 mothers of young male stutterers.	15 pairs of parents of stutterers.
30 controls, matched for age, education, size of family, socioeconomic status, religion, psychological guidance, education of spouses.	15 pairs of parents of nonstutterers, matched for socioeconomic status, age, education, and age of their children.
Significant differences in the pattern of responses. Chi-square analysis yielded a value greater than the .01 level of confidence.	Parents of stutterers and parents of nonstutterers did not differ significantly in the goal-setting behavior for themselves. No statistically significant differences occurred in their estimates of performance following either success or failure.
Mothers of young male stutterers reject their children covertly far more but overtly far less than do the mothers of normal speakers. Mothers of stutterers accept their children covertly less and overtly only slightly less than do the mothers of normal speakers. Mothers of stutterers reject their children more than they accept them while mothers of normal speakers accept their children more than they reject them.	Findings do not support hypothesis that there are differences between parents of stutterers and parents of nonstutterers in the goals they set for themselves on a motor task.

Darley (1955) used the Stanford-Binet and the Wechsler, and found no difference from population norms.

Schindler (1955) compared 126 stuttering Iowa school children with double that number of matched controls, finding a significant lower mean IQ for stutterers, with an average of one

TABLE 7	(continued)
Instrument	Seven family characteristics were assessed from the data supplied by mothers through interview. They were concerned with social class and social mobility, mother's age at marriage and at birth of the child, father's age, family size, and sibling rank.
Investigator	Andrews and Harris, 1964
Subjects	80 stutterers. Ages: 10–11
Controls	80 normal matched children from similar school and residential environments; this far outweighed the disadvantage of partial matching for intelligence and social class.
Significant Findings	None of the seven items revealed significant differences between the experimental and control groups.
Interpretation	More stuttering children than control children have been socially deprived. More have had to cope with the upheaval and change of role implicit in a one-parent home. Mothers of stutterers gave very similar personal histories to control mothers, but they have significantly poorer school records and significantly poorer work histories. Biologically, the two groups of children seem to be comparable, having had similar developmental histories and achieving similar physical parameters. Stutterers are significantly late in talking, and, when they do talk, they have a much higher incidence of developmental disorders of articulation. A positive family history of stuttering, common among the experimental children, was practically absent in the control families. Psychiatric assessment of the children failed to establish differences between the two groups.

Tape samples of conversational speech; family history information (from structured interviews)	100-item questionnaire (based upon most relevant questions of 250-item personality questionnaire previously given to 490 adult stutterers.
Knepflar, 1965	Robbins, 1965
21 mothers of stutterers; 21 fathers of stutterers.	100 high-school and adult stutterers.
21 mothers of nonstutterers; 21 fathers of nonstutterers. Matched for age, educational levels, number of children per family.	100 college non-stutterers.
Parents of stutterers display more disfluencies than parents of non-stutterers (significant at .025 level). Fathers produce about the same number of disfluencies in their speech as mothers.	Stutterers are very similar to people who do not stutter and are generally exposed to the same home, school, and environmental influences as nonstutterers. Stutterers differed from the controls in greater amount of surgery, more frequent exposure to a second language, experiences with parents and more stuttering relatives.
The results of this study have theoretical implications for those who support the concept of familial diathesis and for those who suggest that the high familial incidence of stuttering is based on cultural factors.	There is a limit to the number and frequency of stress experiences that a child can undergo without evincing neurotic symptoms. When this limit, which varies with the individual, is exceeded, the child is likely to exhibit stuttering or some other nervous symptom.

TABLE 7	(continued)
Instrument	Speech survey: Speech screening examination, structured individual interview, Sheehan Sentence Completion Test.
Investigator	Sheehan and Martyn, 1966
Subjects	32 recovered stutterers, 27 male and 5 female. Ages: 17–56. Mean age: 30.5
Controls	366 normal-speaking college students; 32 active stutterers, 29 male and 3 female. Ages: 17–47. Mean Age: 27.5
Significant Findings	Four out of five recover from stuttering spontaneously. Fewer of those who had received public-school speech therapy recovered from stuttering. Fewer of those who had ever been severe recovered spontaneously. Familial incidence was found to be a factor in the occurrence of stuttering, but not in recovery from it. No differences in reported handedness in stutterers or their families. Improvement attributed to self-acceptance and role acceptance.
Interpretation	Spontaneously recovered stutterers comprise a new and unexplored research population. Future formulation of the onset and development of stuttering will have to take into account the predominant nonpersistence of stuttering in most cases in which it develops. Results of previous studies on stuttering are suspect since they are based on data gathered on only one-fifth of those who had ever had the problem.

year retardation in oral reading skill. A marked similarity between groups on other measures was noted.

In recent years, studies comparing stutterers and nonstutterers on IQ dimensions have appropriately dwindled. Most investigators have come to agree with Johnson (1946; Johnson *et al.*, 1967) and with Darley (1955) that there are no demonstrable differences.

Although it is often asserted or assumed that stutterers are superior in intelligence, assertions in the opposite direction have not been lacking. Van Riper (1963b) related that there are more stutterers among mentally retarded than among the normal population, reporting a figure of 20 percent. The one-in-five figure is incorrectly attributed to Gens (1951), who in the cited reference had not gone beyond saying, "We may investigate the rather high incidence of stuttering in mongoloids and relate it to the many theories of stuttering."

Nothing that we know about the social psychology of stuttering should be especially predictive of intelligence as a factor in the disorder.

The puzzling statistic cited by Van Riper partly motivated a recent study by Sheehan, Martyn, and Kilburn (1968). In a speech examination and interview survey of 216 institutionalized at Porterville State Hospital in California, only 26 normal speakers were found. Eighty-three had no speech; delayed speech and articulation made up the bulk of the sample. Only one stutterer was found in this population, along with one clutterer. It should be noted that over one third of the Porterville group did not have enough speech to be judged stutterers. The results of the Sheehan, Martyn, and Kilburn study are corroborative of those of Holmes and Pelletier (1967). Using the category "rhythm disorder" they found a ratio of stutterers not significantly higher than that in the general population.

To check on the possibility that the Porterville patients may have been atypical in some fashion peculiar to that setting, a further survey was undertaken at Camarillo State Hospital in California. The Camarillo mentally retarded were older than those at Porterville and differed in some other demographic characteristics. Martyn, Sheehan, and Slutz (1969) conducted individual diagnostic speech examinations on a larger sample of 346 Camarillo retarded. The results are in close agreement with the Porterville data, and only three stutterers were found —just about what would be expected from the national incidence of stuttering.

Thus, assertions that stuttering appears more frequently among the retarded, or relates to either end of the distribution of intelligence, appear totally unfounded. Again, the result on the intelligence studies is that stutterers are like other people except for the specific problem called stuttering.

TABLE 8	MMPI STUDIES OF STUTTERERS
Instrument	MMPI
Investigator	Pizzat, 1949
Subjects	53 stutterers.
Controls	Test norms.
Significant Findings	Mean profile of stutterers somewhat elevated when compared with test norms.
Interpretation	

VARIED PERSONALITY STUDIES

The personality tests that have been used to assess stutterers have shifted with changing styles in personality assessment. For this reason, direct comparison of the earliest and most recent studies is usually not possible. In Table 13, results on varied personality measures are summarized, from McDowell (1928) and Johnson (1932) through Brown and Hull (1942), and Brutten (1957), to Trombly (1965) and Knabe, Nelson, and Williams (1966).

MMPI	MMPI
Thomas, 1951	Dahlstrom and Craven, 1952
29 stutterers.	100 college stutterers.
Test norms.	Nonstuttering controls: 100 college students; 1,763 psychiatric patients; 3,996 college students seeking counseling help; 618 test norms.
Mean profile somewhat elevated for stutterers when compared with test norms, but well within the range of adjustment.	Stuttering group showed a high degree of heterogeneity. Significant differences between stutterers and between norms and college group, but no significant differences between stutterers and university counselees. No significant relationship found between MMPI scores and stuttering severity.
	As a group, the stutterers differ from the test norms and typical college students in their adjustment patterns. They are not as severely maladjusted as general psychiatric cases and most closely resemble other college students with problems.

Taken together, the studies in Table 13 indicate slight adjustment difficulties of stutterers revolving around the speech situation, and the studies support the conception that those slight differences that can be found are results rather than causes of stuttering. Any one of the authors might of course reject this conclusion. For more precise statements of their views, the original sources should be consulted.

Even though Table 13 conglomerates studies using very different instruments and tapping diverse dimensions, it necessarily omits many other studies that might have merited in-

TABLE 8	(continued)
Instrument	MMPI-derived Anxiety Measures: Welsh's Anxiety Index; Taylor's Manifest Anxiety Scale; Modlin's Neuroticism Scale; Janda's Expressor-Repressor Ratio
Investigator	Boland, 1953
Subjects	24 adult stutterers.
Controls	24 adult nonstutterers.
Significant Findings	Measures of "neuroticism" did not differentiate stutterers from nonstutterers. Stutterers tended to express anxiety overtly. Level of chronic anxiety significantly higher in stutterers (.05). Low correlation between measure of general anxiety and speech anxiety.
Interpretation	Stutterers appear to have preference for expressing anxiety overtly. Speech anxiety and general anxiety may be relatively independent.

clusion. As with the other tables of this chapter, a large "et cetera" should be added.

TIME DIMENSION STUDIES

Time pressure is an important variable in stuttering, for it is through the time dimension that all manner of interpersonal interactions are expressed. In the words of the poet, there is a time to speak and a time to remain silent. When it is his time to speak, the stutterer must deliver the word promptly or

Short Form MMPI	MMPI (Taylor Anxiety Scale)
Walnut, 1954	Frederick, 1955
38 stutterers, 20 male and 18 female. Ages: 15–20	63 stutterers, 51 male and 12 female. Ages: 18 and over
52 normals; 25 crippled students; 26 students with cleft palates. Ages: 15–20	36 nonstutterers, 24 male and 12 female.
All groups were well within the normal range of personality. Stuttering group showed significant differences toward the poor adjustment end of the Depression and Paranoid Scales. Stutterers reacted abnormally to speech and speaking situations.	Female stutterers significantly more disturbed than male stutterers: High anxiety stutterers differ from low anxiety stutterers in their reactions to reward and punishment.
Data does not indicate whether stuttering precipitated abnormal personality or vice versa, since "pathological" groups showed no significant personality deviations.	Stutterers do not necessarily have common psychodynamics despite apparent commonality in presenting symptom.

reveal himself in the stutterer role he typically attempts to conceal. Yet ironically, stutterers tend to internalize time pressures they have experienced from others, to put pressure on themselves, and to operate from a built-in time pressure system. The stutterer hurries himself in a way that becomes so obvious that even the casual listener invites the stutterer to slow down, to take it easy. Unfortunately, like the command to relax, such suggestions tend to have the opposite effect. It is interesting that in accounts and studies of recovery from stuttering, slowing down successfully is one of the frequent reports of those

TABLE 8	(continued)
Instrument	MMPI
Investigator	Lanyon, 1966
Subjects	25 severe stutterers who were rated for severity before and after a year of continuous therapy.
Controls	None.
Significant Findings	Analysis of MMPI profiles revealed that the Es (ego strength) scale was positively related to improvement and the F (deviant responses) scale was negatively related to improvement.
Interpretation	Differences in the findings for psychotherapy and for stuttering therapy were interpreted as due to differences in the nature of these therapies.

who are able to recover without formal treatment (Sheehan *et al.*, 1957; Wingate, 1964; Shearer & Williams 1965; Sheehan & Martyn, 1966; Martyn & Sheehan, 1968).

Against this background, studies involving the time dimension in stuttering come to have a special import. In a 1946 study directed by Van Riper, Sheehan carried out a phonetic analysis of 500 stuttering blocks, 25 each from 20 adult stutterers. The vast majority of the blocks were of one, two, and three seconds duration—strikingly short in view of the monumental handicap that is erected upon such brief interruptions in the forward flow of speech.

Ringel and Minifie (1966) compared stutterers and normal speakers on time estimation, finding that severe stutterers had greater difficulty monitoring the passage of time during communicative activity, and that time factors are important in stuttering behavior.

Reaction time of stutterers and controls was studied by Font (1955) and Adams and Dietz (1965), and stutterers were found to be similar to controls. In a study specifically designed to investigate time pressure, Stunden (1965) presented a word-association list to 18 stutterers and to matched controls. He found no significant differences in number of contrasting adjectives.

However, Stunden (1965) also found that adaptation was significantly retarded by time pressure.

SHOULD THE SEARCH CONTINUE?

So concludes our procession of personality studies, at least from this point on the reviewing stand. Although the parade will no doubt continue, its goal, the search for simple personality differences, is likely to be illusory. Although investigations into specific dimensions such as prognosis or time pressure may be promising, we find words written in 1962 prophetic and worth repeating today.

> *Any future study which reports personality differences between stutterers and nonstutterers should be considered suspect. Such reports in the past have almost without exception proved to be due to methodological error . . . Perhaps the search for basic personality differences between stutterers and nonstutterers has gone far enough, sapped enough creative potential, and should end. (Sheehan, 1962)*

If there are no reliable differences between stutterers and nonstutterers that hold up on repeated samples, why do so many people continue to search, and why do they continue to report differences where none exist? The answer here appears to lie not in the personality problems of stutterers but in those of the investigators. In the following section, we consider the personality projections of the investigators themselves.

STUTTERING AS A PROJECTIVE TECHNIQUE

The problem of stuttering itself has become a projective technique for many investigators. Too often the stutterer has served as inkblot for biased and undisciplined experimenters, or even worse, for "authorities."

Comparative studies have demonstrated no differences between stutterers and nonstutterers. Therefore when an individual claims certain personality characteristics in stutterers, he is not drawing from scientific evidence, but from his own need system. Just as an inkblot elicits projections, so does the problem of stuttering elicit idiosyncratic projections. Hostility? De-

TABLE 9	MMPI COMPARISONS OF PARENTS OF STUTTERERS
Instrument	MMPI
Investigator	Grossman, 1952
Subjects	42 parents of child stutterers.
Controls	42 parents of child nonstutterers.
Significant Findings	Statistically significant difference indicates that stutterers' parents interpret MMPI items more atypically.
Interpretation	No significant difference in pattern analysis.

pendency? Sexual conflicts? Separation anxiety? Maternal deprivation? Any of these allegations are essentially idiosyncratic, concept-dominated projections of the investigator. It would be revealing to study the relationship between the investigator's personal problems and those he imputes to the stutterer. Want to know the personal conflict areas of a nonstuttering speech pathologist? Find out what he projects onto the stutterer!

Minnesota Scale of Parents' Opinion	MMPI
Grossman, 1952	Goodstein and Dahlstrom, 1956
42 parents of child stutterers.	224 parents of stutterers.
42 parents of child nonstutterers.	223 parents of nonstutterers.
Stutterers' parents place less emphasis on active as opposed to passive social participation and responsibility of child and showed markedly low ability to interpret efficiently the desirability and undesirability of specific child behavior-traits and their influence upon the child's social and emotional adjustment.	Control parents had significantly higher mean scores on the K and Do scales; experimental parents had a significantly higher mean score on the A scale. There was no significant difference between the two groups on the high-point codes nor on the T scores above 70.
	Performances of the 2 groups were not significantly different from each other or from the expected performance of psychiatrically normal persons. Results support the notion that such attitudes and adjustments of the parents as may be involved in the etiology of stuttering are probably limited and specific to the speech situation.

It has been charged that the literature on stuttering has been unduly influenced by the circumstance that so many of the writers in it have been stutterers (Wingate, 1965). Not true! The trouble with the literature on stuttering is not so much that stutterers have projected their problems on other stutterers, but that normal-speaking writers have projected their personal abnormalities on the stutterer. After all, even the projections

TABLE 9	(continued)
Instrument	MMPI Cross-validation of earlier study
Investigator	Goodstein, 1956
Subjects	100 parents of stutterers (follow-up parents). Mean age of children: 10.10
Controls	100 follow-up parents from original 200 experimental parents and 200 control parents. Children's Mean age: 5
Significant Findings	Failure to establish any major differences between the follow-up parents and either the experimental or control parents from the initial study. The mean A-scale score (from Taylor Manifest Anxiety Scale) of the follow-up group was between that obtained from the two original groups.
Interpretation	The responses of the follow-up group were not significantly different from those of the two earlier groups, and confirm the conclusions of the prior study that the etiology of stuttering is not related to severe psychopathology on the part of the stutterers' parents.

of a stuttering writer should be valid for his own case. The same cannot be said for the projections of others who may have all kinds of problems except stuttering.

THE PERSONALITY ORIGINS OF STUTTERING: A PUZZLE

As this review has shown, there are no demonstrable differences between stutterers and nonstutterers, child or adult, or between their parents. Since stuttering varies with the social-psychological situation, what are its social and personality origins? How are beginning stutterers different? How are their parents different? Here is a real puzzle, something on which we need imaginative research. The effort is complicated by sparseness of sensitive research tools with children.

Either (1) the experience of stuttering makes the person more like a normal speaker, so that any early differences disappear; or (2) stuttering children are not different to begin with, for the experience of growing up as a stutterer should increase rather than decrease any differences originally present.

In the adult population, where we really have ample studies, we find that the alleged deviations don't hold. Therefore, the whole notion that the stuttering child is deviant becomes suspect. In this connection, there are studies such as Johnson's which have shown that we really can't differentiate which of a group of 100 children are stutterers on any basis other than the stuttering behavior itself.

THE RANGE OF DIAGNOSIS
IN STUTTERING

The relation of stuttering to severe personality breakdown or decompensation is worth studying. The relation of stuttering to personality when it is a relatively minor part of the clinical picture is equally worth studying. Suggestions for further study along these lines, especially considering psychological subtypes in stuttering and the concept that the stuttering is not homogeneous, may be found in Chapter 8, "Research Frontiers." Our survey of the results of personality tests has clearly shown that the concept of a single personality type in stuttering is a fallacy. The notion is probably fallacious in many other disorders as well.

The apparent lack of correspondence between speech behavior and personality dynamics requires explanation. If clinical entities are defined in terms of overt behavior, as is the case in stuttering, then no common set of dynamics can be found. This is probably true all the way up and down the range of psychiatric diagnosis, from those with delusions, those with sexual problems, those with psychopathic behavior, those showing compulsions, those showing headaches, ulcers, anxiety attacks, and so forth.

AVENUES IN AND OUT OF STUTTERING

It is probably a basic fallacy to expect that because the resulting behavior is the same, the underlying dynamics are neces-

129

TABLE 10	CALIFORNIA PERSONALITY STUDIES
Instrument	California Test of Personality
Investigator	Powers, 1944
Subjects	Junior high school stutterers.
Controls	Junior high school nonstutterers.
Significant Findings	No significant difference between two groups in self-adjustment or in total adjustment. Some tendency toward significant difference in social adjustment.
Interpretation	Since no significant difference was found between the groups on the total adjustment score, it may be justly said that stutterers and nonstutterers in junior high school tend to be equally well adjusted.

sarily going to be the same. Or that the route for getting there is the same.

There appear to be many roads leading to Rome and to neurosis; each neurosis seems to have many avenues leading to it and from it.

In the etiology and treatment of stuttering, it is clear that there are several probable avenues in and several probable avenues out. Stuttering is a behavior related to a whole range of psychological dynamics, not just to one. Stuttering is to a high degree *role-specific* behavior. Stuttering is not a unitary disorder, but seems to capture within it different varieties or subtypes (Sheehan, 1958b; 1968). Stutterers may be of widely differing types: exteriorized or interiorized; explicit or implicit; aggressive or passive; outgoing or introverted. Whatever subcategories we might choose, these in themselves are different behaviors and suggest different underlying processes or dy-

Guilford's Inventory of Factors STDCR	California Test of Personality (Adult Form A)
Richardson, 1944	D. W. Perkins, 1947
30 stutterers, 22 male and 8 female. Ages: 17–48. Mean age: 27.8	75 adult stutterers.
30 nonstutterers, matched for age, sex, college experience, and decile rating for mental ability.	None.
Most significant differences in R, followed by S and then D.	
Stutterers are less happy-go-lucky, more socially introverted, and more depressed.	Problems of young adult stutterers fell consistently within areas of self-reliance, feelings of personal worth, nervousness, social skill, and social standards.

namics. The term "stuttering" includes endless variety in "symptoms" and covers a wide range of expressive behaviors. Perhaps, then, it should come as no surprise that stutterers do not show a common personality pattern, and that in group studies stutterers cannot be distinguished from normal-speaking controls.

PSYCHOTHERAPY FOR WHAT?

Part of the puzzle resulting from our survey of personality studies is this: If the stutterer is like everybody else to begin with, what does he need psychotherapy for? A basic aim of psychotherapy is reconstructive personality change or "corrective emotional experience." Psychotherapy may be defined in terms of developing better interpersonal relations. Now, if the stutterer's interpersonal relations, or his ego strength, or

131

TABLE 10	(continued)
Instrument	California Test of Personality
Investigator	Schultz, 1947
Subjects	20 stutterers. Mean age: 29. Mean IQ: 113.5
Controls	Test norms of CTP and case histories of 239 diagnosed neurotics.
Significant Findings	Stuttering group as a whole had median percentile of 25 on CTP.
Interpretation	Stutterers and psychoneurotics have many common symptoms.

his psychodynamics, or his psychosexual development, or his personality traits cannot be shown to be different, then why should he need psychotherapy?

To say that stutterers need psychotherapy or can profit from it is like saying people need psychotherapy or can profit from it. As Wendell Johnson reminded us, stutterers are people. If we are to recommend psychotherapy routinely for stuttering, we may as well tap each person we meet on the street and recommend psychotherapy routinely. We would have just as much justification for doing so. In fact, since the incidence of psychosis is apparently lower in stuttering, we might be better justified in randomly tapping the man in the street for psychotherapy than we would be in recommending that stutterers *ipso facto* receive psychotherapy.

Though stutterers do not need psychotherapy just because they are stutterers, they seem to profit from a program integrating psychotherapy with speech therapy (Sheehan, 1954a; Chapter 7, this book). More precisely, a role-taking psycho-

California Test of Personality	California Test of Personality
Elliott, 1952	Horlick and Miller, 1960
141 children with speech deviations. Grades 1–4, 4–6	26 stutterers; 26 hard-of-hearing nonstutterers. Enlisted male military personnel.
Test norms.	Standardization group.
Pearson r for degree of speech deviation and percentile rank on total adjustment score close to zero for both groups.	Wide variations in intragroup performances were noted. No one characteristic pattern of adjustment for either group could be identified.
Safe to assume no correlation.	Clinical observations and findings are not in agreement with previous investigations attributing specific characteristics to the hard of hearing.

therapy, involving specialized procedures spelled out elsewhere in this book, is recommended as the treatment of choice. Like the rest of us, the stutterer is changed through experience, through doing things.

References

References that are listed here only by author and year of publication appear in complete form in the Bibliography.

Abbott, T. B. (1957)

Adams, M. R. and Dietze, D. (1965)

Andrews, G., and Harris, M. (1964)

Aron, M. L. (1962)

Aten, J. L. (1961) A study of the influence of aggressive stimuli upon the perceptual response thresholds of stuttering and nonstuttering children. Ph.D. dissertation, University of Washington, Seattle.

Atkinson, J. (1958) *Motivation in fantasy, action, and society.* New York: Van Nostrand.

TABLE 11	VARIED MOTOR STUDIES
Instrument	Mahler-Elkin Test
Investigator	Eisenson and Pastel, 1936
Subjects	30 male stutterers. Ages: 10–16
Controls	30 male nonstutterers.
Significant Findings	Statistically significant differences in the groups showed that the stutterers slowed down in their tasks more than the nonstutterers and made more errors while working.
Interpretation	Stutterers perseverate more than nonstutterers. The perseveration is an indication of a resistance to change and lack of adaptability on the part of stutterers.

Atkinson, J. (1967) *The psychology of motivation.* New York: Van Nostrand.

Bardick, R. A., and Sheehan, J. G. (1956) Emotional loading as a source of conflict in stuttering. *American Psychologist, 11,* 391.

Bearss, M. L. (1951) An investigation of conflict in stutterers and nonstutterers. *Speech Monographs, 18,* 237. M.S. dissertation, Purdue University, 1950.

Bender, J. F. (1939) *The personality structure of stuttering.* New York: Pitman.

Berlin, C. (1960)

Cards prepared for Tachistoscope exposure	Serial Movement Learning Tasks
Eisenson and Winslow, 1938	Hill, 1942
15 stutterers.	10 stutterers, 7 male and 3 female. Ages: 18–30
20 nonstutterers.	20 nonstutterers, 10 male and 10 female. Ages: 18–30
Nonstutterers saw more colors than stutterers on the average, and were more variable. No difference between stutterers and nonstutterers on average number of omissions on cards. Statistically reliable difference was found indicating that stutterers did perseverate considerably more frequently.	Perseveration of reactions found in all subjects of all groups. No significant differences found between normal-speaking and stuttering groups in the nature or amount of abnormal behavior following interruption of task, but stutterers' reactions were slower and more prolonged.
Stuttering is a manifestation of the perseverating tendency, which, at least in part, causes the stutterer to stutter as his normal way of speaking.	While there is a general tendency of perseveration for all subjects, the slower performance-speed of stutterers indicates a difference between stutterers' and normal speakers' ability to learn serial muscle activity.

Berlinsky, S. L. (1954)

Bernhardt, R. B. (1954)

Bloodstein, O. N. (1961b)

Bloodstein, O. N., Jaeger, W., and Tureen, J. (1952)

Bloodstein, O. N., and Schreiber, L. (1957)

Boland, J. L. (1953)

Broida, H. (1962) An empirical study of sex-role identification and sex-role preference in a selected group of stuttering male children. Ph.D. dissertation, University of Southern California, Los Angeles.

Brown, S. F., and Hull, H. C. (1942) A study of some so-

135

TABLE 11	(continued)
Instrument	Oseretsky Tests of Motor Proficiency
Investigator	Kopp, 1946
Subjects	50 stutterers. Ages: 6 1/2–15
Controls	Test norms.
Significant Findings	26% of the children showed severe retardation, 46% were classified as "motor idiots," only 3 were "normal," and 1 scored superior. 92% failed in all tests of synkinetic movements.
Interpretation	Tests reveal a global uniform deficiency of the motor functioning of the stuttering children.

cial attitudes of a group of 59 stutterers. *Journal of Speech Disorders* 7, 323–324.

Brutten, E. J. (1951)   Anxiety as a personality factor among stutterers. M.A. thesis, Brooklyn College.

Brutten, E. J. (1957)

Buscaglia, L. F. (1962)   An experimental study of the Sarbin-Hardyck Test as indexes of role perception for adolescent stutterers. Ph.D. dissertation, University of Southern California, Los Angeles.

Burleson, D. E. (1949)   A personality study of fourth, fifth, and sixth grade stutterers and nonstutterers based on the Bender Visual Motor Gestalt Test. M.S. dissertation, University of Pittsburgh.

Calamaras, P. (1964)   An investigation of the degree of tolerance of ambiguity of male stutterers ranging in age from ten to seventeen years. Ph.D. dissertation, New York University, New York.

Carlson, J. J. (1946)   Psychosomatic study. III. *American Journal of Orthopsychiatry, 16,* 114. (Part of J. L. Despert's study.)

Carp, F. M. (1962)

Mira Myokinetic Test; Bender Visual Motor Gestalt Test; Figure Drawing Test	Einstellung-Effect Problems (motor-mechanical, numerical, and oral test).
Wilson, 1951	Solomon, 1952
50 adjusted stutterers.	Male college stutterers.
50 maladjusted stutterers.	Male college nonstutterers, matched for age, education level.
Both groups have in common a certain motor ineptness as revealed by these tests.	Stutterers manifested significantly more rigidity of behavior in an oral situation than the nonstutterers.

Christensen, A. H. (1952)

Cohen, J. G. and Edwards, A. E. (1965) The extraexperimental effects of random sidetones on stutterers. Proceedings of the annual convention, American Psychological Association.

Curlee, R. F. (1967) An experimental study of the effect of punishment of the expectancy to stutter on the frequency of subsequent expectancies and stuttering. Ph.D. dissertation, University of Southern California, Los Angeles.

Dahlstrom, W. G. and Craven, D. (1952) The MMPI and stuttering phenomenon in young adults. *American Psychologist*, 7, 341.

Dahlstrom, W. G. and Welsh, G. (1960) *An MMPI handbook, a guide to use in clinical practice and research.* Minneapolis: University of Minnesota Press.

Darley, F. L. (1955) The relationship of parental attitudes and adjustments to the development of stuttering. In W. Johnson, ed., *Stuttering in children and adults.* Minneapolis: University of Minnesota Press.

Despert, J. L. (1946) Psychosomatic study of 50 stutter-

137

TABLE 11	(continued)
Instrument	Ten tests selected from three perseverative areas: alternating motor area, dispositional area, and the sensory area. Test of general intellectual ability.
Investigator	King, 1954
Subjects	80 stutterers, 72 male and 8 female.
Controls	137 nonstutterers, 82 male and 55 female.
Significant Findings	When all tests viewed collectively, 17 comparisons showed that stutterers indicated a greater amount of perseveration. A perseverative general group factor does not seem to exist in either male or female nonstutterers.
Interpretation	Stutterers demonstrate significantly more perseveration tendencies generally than nonstutterers and are significantly more perseverative on specific tests which demand a contiguous change of set.

EEG	Oseretsky Tests of Motor Proficiency
Murphy, 1953	Finkelstein and Weisberger, 1954
30 stutterers, alpha index 50% or higher.	15 stutterers. Ages: 4–10
30 nonstutterers, alpha index 50% or higher.	15 nonstutterers, matched for age, sex, and laterality.
a) During frustration, stutterers show no significant interhemispheric difference while controls show differences significant at 10%. b) Cortical disruption during frustration significantly greater in stutterers when like hemispheres between groups are compared. c) Both groups show least recovery in dominant hemisphere. d) Stutterers recovered cortical equilibrium to a markedly smaller degree (1%) than controls. e) In both groups, each hemisphere showed significant differences (1%) between rest and frustration. f) Stutterers' cortical behavior during recovery corresponded to state of frustration; nonstutterers to resting state.	As a group, the stutterers were slightly though not significantly superior to the controls in 5 of the 6 tests.
	Stutterers are not retarded in motor proficiencies, but tend to be slightly superior to nonstutterers in such abilities.

TABLE 11	(continued)
Instrument	Pursuit Tasks performed under stress conditions of electric shock; Saslow Screening Test (to measure chronic anxiety level)
Investigator	Berlinsky, 1954
Subjects	14 stutterers.
Controls	14 nonstutterers, matched for age.
Significant Findings	Stutterers and nonstutterers did not differ in level of anxiety as measured by Saslow Screening Test. Frequency and kinds of stuttering varied significantly for stutterers between experimental conditions. Anxiety measures showed a different pattern of relationship for stutterers and nonstutterers. Stutterers showed greatest anxiety under conditions of "anxiety with no speech allowed."
Interpretation	Stuttering is a symptom of an internal maladjustment which increases when the stuttering symptoms cannot be expressed. Stuttering acts as a cathartic activity relieving the anxiety of the stutterer. The stuttering is inferred to be the cathartic activity, not the speech itself.

ing children. *American Journal of Orthopsychiatry, 16,* 100–113.

Dollard, J., *et al.* (1939) *Frustration and aggression.* New Haven: Yale University Press.

Duncan, M. (1949) Home adjustment of stutterers versus nonstutterers. *Journal of Speech Disorders, 14,* 255–259.

Eastman, D. F. (1960)

Eisenson, J., and Pastel, E. (1936) A study of the perseverating tendency in stutterers. *Quarterly Journal of Speech, 22,* 626–631.

Colorimetric Technique (measure of palmar sweating)	Keystone Tachistoscope; case histories
Brutten, 1957	Franks and Rousey, 1958
33 stutterers.	20 stutterers, 16 male and 4 female. Mean age: 9.4
33 nonstutterers, matched for age, sex, educational level.	20 nonstutterers, matched for age, race, IQ, vision, and hearing.
Stutterers not significantly more anxious than nonstutterers in a nonverbal situation. Stuttering and anxiety adaptation were highly similar in decremental form and slope. Expectancy and anxiety adaptation covaried for stutterers but not for nonstutterers.	No significant differences between groups in visual and perceptual abilities, nor in signs of brain damage or emotional disturbance.
Stutterers are not generally more anxious than nonstutterers unless they are in situations involving "noxious cues of verbal intercourse." Stuttering and expectancy-response patterns of stutterers indicate that anxiety is antecedently associated with those cues.	Results fail to substantiate inferences that a disorganization exists in stutterers similar to that found in known brain-damaged persons, and refute theories pointing to visual disturbance in stutterers' thought processes.

Eisenson, J., and Winslow, C. (1938) The perseveration tendency in stutterers in a perceptual function. *Journal of Speech Disorders, 3,* 195–198.

Elliott, J. C. (1952) Personality traits of school children with speech deviations as indicated by the California Test of Personality. *Speech Monographs, 19,* 158. Abstract of M. A. thesis, University of Michigan, 1951.

Fenichel, O. (1945) *The psychoanalytic theory of neurosis.* New York: Norton.

Fiedler, F. E., and Wepman, J. M. (1951)

141

TABLE 11	(continued)
Instrument	Two-Switch Electromaze
Investigator	Kapos and Standlee, 1958
Subjects	15 male stutterers. Ages: 18–30
Controls	15 nonstutterers, matched for age and sex.
Significant Findings	No significant differences observed in third order indices of behavioral stereotype.
Interpretation	Greater perseveration of stutterers in fixed speech pattern does not imply greater general rigidity.

Finkelstein, P., and Weisberger, S. E.   (1954)

Fitzpatrick, J. A.   (1959)   An investigation of the body image in secondary stutterers revealed through self-drawings. Ph.D. dissertation, University of Denver.

Font, M. M.   (1955)   A comparison of the free associations of stutterers and nonstutterers. In W. Johnson, ed., *Stuttering in children and adults*. Minneapolis: University of Minnesota Press.

Franks, B. B., and Rousey, C. L.   (1958)   Visual perception of stutterers and nonstutterers. *Child Development, 29*, 445–447.

Four-Switch Electromaze	Ten tests of perseveration; one group intelligence test
Kapos and Standlee, 1958	King, 1961
16 stutterers. Ages: 17–29	72 male stutterers.
16 nonstutterers, matched for age and sex.	82 male nonstutterers.
No significant differences observed in second-order indices of behavioral stereotype.	On five of the tests, results showed stutterers significantly more perseverative than nonstutterers. One test indicated nonstutterers were more perseverative than stutterers. Stutterers were more perseverative on activities that demanded a contiguous mental or mental-and-motor change of set.
Stutterers in general do not have a greater general behavioral rigidity than nonstutterers.	It was suggested that stutterers were penalized more severely on mental-motor change of set by their anxiety and emotional tensions. The evidence did not support the hypothesis of any influence of a broad underlying factor of perseveration in stutterers' test results.

Frederick, C. J. (1955) An investigation of learning theory and reinforcement as related to stuttering behavior. Ph.D. dissertation, University of California, Los Angeles.

Friedman, G. M. (1955)

Froeschels, E., and Rieber, R. W. (1963)

Fruewald, E. (1936) Intelligence rating of severe college stutterers compared with that of others entering universities. *Journal of Speech Disorders, 1,* 47–51.

Gens, G. W. (1951) The speech pathologist looks at the mentally deficient child. *Vineland Training School Bulletin, 48,* 19–27.

TABLE 11	(continued)
Instrument	Four Motor Perseveration Tests
Investigator	Martin, 1962
Subjects	52 stutterers. Ages: 8–13. IQ: 80–130
Controls	109 nonstutterers. Ages: 8–13. IQ: 80–130
Significant Findings	No significant differences in perseverative behavior were found between stutterers and nonstutterers as a group; between stutterers and nonstutterers in any of three age subgroups; between male and female stutterers; between male and female nonstutterers; and among stutterers whose stuttering was judged as mild, moderate, or severe.
Interpretation	Young stutterers are not more perseverative than young nonstutterers.

Gildston, P. (1964) Stutterers' self-acceptance and perceived parental acceptance. Ph.D. dissertation, Columbia University, New York.

Glasner, P. J. (1949) Personality characteristics and emotional problems in stutterers under the age of five. *Journal of Speech Disorders, 14,* 135–138.

Glasner, P. J., and Rosenthal, D. (1957)

Goldman, R., and Shames, G. H. (1964a)

Goldman, R., and Shames, G. H. (1964b)

Goodstein, L. D. (1956) MMPI profiles of stutterers' par-

Auditory and Visual Perception Ability Test	Critical Flicker Frequency Device and Sound Localization Test (frequency of displaced auditory responses to in-phase and out-of-phase stimuli)
Froeschels and Rieber, 1963	Kamiyama, 1964
20 stutterers. Ages: 17–30	48 stutterers, 24 male and 24 female.
None.	48 nonstutterers, matched for sex, age, vision, hearing.
Subjects did not show auditory or visual imperceptivity during fluent speech. The greater the severity of stuttering, the greater the imperceptivity during the moment of the stuttering block. Data also indicated that those with greatest imperceptivity showed least improvement in therapy.	No significant differences found between groups or sex subgroups on both measures. Stuttering females had significantly greater number of displaced responses on the sound localization test than stuttering males.
Data suggests relationship between degree of imperceptivity during block and degree of severity of stuttering symptoms.	

ents: A follow-up study. *Journal of Speech and Hearing Disorders, 21,* 430–435.

Goodstein, L. D. (1958) Functional speech disorders and personality: A survey of the research. *Journal of Speech and Hearing Research, 1,* 359–376.

Goodstein, L. D., and Dahlstrom, W. G. (1956)

Goodstein, L. D., Martire, J. G., and Speilberger, C. D. (1955) The relationship between "achievement imagery" and stuttering behavior in college males. *Proceedings (s) Iowa Academy of Science, 62,* 399–404.

TABLE 12	INTELLIGENCE STUDIES
Instrument	Stanford-Binet, Pintner-Patterson Shorter Performance Scale
Investigator	McDowell, 1928
Subjects	61 stutterers.
Controls	61 nonstutterers.
Significant Findings	Mean IQ of stutterers was 99 with a standard deviation of 20.3 and a range of 63–156. Subjects did not differ from controls in IQ or achievement measures.
Interpretation	"The two groups showed a surprising amount of similarity . . . the procedure for corrective work with stutterers . . . would naturally swing toward a marked emphasis on the improvement of speech habits rather than upon the eradication of neuropathic or psychopathic tendencies in the individual."

Grossman, D. J.   (1952)

Haney, H. R.   (1951)

Hill, H.   (1942)   Perseveration in normal speakers and stutterers. M.A. dissertation, Indiana University, Bloomington.

Holliday, A. R.   (1958)

Holmes R. W., and Pelletier, L. P.   (1967)   *Pineland hospital speech and hearing survey.* Pownal, Maine. Mimeographed.

Horlick, R. S., and Miller, M. H.   (1960)   A comparative

Ohio State Psychological Examination
Fruewald, 1936
190 stutterers, incoming university students.
Test norms, 100 nonstuttering freshmen.
This group of college stutterers ranks definitely higher in intelligence than the general freshman college population.
Agreement with Travis that the explanation for the superior intelligence found in college stutterers is that "the selective factor at work operates more completely in the case of the stutterer who hesitates to go to college with two handicaps, stuttering and mental dullness."

personality study of a group of stutterers and hard of hearing patients. *Journal of General Psychology, 63,* 259–266.

Ingebregtsen, E. (1936) Some experimental contributions to the psychology and psychopathology of stuttering. *American Journal of Orthopsychiatry, 6,* 630–651.

Johnson, W. (1932) The influence of stuttering on the personality. *University of Iowa Studies: Studies in Child Welfare, 5,* no. 5.

TABLE 12	(continued)
Instrument	Stanford-Binet, Form L
Investigator	Carlson, 1946
Subjects	50 child stutterers. Average IQ: 109 (range 80–130)
Controls	50 nonstuttering children with emotional problems.
Significant Findings	Stutterers rated superior to problem children in verbal material test but below them in nonverbal performances involving visual perception and motor coordination. As a group, stutterers were better readers and showed a higher scholastic achievement but were not functioning up to potentialities.
Interpretation	No direct correlation between stuttering and intelligence.

Johnson, W.   (1942)   A study of the onset and development of stuttering. *Journal of Speech Disorders*, 7, 251–257.

Johnson, W.   (1946)   *People in quandaries*. Chapter 17: The Indians have no word for it. New York: Harper & Row.

Johnson, W.   (1955b)

Johnson, W.   (1961d)

Johnson, W., Young, M. A., Sahs, A. L., and Bedell, G. N. (1959)

Johnson, W., *et al.*   (1959)

Revised Stanford-Binet, Form L (all but 4 oldest); Wechsler-Bellevue Intelligence Scale (four oldest)	Otis Self-Administering IQ Test; Gray's Oral Reading Test
Darley, 1955	Schindler, 1955
50 stutterers. Ages: 2–14. Mean Age: 9.2	126 stutterers (out of 20,976 Iowa school children).
General population norms.	252 nonstutterers (out of the same group), matched for age, sex, race, location.
Chi-square test indicates that there is no statistically significant difference between the two distributions.	Mean Otis IQs of 108 stutterers was 94.9, significantly lower than the mean IQ of 99.5 for the total survey sample. Stutterers showed a mean retardation of approximately one-half year in school placement; nonstutterers showed a little less than one-fourth year difference significant at the 2% level.
Stutterers not different from the general population in intelligence.	Grades 2–5 scores on Gray's Oral Reading Test indicated an average retardation of the stutterers of one year in oral reading skill. There was a marked similarity between the two groups on the organic measures employed.

Johnson, W., et al. (1967) *Speech handicapped school children.* New York: Harper & Row.

Kamiyama, G. (1964) A comparative study of stutterers and nonstutterers in respect to critical flicker frequency and sound localization. *Speech Monographs, 31,* 291. Ph.D. dissertation, University of Wichita, 1963.

Kapos, E., and Standlee, L. S. (1958)

Keisman, I. B. (1958)

King, P. T. (1954)

TABLE 12	(continued)
Instrument	Diagnostic Speech Examination; IQ measures adapted to retardation level.
Investigator	Sheehan, Martyn, and Kilburn, 1968
Subjects	216 institutionalized mentally retarded at Porterville State Hospital, California.
Controls	Survey; test norms.
Significant Findings	26 with normal speech, IQ range of 84–54; 83 with no speech, 70–0; 30 with delayed speech, 70–0; 24 with severe articulation difficulties, 70–24; 45 with mild articulation difficulties, 70–24; 2 aphasic patients, 84–40; 1 stutterer, 54; 1 clutterer, 54–40; 3 voice problems, 84–40.
Interpretation	Stutterers do not differ from nonstutterers along dimensions of intellect. Stuttering is not related to the lower end of the scale any more than it can be shown to be related to the upper end.

King, P. T.   (1961)

Kinstler, D. B.   (1959)

Knabe, J. M., Nelson, L. A., and Williams, F.   (1966)

Knepflar, K. J.   (1965)   A comparative study of fluency in the parents of stutterers and nonstutterers. Ph.D. dissertation, University of California, Los Angeles.

Kopp, H.   (1946)   Psychosomatic study of fifty stuttering children. Round table II: Oseretsky tests. *American Journal of Orthopsychiatry, 16,* 114–119.

Diagnostic Speech Examination, as part of survey; varied IQ measures depending on retardation level of patient

Martyn, Sheehan, and Slutz, 1969

346 older retarded at Camarillo State Hospital, California.

Survey; test norms

74 with normal speech, IQ range of 84–0; 58 with no speech, 69–0; 63 with delayed speech, 69–0; 56 with severe articulation difficulties, 84–0; 66 with mild articulation difficulties, 66–0; 1 cerebral palsy patient, 54–40, 1 aphasic, 39–25; 3 stutterers, 59–25 (1 female, 39; 1 male, 54; 1 male, 69); 1 clutterer, 24–0.

Cross-validating survey corroborates Porterville data from Sheehan, Martyn, and Kilburn. Broadens conclusion that no difference exists in incidence of stutterers among the retarded. The .87 percent is close to the national average.

Krout, M. H. (1936) Emotional factors in the etiology of stammering. *Proceedings of the American Speech Correction Association*, Madison: College Typing Co. Abstract.

Krugman, M. (1946) Psychosomatic study of fifty stuttering children. Round table IV: Rorschach study. *American Journal of Orthopsychiatry, 16,* 127–133.

Kurshev, V. A. (1961)

LaFollette, A. (1956)

Lanyon, R. I. (1966)

TABLE 13	VARIED PERSONALITY MEASURES
Instrument	Woodworth-Cady, Woodworth-Matthew, Kent-Rosanoff Free Association Test
Investigator	McDowell, 1928
Subjects	61 child stutterers.
Controls	61 nonstuttering children, matched for IQ, sex, race, language.
Significant Findings	No significant differences.
Interpretation	Emotional adjustments of stutterers and controls very similar. Need for emphasizing speech rather than eradicating neuropathic tendencies in individual.

Lemert, E. M.   (1962)

Lowinger, L.   (1952)

McDowell, E.   (1928) Educational and emotional adjustments of stuttering children. *Columbia University Teach-*

Woodworth-Cady Mental Hygiene Inventory Test, Childhood and Maturity	Moore-Gilliland Test for Aggressiveness
Johnson, 1932	Templin, 1938
50 stutterers. Ages: 15–34. Mean Age: 21.5	73 college students with defective speech, 53 male and 18 female; 37 with articulatory defects; 15 with voice defects; 19 with rhythm defects. Ages: 15–25. Median Age: 19
400 normal college males; 70 male psychoneurotics.	49 college students with nondefective speech, 45 male and 4 female. Ages: 17–30. Median Age: 20
Stutterers scored significantly lower than neurotics on maturity. Stutterers had significantly more problems on maturity than did the normals.	Normal-speech group more aggressive than defective-speech group. No correlation between aggressiveness and scholarship grades. (Normals tended to have higher grade point average than subjects.)
Stutterers are far from psychoneurotic. Many of their problems in personality are due to restraining and humiliating aspects of stuttering. Burden of proof must rest with those who support the theory that stuttering is or is not a symptom of social and emotional maladjustment.	The speech defective tends to show greater variability in aggressiveness, grade point average, and orientation test scores than controls. The stutterer tends to be more aggressive than the voice defective, and the voice defective more aggressive than the articulatory defective. The more aggressive speech defective tends to be slightly more cooperative in his therapy.

ers *College Contributions to Education.* No. 314. New
   York: Teachers College.
Madison, L. R., and Norman, R. D.   (1952)
Martin, R.   (1962)

TABLE 13	(continued)
Instrument	Minnesota Personality Scale; Speech Attitude Scale (Form F); Speech Experience Inventory (Form C); Personal Inventory Schedules
Investigator	Brown and Hull, 1942
Subjects	59 stutterers. Ages: 17–34
Controls	Test norms.
Significant Findings	Stutterers scored significantly lower in the Speech Attitude Scale and the Speech Experience Inventory than did the norms. Stutterers were rated significantly lower in social adjustment on Part II of the P. I. S.
Interpretation	Of the 5 factors measured by the P. I. S. (morale, social adjustment, family relations, emotionality, economic conservatism), the only part resulting in significant differences were the items concerned with social adjustment.

Martyn, M. M., and Sheehan, J. G. (1968)

Martyn, M. M., Sheehan, J. G., and Slutz, K. (1969)

Mast, V. R. (1952) Level of aspiration as a method of studying the personality of adult stutterers. *Speech Monographs, 19,* 196. Abstract of M.S. Dissertation, University of Michigan, 1951.

May, A. (1968) A study of the presence of normal speaking disfluency in stutterers with high and low listenability ratings. Ph.D. dissertation, Univ. of Calif., Los Angeles.

Meltzer, H. (1944) Personality differences between stuttering and nonstuttering children as indicated by the

Stuttering Attitude Scale; Speech Attitude Scale; Speech Experience Inventory	Adams Personal Audit; Rotter Incomplete Sentences Blank
Tiffany, 1947	Bearss, 1951
28 stutterers. Ages: 7–14	23 male college stutterers.
28 nonstutterers. Ages: 7–14	23 male nonstutterers matched for age and grade.
Marked malattitudes toward stuttering were revealed at the earliest ages tested, but no significant difference was found between stuttering and nonstuttering groups. Scores on the Stuttering Attitude Scale were found to be a function of age with the younger stutterers reacting more unfavorably. A correlation of −.56 was found between age and stuttering attitude scores.	Stutterers and nonstutterers were not differentiable with respect to personality maladjustment as measured by tests. No significant relationship between the judged severity of stuttering and the stutterer's maladjustment score on either of the two tests employed. No significant agreement between the maladjustment scores obtained from the two tests.
Some inconclusive evidence that attitude toward stuttering was a partial function of severity of stuttering.	

Rorschach test. *Journal of Psychology, 17,* 39–59.

Merchant, F. (1952) Psychosexual development of stutterers. Unpublished study cited in G. Blum and H. Hunt, The validity of the Blacky pictures. *Psychological Bulletin, 49,* (1952) 238.

Moncur, J. P. (1952)

Moncur, J. P. (1955)

Murphy, A. T. (1953)

Murphy, A. T. and Fitzsimons, R. M. (1960) *Stuttering and personality dynamics.* New York: Ronald Press.

Perkins, D. W. (1947) An item by item compilation and

TABLE 13	(continued)
Instrument	Word Picture Test of Social Adjustment
Investigator	Spriestersbach, 1951
Subjects	50 male stutterers. Median age: 21.5
Controls	183 nonstuttering college males. Median age: 20.5. 20 male psychotics. Median age:47
Significant Findings	Stutterers differed from the normal males only slightly more than could be attributed to chance. Both the normals and the stutterers differed significantly from the psychotics.
Interpretation	Stutterers displayed mild degrees of social maladjustment, but they more closely resembled the evaluative reactions of the normals than the psychotics.

comparison of the scores of 75 young adult stutterers on the California Test of Personality-Adult Form A. *Speech Monographs, 14,* 211. Abstract of M.A. dissertation, University of Michigan, 1946.

Pitrelli, F. R. (1948) Psychomatic and Rorschach aspects of stuttering. *Psychiatric Quarterly, 22,* 175–194.

Pizzat, F. J. (1949) A personality study of college stutterers. M.S. dissertation, University of Pittsburgh.

Powers, M. R. 1944 Personality traits of junior high school stutterers as measured by the California Test of Personality. M.A. Thesis, University of Illinois.

Quarrington, B. (1953)

Redwine, G. W. (1958) Experimental study of relationships between self-concepts of fourth and eighth grade

Guilford-Martin Inventory of Factors STDCR	Test of Attitude Toward Stuttering
Shames, 1952	Friedman, 1955
27 adult stutterers, 10 with other speech problems.	326 stutterers. Ages: 11–53. Median age: 19.9
Compared subjects before and after therapy.	100 nonstutterers. Ages: 19–52. Median age: 28.8
Factors significantly related to improvement at 10% level: Factor S- social introversion; Factor T- thinking introversion; Factor R- happy-go-luckiness.	No significant difference between the 2 groups in mean attitude test scores. 2 groups showed about the same degree of nonacceptance of stuttering. Stutterers who judged their stuttering as severe made higher scores on the atitude test than those who judged their disorders as mild or average.
Statistically inconclusive.	Some indication of a relationship between severity of stuttering and intensity of the attitude of nonacceptance of stuttering.

stuttering and nonstuttering boys. Ph.D. dissertation, University of Southern California, Los Angeles.

Richardson, L. (1944) The personality of stutterers. *Psychological Monographs, 56,* 1–41.

Rieber, R. W. (1963) Stuttering and self-concept. *The Journal of Psychology, 55,* 307–311.

Ringel, R. L., and Minifie, F. D. (1966)

Robbins, S. D. (1965)

Rosenberg, I. (1961) An experimental investigation of some effects on stutterers on Pacatal-aided group psychotherapy: A comparison of the effects on male adult stutterers of group psychotherapy with and without the tranquilizer Pacatal as an adjuvant. Ph.D. dissertation, New York University, 1961.

TABLE 13	(continued)
Instrument	Rogers Test of Personality Adjustment
Investigator	Darley, 1955
Subjects	50 stutterers. Ages: 2–14. Mean Age: 9.2
Controls	50 controls. Ages: 2–14. Median Age: 9.0
Significant Findings	In none of the five distributions of scores (Personality Inferiority, Social Maladjustment, Daydreaming, Family Maladjustment, and total scores) were the two groups of children found to differ significantly.
Interpretation	Although differences are not statistically significant, there is a tendency for the stuttering children to make higher area and total scores than the nonstuttering children, and more stuttering than nonstuttering children rated "High" in more than one area.

Rosenthal, R. (1966) *Experimenter effects in behavioral research.* New York: Appleton.

Rotter, J. (1939) Studies in the psychology of stuttering. XI. Stuttering in relation to position in the family. *Journal of Speech Disorders,* 4, 143–147.

Santostefano, S. (1960)

Schindler, M. D. (1955) A study of educational adjustments of stuttering and nonstuttering children. In W. Johnson, ed., *Stuttering in children and adults.* Minneapolis: University of Minnesota Press.

Schultz, D. A. (1947) A study of nondirective counseling as applied to adult stutterers. *Journal of Speech Disorders,* 12, 421–427.

Sergeant, R. L. (1962) An investigation of responses of

Maslow Security Index	Anal Trait Checklist; Anal Interest Picture Test
Brutten, 1957	Keisman, 1958
16 stutterers.	30 Stutterers. Ages: 18–45
16 nonstutterers.	30 nonstutterers with functional speech disorders, and 30 normals.
No significant differences found between stutterers and nonstutterers.	Findings largely negative and inconclusive. Stutterers did exhibit significantly greater intraindividual variability in the time taken to rate themselves on anal traits.
Although differences are not statistically significant, there is a tendency for the stuttering children to make higher area and total scores than the nonstuttering children, and more stuttering than nonstuttering children rated "High" in more than one area.	Although findings mostly negative, they provide some qualified support for the postulate that stutterers have anal fixations.

speech defective adults on personality inventory tests. Ph.D. dissertation, Ohio State University, Columbus.

Shames, G. H. (1949) The relationship between the attitude toward stuttering of secondary stutterers and several of their personality characteristics. M.S. dissertation, University of Pittsburgh.

Shames, G. H. (1953)

Shearer, W. M., and Williams, J. D. (1965)

Sheehan, J. G. (1946) A study of the phenomena of stuttering. M.A. Thesis, University of Michigan.

Sheehan, J. G. (1953) Rorschach changes during psychotherapy in relation to the personality of the therapist. *American Psychologist*, 8, 434–435.

Sheehan, J. G. (1954a)

TABLE 13	(continued)
Instrument	Edwards Personal Preference Schedule
Investigator	Wingate, 1962
Subjects	70 male stutterers.
Controls	Test norms.
Significant Findings	Mild to moderate maladjustment in stutterers in the area of social relationships.

Sheehan, J. G.   (1954b)

Sheehan, J. G.   (1958a)

Sheehan, J. G.   (1958b)

Sheehan, J. G.   (1962)   Projective studies of stuttering. In E. P. Trapp and P. Himelstein, eds., *Readings on the exceptional child: Research and theory.* New York: Appleton.

Bell Adjustment Inventory; Berneuter's Personality Inventory; Biographical Inventory; Speech Problem Inventory; Interviews	Witkin Embedded Figures Test (measures ability to cope with complexity); Barron-Welsh Art Scale (measures performance for complexity and asymmetry)
Sergeant, 1962	Calamaras, 1964
210 subjects classified into groups: stuttering, articulation, voice, cleft palate, laryngectomy, normal speaking.	34 male stutterers. Ages: 10–17
Test norms plus comparison of groups in the sample.	34 male nonstutterers, matched for age, intelligence, race, socioeconomic level.
Scores obtained by speech defectives were more variable than normals for scales of manifest anxiety, emotional adjustment, and health adjustment. Mean scores of normals were in direction of better adjustment than speech defective group.	Stutterers and nonstutterers from different age levels differ significantly in their ability to cope with complexity. Stutterers do not differ significantly from nonstutterers in their performance for complexity and asymmetry. The more severe stutterers had a greater preference for complexity and asymmetry than less severe stutterers.
Results indicated that speech-defective persons probably respond differently from normal speakers to items containing words related to talking.	Differences found between the two groups at a younger age are not apparent by the time they enter the 14-to-17 age range.

Sheehan, J. G. (1963) The effect of role commitment on stuttering. Paper presented to International Society for Rehabilitation, Copenhagen.

Sheehan, J. G. (1968)

Sheehan, J. G. (1970) Cross-validation of a Rorschach prognostic study. Unpublished, Univ. of Calif., Los Angeles.

TABLE 13	(continued)
Instrument	34 Multi-Choice items.
Investigator	Trombly, 1965
Subjects	100 stutterers. Mean age: 22.1
Controls	129 Normal speakers. Mean Age: 20.3
Significant Findings	Stuttering tends to increase when the stutterer attaches prestige to the listener or when he evaluates the speaking situation as important.
Interpretation	The variation of fluency within the social context raises questions about the stutterer's concept of himself in relation to others and about his reactions to success and failure. Differing behavior for males and females is noted.

Sheehan, J. G. (chairman), Bleumel, C., Clancy, J., Coleman, W., Frick, J., Johnson, W., Van Riper, C., and Williams, D. (1957) A symposium of recovered stutterers. American Speech and Hearing Association convention, Cincinnati, Ohio.

Sheehan, J. G., and Martyn, M. M. (1966)

Sheehan, J. G., and Martyn, M. M. (1967)

Sheehan, J. G., and Martyn, M. M. (1970)

Sheehan, J. G., Martyn, M. M., and Kilburn, K. L. (1968)

Sheehan, J. G., and Zelen, S. L. (1951) A level of aspiration study of stutterers. *American Psychologist, 6,* 500. Abstract.

Test of Behavioral Rigidity	
Wingate, 1966	
12 male stutterers. Ages: 19–33. Mean Age: 25.6	
12 nonstutterers, matched for sex, age, and educational level.	
Superiority (greater flexibility) of nonstutterers on the Motor-Cognitive Factor is significant beyond .01. Higher scores for normals on Composite Rigidity and Psychomotor Speech attain low level of significance. Nonstutterers endorsed significantly more Social Responsibility Statements.	
Stutterers have less ability to adjust to shifts in familiar patterns and to continuously changing situational demands of a cognitive nature. Evidence contradicts the idea that stutterers have a high, rigid moral code.	

Sheehan, J. G., and Zelen, S. L.   (1955)

Sheehan, J. G., and Zussman, C.   (1951)   Rorschachs of stutterers compared with clinical control. *American Psychologist, 6,* 500.

Silverman, L.   (1952)   The factor of maternal dominance in 10 male stutterers as indicated by the Figure Drawing Test. *Psychology Newsletter, 37,* 1–22.

Snyder, M. A., *et al.,*   (1958)

Solomon, I. L.   (1963)   Aggression and stuttering: An experimental study of the psychoanalytic model of stuttering. Ph.D. dissertation, Yeshiva University.

Solomon, N. D.   (1952)   A comparison of rigidity of be-

TABLE 13	(continued)
Instrument	A series of 10 questions. 5 personal (contained the pronoun "you") and 5 impersonal (did not contain the pronoun "you")
Investigator	Knabe, Nelson and Williams, 1966
Subjects	16 college stutterers.
Controls	16 college nonstutterers, matched for age, sex, academic classification, and as closely as possible on verbal ability.
Significant Findings	It was found that these groups differed significantly only on the measure of fluency, the stutterers being less fluent than the normals.
Interpretation	It is hypothesized that messages of the 2 groups are not perceived with equal fidelity because of the increased disfluency in the stutterers.

havior manifested by a group of stutterers compared with "fluent" speakers in oral and other performances as measured by the Einstellung effect. *Speech Monographs, 19,* 198. Abstract of M.A. dissertation, University of Michigan, 1951.

Speidel, L. M. (1963)

Spriestersbach, D. C. (1951)

Staats, L. C. (1955)

Stunden, A. A. (1965)

Templin, M. (1938) Study of aggressiveness in normal and defective speaking college students. *Journal of Speech Disorders, 3,* 43–49.

Thile, E. L. (1967) An investigation of attitude differences in parents of stutterers and parents of nonstutterers. Ph.D. dissertation, University of Southern California, Los Angeles.

Thomas, L. (1951) A personality study of a group of stutterers based on the MMPI. M.A. dissertation, University of Oregon, Portland.

Tiffany, W. R. (1947) An experimental study in the

growth of speech and stuttering attitudes in children. M.A. thesis, University of Washington. Also in *Speech Monographs, 15,* 1948, p. 210.

Travis, L. E. (1931) *Speech pathology.* New York: Appleton.

Travis, L. E. (1946) My present views on stuttering. *Western Speech, 10,* 3–5.

Trombly, T. W. (1958) A comparative study of stutterers' levels of aspiration for speech and non-speech performance. Ph.D. dissertation, University of Missouri, Columbia.

Trombly, T. W. (1965) Responses of stutterers and normal speakers to a level of aspiration. *Central States Speech Journal, 16,* 179–181.

Trotter, W. D., and Bergman, M. (1957) Stutterers and nonstutterers reactions to speech situations. *Journal of Speech and Hearing Disorders, 22,* 40–45.

Van Riper, C. (1946) Speech pathology, in *Encyclopedia of Psychology.* New York: Philosophical Library.

Van Riper, C. (1963b)

Van Riper, C., ed. (1964)

Wallen, V. (1959)

Walnut, A. (1954)

Wilson, D. M. (1951)

Wingate, M. E. (1962b)

Wingate, M. E. (1964)

Wingate, M. E. (1965) Panel comment at American Speech and Hearing Association meeting, Chicago.

Wingate, M. E. (1966b)

Wyatt, G. L. (1958)

Zelen, S. L., Sheehan, J. G., and Bugental, J. F. T. (1954)

TABLE 14	TIME-DIMENSION STUDIES
Instrument	Phonetic Analysis of Stuttering Patterns
Investigator	Sheehan, 1946
Subjects	20 stutterers from Army Hospital.
Controls	None.
Significant Findings	Most stutterers' blocks are of very short duration, 3 seconds or less. More than 50% of all blocks involve some degree of stuttering on the wrong sound. Stutterers frequently continue to stutter on sounds and words they have already spoken successfully.
Interpretation	Repetition and prolongation are the only symptoms common to all stutterers. Stuttering chiefly a disorder of release, with irrelevancies and crutches used to satisfy the fear and bring about termination of the block.

Kent-Rosanoff free-association test	Reaction time index of associative responses to 118 stimulus words
Font, 1955	Adams and Dietze, 1965
9 college stutterers.	30 male stutterers. Ages: 18–45
49 nonstuttering college students.	30 nonstuttering males, matched for age and education.
No significant difference between reaction times or "usual" response.	Mean scores of both groups maintained approximately the same rank order. Stutterers were significantly slower (.02 level) than controls on all words. Differences between reaction time to the guilt words as compared to other word categories were significantly larger for stutterers. Stutterers were significantly slower than controls on aggression and depression words.
The application of the association test by this method revealed no sharp distinction between the stutterers and nonstutterers.	Although both groups responded to the stimulus words in much the same manner, stutterers appear prone to overreact when exposed to many negative affect-connoting stimuli. The stutterers' generalized slowness may indicate that they were more emotionally aroused by the stimulus words, or that they may have perceived the experimental setting itself as an "affective situation." Findings suggest that guilt may be an important factor in the psychological makeup of stutterers.

TABLE 14	(continued)
Instrument	5 Protensity judging activities: Time estimation of a 10-second period while simultaneously engaged in silence, oral reading, silent reading, listening, and spontaneous speech
Investigator	Ringel and Minifie, 1966
Subjects	11 mild stutterers; 10 moderate to severe stutterers. Ages: 18–26
Controls	11 normal speakers. Ages: 18–26
Significant Findings	Stutterers, regardless of their severity, experienced more difficulty during communicative activities in accurately judging the duration of an elapsed period of time than did nonstutterers. Differences reached level of significance only for severe stutterers. Performances of the mild stutterers were more similar to normals than to moderate or severe stutterers.
Interpretation	Stutterers have greater difficulty monitoring the passage of time during communicative activities than nonstutterers. Time factors are important variables in stuttering behavior.

Word association list (presented under conditions of time pressure and no time pressure)

Stunden, 1965

18 stutterers. Ages: 19–41. Mean Age: 28

18 normal speakers, matched for age, sex and education; 18 highly anxious normal speakers (as measured by one form of the Taylor Anxiety Scale).

Under time pressure, all groups gave a large number of contrasting adjective responses. Differences among groups not significant. In the no-time-pressure condition, stutterers continued to give contrasting adjectives, whereas both groups of normal speakers did not.

". . . the lack of change in the verbal behavior of the stuttering group is related to the presence of a self-defined, personal time pressure set." "Stutterers react to speech situations as if under the constant influence of time pressure."

About the Author EDWIN M. LEMERT, Ph.D., is Professor of Sociology at the University of California, Davis. He is the author of *Social Pathology; Human Deviance, Social Problems and Social Control,* and of several monographs and numerous articles on deviance and social problems, including forgery, alcoholism and paranoia. A colleague has described Lemert as a sociologist-anthropologist with a psychological point of view; this reflects the breadth of his interests in cross-cultural research. His field work on stuttering has been with Northwest Coast Indians, Polynesians, and Japanese.

About the Chapter The relationship of stuttering to culture, the characteristic of the problem in primitive groups and in our own society, is a facet of stuttering that has never been subjected to authoritative sociological scrutiny. Dr. Lemert's discovery of stuttering—and words for it—in American Indian tribes ranks as a major breakthrough in our understanding of the disorder. In this chapter he brings his unusually rich background into focus with an insightful sociological perspective.

4

SOCIOLOGICAL
PERSPECTIVE

EDWIN M. LEMERT

4

Sociologists have long been concerned with human abnormalities such as blindness, deafness, accident and disease, disabilities due to birth anomalies, drug addiction, crime, and mental disorders. Yet speech defects, stuttering among them, have attracted scant attention among writers and investigators in this field. This in itself may be a significant datum, indicating the nondramatic nature of stuttering in comparison with other human abnormalities. The fact that stuttering is not socially harmful also may help explain its neglect by social scientists, as it explains the humorous light in which speech defectives are generally regarded by other members of society. Social scientists have been content to leave the stutterer to the "speech correctionists" or to the clinical psychologists, with the assumption that the stutterer merely has faulty speech habits or at most suffers from a personality disorder of which stuttering is a symptom.

Recent decades have seen a renewal of interest in abnormal behavior by both sociologists and anthropologists. Much of this interest has centered on problems of definition and the meaning of abnormal behavior—or deviant behavior, as it is termed by many writers today. At the same time, concern with social and cultural factors in the etiology of deviance has been stirred by efforts to formulate systematic theories of social structure, social action, and social control (Lemert, 1967). Psychiatrists, medical researchers, and epidemiologists have given additional impetus to sociological studies of human deviations.

CULTURE AND STUTTERING

One of the chief concepts in the intellectual stock-in-trade of sociologists and anthropologists is that of culture. Unfortunately, this term is often abused and frequently reified or converted into an explanatory concept, as if it were a causative entity, like "instinct" or "heredity." With care the concept can be used most appropriately as an orientation to a body of data. It refers to forms of human behavior which are patterned and which are cumulative through time, i.e., which have an ongoing existence independent of biological individuals in whose neural systems they are carried. It includes directly observable behavior and also such items as values, norms, themes, meanings, and sentiments, which are inferences or higher-level abstractions from the sense-observable data of human behavior.

Whether the culture concept can help explain stuttering and provide clues to its treatment is largely a question for research. At the very least, the comparison of abnormal and deviant behavior in different cultures should be helpful in shedding light on the part played by biological factors in producing stuttering. If cultures can be found in which there is neither current incidence of stuttering nor historical evidence of stuttering, then the notion of a genetic basis for stuttering can be summarily set aside. The alternative would be to conclude that whole populations or races differ in their biological potentialities for stuttering, which, within the scope of present knowledge concerning race, does not seem tenable.

In a "cross-cultural" survey Bullen (1945) came to the conclusion that in some preliterate societies—including the Navaho, the Polar Eskimo, and New Guinea tribes—stuttering is rare or nonexistent, and that where it did occur it appeared to be the result of acculturation. These conclusions, however, were based upon rather cursory reports and thin data at best. For at least one of the Navaho societies there is counterevidence that stuttering does exist and that there are linguistic concepts for defining the disorder (H. Hoijer, personal communication). Johnson (1944) and Snidecor (1947) reported an absence of

173

both stuttering and linguistic definition of stuttering among the Bannock and Shoshone Indians of Idaho. From this they generalized that stuttering was absent among the American Indians. Yet as early as 1915 Sapir had recorded the presence of stuttering as a speech defect among the Nootka Indians of the West Coast of Vancouver Island and also described rather complex language adaptations which culturally acknowledged it as a status attribute of the deviant speaker. Stuttering and its linguistic recognition was discovered among the Quileute Indians, in the State of Washington, by Frachtenberg in 1920.

Lemert (1952, 1953), in a systematic effort to test the theories of Johnson and Snidecor, found numerous cases of stuttering and strong evidence that it existed aboriginally among the following tribes of the Northwest Pacific Coast: Gulf of Georgia Salish, Kwakiutl, Haida and Tsimshian. Joseph and Murray (1951) tell of stuttering among the Chamorros and Carolinians on Saipan. Data showing the occurrence of stuttering among Brazilian tribes has been supplied by Hohenthal (personal communication), who has done extensive field work among the Fulnio on the Pernambuco River. Aron (1962) has reported the occurrence of stuttering and its linguistic recognition among Bantu school children. Finally, Lemert (1962) described culturally recognized stuttering in a number of Polynesian societies, as well as a relatively high incidence among Japanese in Hawaii and in their homeland. Tamai *et al.* (1962) also discuss stuttering among the Japanese.

In contrast to these findings, Stewart (1960) suggests that the Ute are a nonstuttering people who also lack linguistic concepts for defining the disorder. His data come from reports of others and from his own interview sample of thirty Ute families in northeastern Utah. Whether his research data are valid for the entire population of Utes, whose ethnography has been little studied, must await further inquiry. Meantime, honesty compels admission that data on the cultural distribution of stuttering are spotty and, save in one or two instances, are not the result of systematic inquiry by persons trained in its recognition. Kluckhohn's earlier conclusion (1954) still seems apropos: "No single unequivocal case of the absence of stuttering among a people has been found." Kluckhohn goes on to say that "biological or idiosyncratic life history factors can be productive of stuttering in all cultures." But this is a rather large speculative leap from the somewhat shaky premise that because such cases haven't been found they won't be found, and such a conclusion does little to settle the question whether biological factors actually do enter into the etiology of stuttering—it simply admits the possibility. As an informed guess, however, Kluckhohn's point should not be disregarded.

What seems capable of firm statement at this time is that stuttering does occur in preliterate societies and that it occurs apart from the influence of acculturation. It is also reasonably certain that stuttering varies in its incidence from culture to culture. This, coupled with the knowledge that language and expressive behavior are important aspects of culture, makes it plausible that culture in some manner contributes to the genesis of the disorder. Just how culture asserts its influence to induce stuttering can only be a matter for interpretation. Three hypotheses suggest themselves: (1) stuttering is a pattern of behavior directly learned from others; (2) culture exerts stress upon the individual, either through competition or conflicting demands, in such a way as to disrupt speech coordinations; (3) culture operates through values or themes as part of a sociopsychological process which produces stuttering.

Most clinical workers probably will reject the first hypothesis on the grounds that stuttering is never the resut of imitation. However, it is interesting to note that among the Nootka Indians dialectical differences in related tribes are looked upon and reacted to as speech defects when they occur in the speech of fellow tribesmen. According to Sapir, the northernmost Nootka, the Chickleset, were said to be all stutterers and were imitated in jest by other Nootka tribes. This was never verified, but Thalbitzer (1904) reported a field investigation in which this kind of diffusion of speech abnormalities was discovered to have taken place among the West Greenland Eskimos. Tenuous as these data are, they nevertheless suggest that what Bluemel (1932) has called "primary symptoms" of stuttering may fall within the range of speech behavior that cultures can capitalize on and incorporate in their linguistic systems.

From Sapir's discussion of consonantal play comes a research lead into some of the more subtle aspects of the processes that originate cultural definitions and patterns of reaction to persons with speech defects as well as physical defects and other deviant qualities. Consonantal play consists in either alternating certain consonants with other phonetically related consonants or inserting meaningless consonants or consonant clusters into the body of the word. The Nootka Indians typically incorporated such play into their language as modes of address to large and small persons, to those with physical defects and stigmata, and also to stutterers. Other American Indians are known to use similar phonetic devices, especially in attributing unpredictable, child-like, or *enfant terrible* qualities to culture heroes and other dramatis personae in their myths and songs. Sapir's summary statement of the problem, for some reason laid dormant in the literature for many years, is well worth noting:

> *The matter of consonantal play to express modalities of attitude doubtless is a fruitful field for investigation . . . and should receive more attention than has hitherto been accorded. It may be expected to turn up particularly in connection with notions of smallness, largeness, contempt, affection, respect and sex differences.*

Stewart (1960) has proposed that culture may structure the uses of consonantal play, reduplication, and diminution in such a way as to affect acquisition of language by children. The extent to which baby talk or a "little language" is utilized in socialization of children in different cultures is held to be of possible significance in the incidence and nonincidence of stuttering. Thus the assertedly nonstuttering Utes are said to employ baby talk reciprocally between children and adults, whereas Northwest Coast Indians use it unilaterally, insisting on proper forms of address by children to adults. Transition to adult speech thus is made more difficult.

Although the hypothesis is an attractive one, Lemert (1962) found it difficult to apply to Polynesian and Japanese societies. Polynesians, among whom stuttering is comparatively rare, make no use of baby talk whatsoever, while Japanese, who have enough stutterers in their population to have developed formal methods of treatment, do commonly use baby talk in teaching language to their children. Furthermore, as Ferguson (1964) shows, baby talk may have multiple functions in primitive societies, not all of which are related to interaction with children. Despite these negative findings, some complexities in the data suggest that clinically oriented speech pathologists may have been too ready to dismiss the structure of language as a possible etiological factor in stuttering.

In general, whatever may be gained from research into such questions, what is presently known seems strong in support of the proposition that dysrythmic speech is culturally defined and that the essence of stuttering is attitudinal. But it does not follow that attitudinal expressions and postural sets which elaborate into complex blocks and spasms of a "secondary" nature within the stutterer are the result of direct cultural learning.

The idea that culture conflict and competitive stress are responsible for psychogenic disorders is an appealing one, but as a general proposition it has been pretty well disposed of by Beaglehole (1940), who showed that the individual in a society is never exposed to the complexities and conflicts of the culture as a whole. Consequently, it is necessary to consider social structure as well as culture in order to know what classes of persons at what points in time and space are faced with conflicts of cultural origin. It would appear from generally accepted knowledge of the disorder in American society that culturally induced stresses in parental and child roles which arise in the early years of the child's life are the most significant ones in the genesis of stuttering. Lemert found this to hold true without exception for stutterers he contacted and interviewed in Northwest Coast Indian societies. It was further documented in stories he had asked teen-agers in the Port Alberni Indian school to write on the subject "A Person Who Couldn't Talk Right." Nine of the ten stories dealt exclusively with small children struggling to learn to talk, the majority of whom showed symptoms of stuttering. The historical recollections of Indian informants about fathers or grandfathers who stuttered likewise pointed to early childhood as the period when the speech difficulty first appeared.

One of the distinctive features of the Northwest Coast Indian cultures was the high standard of childhood decorum and the expectation of early participation of the child in dance, song, and speech rituals. The expectation that children be like "little adults" was strong, and the regard for the "good name" of the child's family was ubiquitous. When these are considered in the context of a thematic emphasis upon competition, it becomes possible to say that these cultures were favorable environments for the development of stuttering. And, the reported absence or low incidence of stuttering among the Ute, Bannock, and Shoshone Indians may be related to the comparative freedom of their children from anxiety-inducing adult expectations. A fair conclusion from this line of reasoning is that primitive societies with structures most nearly resembling our own are likely to generate a high incidence of stuttering.

The social structuring of sex roles also may be said to effect the way in which cultural pressures impinge upon individuals to maximize or minimize their likelihood of stuttering. Henry

177

(1940), while not specifically commenting on stuttering, reports that among the Pilega Indians of South America girls displayed more severe speech disturbances than boys. This he interpreted as a function of what he termed an "anti feminine" culture which led to rejection of girl children. In the Fulnio village studied by Hohenthal two persons were described as having speech disorders; both were women, one was a stutterer. If these findings are indicative, they run counter to our own culture, where stuttering, according to a number of studies, is much more frequent among men. Rose (1943), drawing upon Orton (1937), has speculated that speech disorders are more likely to develop in a cultural area in which "collective importance is attached to language functioning as a symbol of creative self-expression." He further believes that oratory is equated with masculine achievement in the southern states in our society, with the consequence that men there are more likely to become stutterers than women. Schuell (1946) also gives what is at least an implicit cultural explanation of sex differences in the incidence of stuttering. The possibility of a relatively high incidence of stuttering among females in Japan, reported to Lemert (1962) by informants, tends to be consistent with the cultural imposition of heavy responsibility in their family roles and the comparatively few socially sanctioned outlets or escapes from tension available to them.

Class structure, as well as role differentiation based upon age and sex, may provide a source of investigation into the differential impact of cultural pressures that affect speech co-ordination in children. One hypothesis that readily suggests itself is that middle and upper social classes uphold higher standards of speech performance for children than lower classes. Support for this idea comes from Irwin (1948b), who has collected data to show that speech development is slower among children of laboring class parents than it is among those whose fathers are in professional, business, and clerical occupations. A survey by Schnidler (1955) furnishes some evidence that stutterers more frequently come from families where the parents are in the managerial, professional, and clerical occupations. But Morgenstern's research in England (1956) gives a somewhat different picture—a higher proportion of stutterers were discovered to have fathers or guardians in the semiskilled manual laboring classes.

Even if class differences in rates of stuttering are found to exist, the problem of their significance will remain a formidable one. Presumably, such differences will be a measure or a reflection of variations and preferences in child-rearing practices which in some way are related to stuttering. Some studies, such as Glasner's (1949), point to harsh discipline, threats, shame, humiliation, and corporal punishment, coupled with indulgence and pampering, as qualities of child rearing which may engender stuttering. On the other hand, Moncur (1952) is of the opinion that parental domination as a factor in stuttering may be simply part of a syndrome of factors. It is worth noting here that sociological studies of class variation in child-rearing practices have not proved up the early expectations held out for them. The magnitude of the differences brought out in these researches has not been large, and the differences between subgroups (such as ethnic groups) often has been greater than that between classes.

It may be that socioeconomic status *per se* is less important in accounting for the variable incidence of stuttering in a population than is the group or groups towards which the child's parents are sociopsychologically oriented. This suggests the possible application of what Merton (1957) has discussed as "reference group theory" to further research on this subject. Upward-mobility striving through identification with upper or middle class values, or threats to certain cherished group values, may serve as a more discriminating lead to the discovery of family types with which stuttering is associated. This analysis leads towards the third of our previously announced hypotheses, namely, that culture enters into the genesis of stuttering through the media of values or themes. However, shared values of a culture at best can only be reference points for human action. Furthermore, they are modified in expression by the influence of more specialized, idiosyncratic values within the person. It is also true that values of either kind are expressible only as the situation permits. For these reasons, the more dynamic concept of interaction must be invoked and formulated in some way to throw systematic light on stuttering.

INTERACTION ANALYSIS

From the sociological point of view, the most significant interplay of values in stuttering is that which arises in "self" and "other" interaction. The casting of analysis into this context makes stuttering a phenomenon of social definition, an emergent product of the speaker's behavior and that of his auditors. This has certain advantages over the use of traditional types of learning theory. The most obvious advantage is that it more readily

179

admits meaning as a factor in the process, in contrast to the laws of learning, which tend to be formal and devoid of content. At the same time the adoption of an interactional perspective is not necessarily inconsistent with principles of learning theory and its key notion of reinforcement.

Interaction most realistically should be conceived as taking place within limits. These limits may be biological, sociopsychological, and sociocultural in nature, or interactional products of all three. In this frame of reference the stutterer is seen as an active, choice-making agent who is free to follow alternative modes of adjustment within limits imposed by internal "within the skin" factors and by external situational factors. As choices are made, their consequences become new internal and external limits within which further choices willy nilly have to be made. An important point is that once established, stuttering becomes a set of anticipatory responses which cue differential penalizing responses in others. Stutterers must continually be prepared to normalize strained interaction with normal speakers.

In sociological language, meaningful choices are made of behavior that is incorporated into social roles. This is not to say that the person chooses to stutter or chooses the role of the stutterer. Nevertheless, the so-called secondary adaptations that the individual makes can be regarded in large part as the result of choices, at least in their beginning. Furthermore these secondary manifestations or symptoms of stuttering can be conceived of as efforts, however feckless, to play a given role in a given situation. Van Riper (1957), in speaking of the nature of these symptoms, states that "symbolically, stutterers soil, whimper, bite, gag and recoil from themselves and their listeners as they stutter." Each symptom has its special value and gets its meaning in relation to the role played, and each symptom, through social interaction, reflects upon or becomes part of the stutterer's damaged self-image. Furthermore, once they are acquired, the symptoms act as new limits determining what social roles the stutterer will attempt to play and what roles will be perceived as closed to him. The "success" or "failure" of these adaptations will greatly affect the spread of the stuttering response from one role to another or perhaps bring about stabilization of the deviant speech at some point which is tolerable to the stutterer and to others.

The idea that stuttering in some way is intimately associated with the self has been implicit in a good deal of theorizing about the disorder by speech pathologists. Recently it has entered more explicitly into theory and research, the nature of which has been reviewed by Rieber (1963). Sheehan (1963, 1968), who has done a good deal of research in this area, has proposed that the stutterer's problem may be fundamentally an expression of self–role conflict.

VISIBILITY

One significant feature of stuttering, which bears upon the range of choices available to the speaker, is social visibility, by which is meant the extent to which others perceive and become aware of the deviation. Some stuttering is or can be masked or covered by a variety of devices or "crutches" well known to clinical workers. Some of these tricks miss their mark and actually heighten the social visibility of the stuttering. Others are successful—In sociological terms they offer the deviant speaker the choice of passing himself off as a normal speaker, perhaps as a "strong silent man" or the "taciturn type." This, of course, is much easier to bring off in social situations where interaction is on a casual basis, or with strangers, or where it is highly formalized. Needless to say, this kind of role choice creates problems at the level of self-acceptance, inasmuch as the stutterer is usually well aware of the spurious or artificial nature of his role. Stutterers of this sort often show a great deal of guilt and consciousness of themselves as "phonies." Subjectively, they have self-definitional problems in common with what Lemert (1967) has called the "naive check-forger," who during his check-writing sprees is plagued by the sense of "false" structure to his life. Both of these deviants stand in contrast to the blind person, whose defect generally has such high social visibility that attempted adjustment through spurious roles is not possible.

Where stuttering is highly visible, the speech deviant's choices rest more directly upon the range of roles externally available to him. The problem for the stutterer in American society, if not universally, is that there are so few roles for which adequate speech is not a prerequisite. In greater or lesser degree, stuttering compromises the success with which any role can be played. Only rarely, usually in the role of the clown or entertainer, can the stutterer gain any rewards for public display of his disorder.

Highly relevant to this is that stutterers—unlike the blind, the deaf, the physically handicapped, narcotics addicts, criminals, and other deviants—do not form groups of their own, nor do they develop a subculture. Furthermore, they neither organize nor support therapy groups comparable to Alcoholics Anonymous. Stutterers have no opportunities to adjust through institutionalized deviant roles and to make use of socially acquired techniques and subcultural ideologies for dealing with the rejection and social degradation they experience in society.

Another quality of stuttering, having an important bearing on interaction between the deviant speaker and others, is its intermittency. This characteristic, which is similar to that in certain other forms of deviancy, such as alcoholism, begets an inconsistent reaction from others and in some cases permits or encourages their denial of the problem. It also allows the deviant speaker to dissociate unpleasant self-conceptions. Dichotomous contrasts drawn by parents or others between the deviant's stuttering speech and his speech on "days when he speaks perfectly" may contribute to cleavages in the self-image. Research by Tuthill (1946) and by MacDonald and Frick (1954) has brought out the considerable variation in listener reactions to stutterers so far as identifying their speech as abnormal is concerned. Thus from the "other's" side of the interactional equation there is a further source of confusion in defining the stutterer's role.

These facts, when taken with Porter's finding (1939) that stutterers apparently react to some auditors as "hard" and to others as "easy," emphasize the often subtle nature of the interactions that generate and maintain stuttering. Posture, nonvocal gestures, empathy, and subliminal responses all probably have functions in stutterer–others interaction. Factors of this sort are subcultural in nature rather than cultural. Research is needed to determine their significance in relation to meanings, values, and definitions, which are more clearly cultural in origin.

THERAPY

Sociology is not an applied science, nor does it have practitioners. Consequently, it can have little direct use in interindividual psychotherapy. However, sociologists in recent years have well demonstrated the worth of their discipline by analysis and research into the structure and functioning of clinical treatment and custodial care in the institutional setting of the mental hospital. The distinctive point of view of the sociologist in these research studies has been the attention given to the unanticipated social consequences of formal policy and formal organization. The approach has especially highlighted the informal social organization which often evolves among staff and patients as a response to demands of institutional organization. One of the more promising concepts that has evolved out of this kind of research has been that of the therapeutic community, devised as a typological contrast to the traditional custodial community.

While speech therapy is largely confined to clinics, remedial classes in public schools, commercial schools, and private practice, it seems no less amenable to sociological analysis than mass-treatment institutions for the mentally ill. The same concepts of role, status, interaction, informal organization, and community seem applicable as research tools to such things as clinician-client relationships, clinic organization, and the relation of the clinic to its institutional host. We know, for example, that remedial speech classes often fail of their purpose in public schools because of the invidious status connotations they take on in pupil-to-pupil interaction. The failure of commercial schools for stutterers usually has been explained by reference to the mechanical or "quack" methods they employ, but an equally good case can be made for a sociopsychological explanation of these failures. Therapists in reputable agencies often look at their case failures exclusively from the standpoint of what they "did wrong" as individuals, or blame failures on defective technique. Yet in many such cases it may be more helpful to study their failures as consequences of the form of the social relationship which existed between the therapist and the client. In other cases, failures may result from status problems or extraclinical interaction patterns of which the clinician may be only dimly aware or over which he has little control.

Broadly conceived, present-day clinical procedures seem to be directed towards preventing the growth of self-awareness as a stutterer in cases involving children with dysrythmic or disfluent speech. In adult stutterers, self-confrontation and self-acceptance as a stutterer or non-fluent person appear to be widely held objectives in early and continuing therapy—therapy thus becomes a form of control over a self-and-other symbolic process which is the reciprocal of a social process. If this objective is to be achieved, it means that control will have to extend beyond clinician-client contacts into other significant areas of social interaction and social participation of the deviant speaker. In effect, this is done in many speech clinics. The clinic to a large degree becomes a special speech community, centripetally integrated, with a subculture in which for the first time the stutterer finds his stuttering permissive, socially acceptable, or even socially rewarded. The deviant becomes a part of small-group interaction with others who are undergoing therapy. He or she acquires a special role and status in clinical groups whose functioning, morale, and social control are at least as important in the outcome of treatment as is the more intensive interaction with the clinician.

Undoubtedly the association of speech therapy agencies with other institutions, such as hospitals, remedial schools, public schools, colleges, and universities, carries important symbolic and organizational consequences for those who come under their influence. However, with the present state of our knowledge, these impacts can only be guessed at. Apropos of possible research on the subject, questions might well be raised about the worth of the traditional tendency to organize speech therapy for stutterers under the remote aegis of medicine in conjunction with that for cleft palate, cerebral palsy, and other organically based speech disorders. A large question with many ramifications is whether the objective of working with stutterers should be to "cure" them of an illness or a disease. If not, then we need to re-examine the pertinence of a clinic type of organization, with examining rooms and instrument cabinets, along with the acceptance and application of concepts such as "pathology" and, indeed, "therapy" itself.

A logical extension of this trend of thought raises challenging queries about the nature of the emphasis in current therapy. The estimated number of stutterers in the American population (over a million) makes the uncommitted, thoughtful observer highly dubious that clinics relying upon interindividual therapy can be anything more than pilot-plant agencies. In less temporizing terms, it verges on preposterous to assume that the time-expensive, individualized methods of working with stutterers can ever do more than imperceptibly dent the overall problem. The alternative seems to be the development of administrative therapy somewhat along the lines of administrative psychiatry. A great deal of what is now done in working with the speech problems of small children already seems to be moving in this direction.

The other obvious area for some kind of administrative therapy is in the schools. Yet in contrast to the advances made in clinical psychotherapy for stutterers, the thinking and procedures for dealing with stutterers by administrative methods in the schools remain barren and crudely empirical. Little research has been done on the subject, most probably because the conventional psychological formulations of stuttering as an individual problem are wholly inapplicable to the kinds of problems that arise. It is precisely here, in research into problems of group and institutional controls, that the formulations and concepts of sociology can be more useful.

References

References that are listed here only by author and year of publication appear in complete form in the Bibliography.

Aron, M. L. (1962)

Beaglehole, E. (1940) Cultural complexity and psychological problems. *Psychaitry, 3,* 329–340.

Bluemel, C. S. (1932) Primary and secondary stuttering. *Proceedings of the American Speech Correction Association,* 91–102.

Bullen, A. K. (1945) A cross cultural approach to the problem of stuttering, *Child Development, 16,* 1–88.

Ferguson, C. (1964) Baby talk in six languages, *American Anthrop., 66,* 103–114.

Frachtenberg, L. J. (1920) Abnormal types of speech in Quileute. *Int. J. Amer. Ling., 1.*

Glasner, P. J. (1949) Personality characteristics and emotional problems in stutterer under age five. *Journal of Speech and Hearing Disorders, 14,* 135–138.

Henry, J. (1940) Speech disturbances in Pilaga Indian children. *American Journal of Orthopsychiatry, 10,* 362, 269.

Irwin, O. C. (1948a) The effect of occupational status and of age on sound frequency, *Journal of Speech and Hearing Disorders, 13,* 320–323.

Irwin, O. C. (1948b) Infant speech: The effects of occupational status and age on the use of sound types. *Journal of Speech and Hearing Disorders, 13,* 224–226.

Johnson, W. (1944) The Indians have no word for it: Stuttering in children. *Quarterly Journal of Speech, 30,* 330–337.

Joseph, A., and Murray, V. F. (1951) *Chamorros and Carolinians of Saipan: Personality studies.* Cambridge, Mass.: Harvard University Press.

Kluckhohn, C. (1954) Culture and behavior. In G. Lindsey, ed., *Handbook of social psychology,* Reading, Mass.: Addison-Wesley.

Lemert, E. M. (1952)

Lemert, E. M. (1953)

Lemert, E. M. (1962)

Lemert, E. M. (1967) *Human deviance, social problems and social control,* Englewood Cliffs, N. J.: Prentice-Hall, Chap. 3.

MacDonald, E. T., and Frick, J. (1954) Store clerks' reactions to stuttering. *Journal of Speech and Hearing Disorders, 19,* 206–211.

Merton, R. K. (1957) Social theory and social structure. New York: Free Press.

Moncur, J. P. (1952)

Morgenstern, J. J. (1956)

Orton, S. T. (1937) *Reading, writing, and speech problems in children.* New York: Norton.

Porter, H. V. K. (1939) Stuttering phenomena in relation to size and personnel of audience. *Journal of Speech Disorders, 4,* 323–333.

Rieber, R. (1963) Stuttering and the self concept. *Journal of Psychology, 55,* 307–311.

Rose, J. A. (1943) Diagnosis and treatment of speech disorders. *American Journal of Orthopsychiatry, 13,* 284–289.

Sapir, E. (1915) *Abnormal types of Speech in Nootka.* Department of Mines, Ottawa, Canada. Memoir 62.

Schnidler, M. D. (1955) A study of educational adjustments of stuttering and non-stuttering children. In W. Johnson and R. R. Lentenberger, eds., *Stuttering in children and adults.* Minneapolis: University of Minnesota Press.

Schuell, H. (1946) Sex differences in relation to stuttering. I. *Journal of Speech and Hearing Disorders, 11,* 277–298.

Sheehan, J. G. (1963) The effect of role commitment on stuttering, *American Psychologist, 18,* 401–407.

Sheehan, J. G., (1968)

Sheehan, J. G., Hadley, R., and Gould, E. (1967)

Snidecor, J. C. (1947) Why the Indian does not stutter. *Quarterly Journal of Speech, 33,* 493–495.

Stewart, J. L. (1960)

Tamai, S., Dendo, T., Kobayashis, and Umegaki, M. (1962) Studies of stuttering children, *Journal of Mental Health, Chiba, 10,* 72–83.

Thalvitzer, W. (1904) A phonetical study of the Eskimo language. *Meddelelser om Grönland, 31,* 178–180.

Tuthill, C. E. (1946) A quantitative study of extensional meaning with special reference to stuttering. *Speech Monographs, 13,* 2.

Van Riper, C. (1957) Symptomatic therapy for stuttering. In L. E. Travis, ed., *Handbook of speech pathology.* New York: Appleton.

Zelen, S. L., Sheehan, J. G., and Bugental, J. F. (1954)

About the Author WILLIAM H. PERKINS, Ph.D., is Professor of Communicative Disorders and Otolaryngology, and Executive Director, Las Floristas Speech Clinic for Children at the University of Southern California. He is a fellow of the American Speech and Hearing Association, with a Certificate of Clinical Competence in Speech. Dr. Perkins was assistant editor in charge of articles of *Asha* from 1962 to 1967, and since 1962 a consulting editor for the *Journal of Speech and Hearing Disorders*.

About the Chapter All behavior has a physiological side, and stuttering has also been approached from this vantage point. Investigation into the physiological side of stuttering, largely under the pioneering influence of Dr. Lee Edward Travis at the University of Iowa, contributed greatly toward establishing speech pathology on a scientific footing. As this chapter reveals, the substantive rewards of physiological inquiry into stuttering have been comparatively meager.

In 1944, after most of the pioneering studies were completed, Dr. Harris Hill concluded: "An agent in the form of an inner condition . . . is still as distant from discovery as it was 4,000 years ago." A decade later Dr. Wendell Johnson summarized his impressions: "As the years passed, the search for the flaw in the physical makeup of the stutterer changed by degrees from a swift scurry to a slow meander." Compare these conclusions with those of Dr. Perkins, whom Dr. Travis nominated as contributor for this chapter.

5

PHYSIOLOGICAL
STUDIES

WILLIAM H. PERKINS

5

Implicit in much of the physiological work that has been done on stuttering is the conviction that stutterers are different from nonstutterers along some organismic dimension. Often, the fact of stuttering has been taken as evidence that different physiological processes operate in stutterers and nonstutterers, *ergo*, stutterers must be different in some basic organic respect.

The attempt in this critical analysis is to interpret the evidence in terms of the limitations imposed by the research designs. This means, for example, that results of descriptive studies will not be considered adequate to support causal statements but may be considered suggestive of relationships. At best, descriptive studies control the conditions of observation; they do not provide for experimental manipulation of variables. Without experimentation—the most powerful research approach to obtaining definitive answers—statements of causal relationships must, indeed, be weak. On the other hand, the major questions to which the research has been explicitly or implicitly addressed (usually the latter) will be stated in terms of the causal answers sought. These questions provide an organizational framework for the chapter; the evidence is assessed for each to determine the best available answers. The questions posed are the following.

1. What conditions predispose onset of stuttering?
2. What conditions precipitate early evidence of stuttering?
3. What conditions precede instances of stuttering?
4. What conditions occur during instances of stuttering?
5. What conditions follow instances of stuttering?
6. What conditions perpetuate stuttering?
7. What conditions reduce stuttering?

REVIEW AND ANALYSIS

What Conditions Predispose Onset of Stuttering?

The data related to the idea that an organic variant provides fertile soil from which stuttering can grow are numerous and varied.

Sex Ratio Milisen (1957), in a review of the reports of incidence of stuttering, (Bills, 1934; Burdin, 1940; Mills & Streit, 1942; Root, 1925; White House Conference, 1931), found survey results ranging from 2.2:1 to 5.3:1 greater frequency among males than females. Weinburg (1964) even found not only a normal incidence of stuttering among blind and partially sighted children, but also a typical 4:1 sex ratio. This ratio compares with the 4:1 reported by West (1943), 4.4:1 by Morgenstern (1956), and 4.5:1 by Carroll (1965). A curious pattern can be discerned from these reports (especially from Carroll's recent study of 1958 stutterers in the Los Angeles City Elementary Schools): girls begin to stutter at a later age than boys and remain rather steady in number through the grades; boys start younger, peak at the fourth and fifth grades, and then decline in frequency in the sixth grade. That stuttering is primarily a male disorder is clearly demonstrated; that this is evidence of some diathesis is a possible, even tempting, conclusion.

Although Bryngelson and Clark (1933) found what they considered to be indications that left-handedness is a sex-linked characteristic most often transmitted from the male through the female and back to the male, this link to stuttering is too tenuous to be meaningful. Schuell (1946), in her extensive review of the literature on sex differences in stuttering, reached the conclusion (still in vogue) that the male child, whose physical, social, and language development proceeds at a slower rate than that of the female, encounters more unequal competition, consequently more frustrations, more insecurity, and as a result more hesitancies in speech. Although Schuell's is certainly a tenable interpretation it does not rule out the

191

possibility of an organic variant that predisposes boys more than girls to stuttering.

Audition Several probes have been made into the auditory system as a possible site of difference between stutterers and normal speakers. Gregory (1959, 1964b), in a study of the neurophysiological integrity of the auditory feedback system in stutterers, found no difference between them and normal speakers on the binaural in-phase and out-of-phase median-plane localization tests at different intensities and frequencies. Likewise, Shearer and Simmons (1965) reported no difference in the activity of the middle ear muscles during speech of normal speakers and stutterers. Schilling and Biener (1959) thought that bilateral threshold differences they detected in 26 out of 112 stutterers were diagnostic clues of organic central disturbance, but, of course, drawing such a casual inference is scientifically perilous.

An intriguing and prospectively substantial lead (a rarity to be sure) has been developed over the last dozen or so years by Stromsta (1958, 1959, 1964). Initially, he demonstrated that stutterers differ from nonstutterers with regard to the relative phase angle of bone-conducted speech sound-energy. His evidence suggested that the phase discrepancy increases more for stutterers than for normal speakers as fundamental frequency decreases, suggesting further that less discrepancy would occur in the female voice than in the male. He then showed that as the frequency of a masking signal was decreased, the fundamental frequency of the voice increased and concurrently stuttering was reduced. Stromsta considers this further suggestive evidence of a connection between vocal pitch and stuttering. Next, he partially confirmed an earlier finding by Vannier *et al.* (1954) that phonation could be arrested by distortion of auditory side-tone. Then he investigated the localization of a sound image on a midsaggital plane and found that stutterers located sound images at different subjective sites than nonstutterers. He has also pursued central nervous system (CNS) correlates of these differences; these results will be discussed later under "CNS Functions."

Stromsta's work catches our interest if for no other reason than that he may be ferreting out a basis for the fact that there are more male than female stutterers—one of the few facts about stuttering that does not fit easily within a learning paradigm of the problem. The conclusion to be inferred from his work is that stuttering is something that happens because of a somatic condition. Before this conclusion will be persuasive, though, he will have to account for the stutterer's normal speech as well; that is, if phase-angle discrepancy is the mechanism of his stuttering, then what is the mechanism of his fluency?

Twinning Studies of stuttering and twinning point to the likelihood that stuttering occurs relatively more frequently among twins and in families in which twinning occurs (Berry, 1937b, 1938a). This finding is corroborated by the report of Nelson, Hunter, and Walter (1945) who studied 200 twin pairs and found stuttering in about 20 percent of them. It is also supported to some extent by Graf (1955), who collected questionnaire responses from schools and from parents of 553 pairs of twins. She found that 1.9 percent of the 1104 twins stuttered, which is slightly higher than the percentage in the general population. These reports could indicate a hereditary factor, but the differences are not consistently large enough to be convincing. Moreover, Carroll (1965) found no difference between twins and nontwins in the 1958 stutterers he studied, and Koch (1966), in a study of 90 pairs of twins, concluded that stuttering and twin zygosity are not significantly related.

Familial Incidence Wepman (1939) matched a group of 250 stutterers with 250 nonstutterers for age, sex, and social environment. He found instances of stuttering in 68.8 percent of the families of stutterers and in only 15.6 percent of the matched-group families. West, Nelson, and Berry (1939) studied 204 families of stutterers and reported that stuttering ran in 50 percent of them for several generations. The same results were also reported by Nelson (1939b). Freund (1952) questioned 121 stutterers and their relatives about stuttering and cluttering. The operational distinctions between these two behaviors were not specified, but 74 percent of the stutterers' relatives were reported to stutter. Johnson (Johnson *et al.*, 1942), too, found that stuttering had occurred four times as frequently in the families of stutterers as of nonstutterers. Carrall (1965), however, using school records for the 1139 stutterers for whom evidence was available, found only 14.6 percent who were reported to have parents or siblings who stuttered. An even bigger blemish on this unsullied picture of familial incidence is the finding (Sheehan & Martyn, 1966) of no difference in incidence of relatives who stutter among the families of active stutterers, recovered stutterers, and an equivalent group of normal speakers.

Stuttering may well be a familial disorder. That this demonstrates a genetic transmission factor is another matter. Nelson (1939) stated that stuttering frequently appears in children of stuttering parents with whom the children have had little if any contact. If her observation is valid, it would be a strong argument in favor of a hereditary link in the transmission of stuttering. On the other hand, Berman and Train (1940) point out that the nature of the occurrence of stuttering in families from generation to generation does not follow Mendelian laws. Gedda, Branconi, and Bruno (1960), after studying two pairs of monozygotic twins and four pairs of dizygotic twins, found no evidence of sex-linked transmission of stuttering. Along similar lines, Gray (1940) studied Iowa and Kansas branches of a stuttering family and found eleven who had stuttered and sixteen who had not in the Iowa branch as contrasted with one stutterer and sixteen nonstutterers in the Kansas branch. Rotter (1939), after finding a greater number only of children, fewer middle children, and a greater age difference between stutterers and their siblings, inferred that the problem could be more the result of pampering than of heredity.

An explanation of familial incidence of stuttering is fraught with uncertainty. It could be a genetic problem, but it could just as well result from the perpetuation from one generation to the next of a psychological climate conducive to stuttering. Another persuasive possibility suggested by Sheehan and Martyn (1967) is that families of stutterers may be more likely than families of nonstutterers to search out and report stutterers in their ancestry. They called this tendency *differential preliminary search,* and noted that it was especially likely in the case of stuttering, since the problem is known to run in families. The evidence that we have seen is not sufficiently convincing to *require* one explanation or another, but the hereditary explanation seems less likely.

Diabetes One of the bits of folklore about stuttering is that diabetics are immune to it. If this were so, it would suggest that some physiological condition is crucial to the prevention of stuttering. By inference, lack of that condition might be essential to its development. Although we have not encountered any stutterers who were known to be diabetics, the occurrence of stuttering in the general population is low enough (about 1 in 100) that several thousand diabetics should be surveyed before we can conclude that diabetics do not stutter. West (1958) has come closest to providing this evidence. He examined the records of diabetics in one of the hospitals that originally experimented with insulin treatment. No instances of stuttering were reported. A physician who had interviewed each case was "positive" that no stutterers were among them. By contrast, we know a physician who says he has encountered diabetics who stutter. Although this type of evidence does not firmly establish the relationship between diabetes and stuttering, the connection is one of the most suggestive leads we have for pursuing the idea of an organic variant.

Epilepsy West (1958) has proposed a parallel between stuttering and epileptiform seizures. This parallel is corroborated by some research. Berry (1937a) compared the medical records of 430 children who stuttered with those of 462 who did not and found that 36 stutterers as against 12 nonstutterers had suffered from epilepsy or convulsions prior to the age of five. Harrison's (1947) study of sixty epileptics also supported this position, in that stuttering was found 36 times as frequently as in the general population, disturbed laterality five times as frequently and twinning three times as frequently.

West contends that stutterers are convulsion-prone and that they are linked to epilepsy and diabetes mellitus through the role of blood sugar. The diabetic is thought not to be convulsion-prone because insulin and blood sugar are inversely related and the diabetic tends toward hyperglycemia whereas the epileptic tends toward hypoglycemia.

The evidence related to this formulation is varied. Palasek and Curtis (1960) administered lactose placebos to nine stutterers and found a statistically nonsignificant tendency for stuttering to be reduced. Then, too, Glaser (1936) reported the responses of nineteen endocrinologists to a questionnaire inquiry into the relationship of stuttering to endocrine malfunction. Six reported stuttering associated with hyperinsulinism and thyroid insufficiency. Kopp (1934), on the other hand, compared 49 stutterers with 23 nonstutterers and found significantly higher blood sugar content in the stutterers. Johnson, Stearns, and Warweg (1933) took blood samples from fifteen male stutterers after eating, resting, and stuttering. The blood sugar level in all samples was not indicative of disease. In fact, Moore (1959) hypnotized 12 stutterers, asked them to talk about pleasant and unpleasant memories, and then took blood samples. With one exception, blood sugar decreased rather than increased with unpleasant memories even though all of the subjects stuttered more. Although stutterers may be convulsion-prone, blood sugar

195

level has not been clearly demonstrated as the link between their stuttering and any proclivities they may have to epilepsy.

Laterality   Results from laterality studies fall into two contradictory groups. Bryngelson (1935, 1939, 1940; Bryngelson & Clark, 1933; Bryngelson & Rutherford, 1937; Fink & Bryngelson, 1934) has been responsible for the most convincing suggestion that sidedness is an etiological factor in stuttering. His work about three decades ago was supported by that of Travis (1931; Travis, Tuttle, & Bender, 1936), Quinan (1921), and Van Riper (1935). Bryngelson's findings are mainly from 700 stutterers whom he interviewed (1935) and from two sets of matched groups of stutterers and nonstutterers, one with 74 in each group (Bryngelson & Rutherford, 1937) and the other with 78 (Bryngelson, 1939, 1940). Curiously, he used more females than males in his matched groups. Whether this unusual distribution contributed to his findings cannot be ascertained. His major findings were that stutterers, if anything, are less likely to be left-handed than nonstutterers but are four to twelve times as likely to be ambidextrous and to have had their handedness shifted.

The work of Johnson and his group (1955; Johnson & Duke, 1936; Johnson & King, 1942), Van Dusen (1939), Heltman (1940), Daniels (1940), and Spadino (1941) contrasts sharply with the work supporting laterality differences. With the exception of Van Dusen's (1939) finding of a laterality difference only in strength and usage, none of these investigators found significant differences in the laterality of stutterers and nonstutterers. Why these two groups of investigators who worked at about the same time have produced such divergent results is puzzling. Granted that the statistical inferences drawn in those days were naive by present standards, Bryngelson has reported results on a very large sample of stutterers, and this lends credence to his position. Yet opposing his findings are several independent studies of respectably large samples that are persuasive by virtue of consensus. Persuasion approaches conviction with the report of Sheehan and Martyn (1966) that handedness, whether left, right, changed, or ambidextrous, does not differentiate among recovered stutterers, active stutterers, and normal speakers; for that matter, neither does a history of left-handedness in the family. As these researchers stress (1967), handedness is only one aspect of sinistrality or laterality, but, they conclude, "Whatever is sinister about the stutterer, it does not appear to show up in his hand usage."

Speech Motor Performance West (1929) reported that the stutterers he studied were slower than nonstutterers in their rate of repetitive movement of mandible and eyebrows. A few years later Blackburn (1931) had similar findings for voluntary rhythmical control of the diaphragm, tongue, lips, and mandible, as did Hunsley (1937) in his comparative investigation of twenty stutterers and twenty nonstutterers. They concluded that stutterers were inferior to normal speakers in control of speech structures for nonspeech activities. Strother and Kriegman (1943) showed no difference, though, with matched groups of fifteen stutterers and fifteen normal speakers in diadochokinetic rate for lips, mandible, tongue, or fingers. Strother (1944) also found the same lack of difference when he tested the same structures for rhythmokinesis. If anything, the stutterers were slightly superior in both studies. Additional studies of various nonspeech motor functions of oral structures—e.g., by Cross (1936), Palmer and Osburn (1940), Seth (1934), and Spriestersbach (1940)—merely confirm the impression that any difference in these motor skills between stutterers and nonstutterers is either slight or nonexistent.

General Motor Performance The general motor performances of stutterers range from almost normal to grossly inferior. The greatest discrepancy is between Kopp's (1943) results on the Oseretsky Tests of Motor Proficiency and Finkelstein and Weisberger's (1954) replication of her work. Whereas they found their fifteen stuttering children slightly inferior, Kopp reported profound motor disturbances for her group of 450. Schilling (1966) reports several German studies (Böhme, 1965; Schilling, 1959; Schilling & Krueger, 1960; Schilling & Schilling, 1960; Schlange, 1961; Schonharl & Bente, 1960; Wegener, 1963), interpreted as indicating brain injury in early childhood of stutterers, that are supportive of Kopp's results. In fact, Schilling suggests from his evidence (1962) that stutterers with damage in the brain stem and a pathological electronystagmogram show monotony within vowels, those with damage in the cortex show monotony within sentences, and those without brain damage show normal speech melody. In standardized motor test performances (Bilto, 1941; Westphal, 1933), in bimanual activities (Cross, 1936), in breathing and eye movement during silent reading and reasoning (Murray, 1932), in eye movement during oral and silent reading (Kopp, 1943), and in finger control (Rotter, 1955), stutterers have been found slightly-to-definitely inferior. Only Ross (1955) reported nor-

197

mal performance for them and this was on psychomotor tests of speed, memory, and integration. Conservatively, we can see the smoke from these results, if not the fire. Some may be tempted, as apparently the medically oriented Europeans are, to see convincing proof of brain damage, especially in the motor system of the majority of young stutterers. Before we join in fanning these sparks into a full-blown organicist's conflagration, we will want to see the evidence from more than *ad hoc* clinical observations. Where such evidence exists, sizable differences have not been found. As matters stand, we cannot determine whether the motor deficiencies that have been observed are a cause or a consequence of stuttering.

Perseveration Essentially the same ambiguity prevails with interpretations of the work on perseveration. Eisenson (1958) theorized that over 50 percent of stutterers are constitutionally predisposed toward perseverative behavior. He cites as evidence the perseverative tendencies of adult stutterers on alternating or nonalternating motor or sensorimotor tasks (Eisenson, 1937; Eisenson & Pastel, 1936; Eisenson & Winslow, 1938; King, 1953). Additional evidence is offered by Lightfoot (1948), who found greater perseveration in serial identification of colors by severe than by mild stutterers or nonstutterers. Hill's (1942) work on motor repetitions and prolongations, and Goldsand's (1942) on sensory perseveration, are also supportive. Opposed to Eisenson's thesis is the work of Sheets (1941) on visual perseveration and of Gold (1941) using the same experimental design with auditory stimuli. Neither found significant differences between stutterers and nonstutterers.

Two reasonably definitive studies were done subsequently that resolve these apparent contradictions. King (1961) administered to 72 adult stutterers and 82 nonstutterers ten tests to measure sensory, dispositional-rigidity, and alternating-activity perseveration. He found that the only tests on which stutterers perseverated significantly more were the alternating-activity and the sensory tests that required continuous, rapid change of set. These are the same types of performances in which stutterers were found to be perseverative in the earlier investigations. King speculated that these tests are difficult for stutterers if they overreact, become rigid, and are thus blocked from performing alternating-motor acts or from changing set rapidly. In fact, Lightfoot (1948), in discussing possible reasons for the perseveration he observed in stutterers, remarked that they seemed reluctant to make incorrect responses. "Such behavior may be compared with that of the amateur typist who tries to type an important document with several carbons. Every stroke of the key constitutes a minor crisis, a thing to be checked and double-checked before being acted upon."

The other definitive study was done by Martin (1962). He reasoned that if over 50 percent of stutterers are organically predisposed to perseverate, as Eisenson believes, then young stutterers should exhibit the same perseverative tendencies as adults. He gave four motor perseveration tests to 161 children between eight and thirteen years of age, 52 of whom were stutterers. He found no differences in any respect whether based on stuttering, severity, age, or sex. This does not accord with a constitutional predisposition to perseverate.

Allergy Association of stuttering and allergic diathesis is suggested by the two studies that have been done on the question. Kennedy and Williams (1938) reported 52 out of 100 stutterers from five to fourteen years of age with a personal history of allergy and 95 with allergy in the family history. They did not use a control group so their results are difficult to interpret. In view of Card's (1939) findings that 62 percent of 104 nonstutterers had allergy in their families and his report that 53 percent of college students normally have positive allergic reaction, the Williams and Kennedy study may not be indicative of an unusual extent of allergy among stutterers. Card, however, found in his matched group of 104 stutterers that 102 had noticed allergies in themselves or their families. Forty of the 102 were tested for allergy; all reacted positively, the degree being usually proportional to the severity of stuttering. The dimensions of these investigations are too loosely defined to provide confidence in their results. Even if allergy and stuttering are associated, we do not know whether they are connected causally, through a common diathesis, or whether they are connected through reactions to a common pattern of environmental stress.

Developmental History Berry (1938b) compared the birth records of 430 children who stuttered with those of 462 who did not. She found among stutterers a far higher incidence of infectious diseases of the respiratory system that involve high fevers and of their possible sequelae; epilepsy, convulsions, and encephalitis. In general, Travis (1931) and Despart (1946) reported similar findings. Berry also noted in another study (1938c) of the birth records of 227 stutterers and a similar number in a control group that aside from stutterers being late in the acquisition of speech, the only difference was in the greater number of mothers of stuttering children who had had thyrotoxicosis and exophthalmic goiter during pregnancy. Her report that no significant differences were found in conditions of birth was corroborated by Boland's (1951) data (although he interpreted them with a correction factor that produced a difference) and by Johnson's report (Johnson *et al.*, 1942) of no difference in birth, development, or speech onset. Johnson did find a few more diseases and injuries among stutterers, which seems to be about the only early-history factor that appears in the studies with any consistency.

Psychosis The impression that psychotics do not stutter is also not well founded, as the evidence of Barbara (1946), Freund (1955) and Pitrelli (1948) bears out. The incidence seems to be in the range of expectation for the normal population, with the exception of Freund's report of three times the number of stutterers among 149 ambulatory schizophrenics as in the general population. Although any connection that might exist between psychosis and stuttering could be entirely psychogenic (Barbara; Pitrelli), the possibility of the operation of an organic variant cannot be ruled out, which is the reason for including this section.

CNS Functions In the United States, the early electroencephalographic investigations of stuttering were developed around the Orton-Travis theory of cerebral dominance and sought evidence concerning the incidence of bilateral brain-wave asymmetry in stutterers and nonstutterers. Travis and Knott (1936, 1937) found small unsystematic bilateral differences during silence that were correlated with severity of stuttering, and Douglass (1943) showed differences that distinguished stutterers from nonstutterers physiologically only in unilateral alpha blocking in the two hemispheres. Knott and Tjossem (1943) repeated and confirmed the Douglass finding. Lindsley (1940) also recorded similar results in the brain waves of two adult stutterers that were compared with those of 65 nonstuttering children. Along a slightly different line, Freestone (1942) indicated greater alpha activity among stutterers, especially during stuttering. More recently, Umeda (1960) found in six out of ten stutterers irregular EEG tracings that correlated with the severity of their defective speech.

The contrasting evidence is reported by Scarbrough (1943), by Rheinberger *et al.* (1943), and recently by Fox (1965, 1966).

The condition under which Scarbrough found no difference between the brain waves of stutterers and nonstutterers involved minimum activity. The subjects reclined and did not speak, whereas in the other experiments in which differences were found the subjects were recorded during both speech and silence. The differences in results from these studies, then, could be the consequence of recording brain waves when the subjects were asked to do nothing but relax and be silent and recording them when the period of silence was preceded by speech and stuttering. Fox, on the other hand, compared electronically analyzed EEG correlations from right and left hemispheres of thirteen stutterers who were paired with nonstutterers matched for sex, age, handedness, and imitative simulation of the stuttering pattern. After comparing them with their eyes open and closed under conditions of silence, stuttered speech, and nonstuttered speech, she found a strong possibility that stuttering behavior, whether simulated by nonstutterers or produced by stutterers, is disruptive of the EEG display; the differences that do occur are probably the result of behavior and not of interhemispheric covariability.

Electroencephalographic research in stuttering is like a cat with nine lives: each time it seems to have been laid to rest it springs forth afresh with renewed life and vitality. Stromsta (1964) undertook an EEG analysis to determine if CNS correlates of auditory phase-angle differences could be detected. From several promising theoretical leads he obtained harmonic analyses of correlograms of EEG potentials of 15 stutterers and 15 nonstutterers under conditions of silence and wakeful relaxation while seated comfortably in a darkened room with eyes closed. He found that the groups could not be differentiated by comparing autocorrelograms (EEG signals from one hemisphere), but could be distinguished on the basis of crosscorrelograms (bilateral signals).

When the differences among stutterers and nonstutterers are viewed collectively—in terms of sex ratio, audition, twinning, familial incidence, diabetes, epilepsy, laterality, motor coordination, perseveration, allergy, developmental history, psychosis, and CNS functions—we must recognize the possibility of a constitutional predisposition to stuttering. To take this conclusion seriously, however, would be risky on several counts. For one thing, no factor or combination of factors has been reported as consistently present in all or most instances of stuttering. If organic variants are operative, they would presumably be effective continuously, at least from moment to moment.

Yet, stuttering varies so much from moment to moment, hour to hour, day to day, and year to year, that to explain these variations as evidence of an abiding physiological deviation is troublesome.

When the spotlight of investigation was on the *person* who stutters, constitutional predisposition theories were rampant. Searchers were sniffing for evidence of dysphemia, spasmophemia, strephosymbolia, cerebral dominance—in fact, for any somatic variant that could distinguish stutterers from nonstutterers. As we have seen in this review of what was turned up in the search, sizable differences would be reported by one investigator only to be contradicted by the next. Interestingly, the sizes of the differences have been inversely proportional to the rigor of the observations and inferences. Successful replication has not distinguished attempts to delineate stutterers from nonstutterers.

As the focus of research has shifted from the person of the stutterer to his defectively disfluent speech behavior, stricter definitions of what he actually does that is defective have begun to evolve. Specific descriptions of observed phenomena, particularly stuttering, are either nonexistent or vague in most of the literature reviewed for this section. This leaves open the possibility that the label "stuttering" has been applied to a variety of behaviors for which it would be inappropriate. When the stutterer's behavior is made explicit, then observations, physiological and otherwise, become relatively stable. In fact, judging from the two studies (Fox, 1965; Williams, 1955) in which nonstutterers have simulated the oral performance of stutterers, both groups have produced the same physiological results—results that under other conditions have been viewed as evidence of a constitutional predisposition. All of which suggests strongly that the only thing different about the stutterer is what he does.

What Conditions Precipitate Early Evidence of Stuttering?

The evidence of precipitating as distinct from predisposing conditions for the onset of the problem of stuttering is somewhat limited. We have selected for this section those investigations in which stuttering has been observed to begin or to vary subsequent to the reported changes in the physiological condition.

Handedness Change Johnson and Duke (1935), Milisen and Johnson (1936), and Fagan (1931) reported onset of stuttering following change of handedness. Fagan concluded from his nine left-handed and four ambidextrous cases who began to stutter within a year after their handedness was shifted that such changes were definitely linked to stuttering. Johnson and Duke were more cautious, however. They studied histories of 16 cases ranging in age from five to seventy-one and found evidence of a temporal relation between stuttering and change of handedness. The reports of such factors as disease and emotionality prior to onset of stuttering led them to limit their conclusions. We would add to their caution the problem of accuracy of historical reports and the possibility of coincidence of age of onset of those studied, age of handedness shift, and peak age of onset (around three) for the majority of stutterers (Johnson & King, 1942).

Heltman (1940), utilizing Daniels's (1940) data, concluded that the likelihood of change of handedness affecting stuttering is slight. Of 1594 college students checked, 77 had been shifted from left to right. Of these 77, only one, or 1.3 percent, stuttered; this does not differ significantly from the 1.1 percent normal incidence of right-handers who stutter or from the 1.3 percent of the 1594 students who stuttered.

Disease Some evidence supports the notion that disease tends to precipitate stuttering (Berry, 1937a, 1938c; Goda, 1961; Travis, 1931). West, Nelson, and Berry (1939) reported that 16 to 20 percent of 204 cases began to stutter immediately after recovery from infectious disorders of the respiratory system accompanied by high fever. Johnson (Johnson *et al.*, 1942), however, compared 46 stutterers with a matched group of nonstutterers, median age was four years and two months, and found practically no difference in incidence of disease.

Miscellaneous Two physiological reports are available on unrelated questions. These reports stand alone without verification, and consist of uncontrolled observations of a few cases. Arend, Handzel, and Weiss (1962) found two persons who developed stuttering concurrent with dysphasia from damage in the motor speech area; their stuttering subsided as the dysphasia improved. Gordon (1928), an endocrinologist, reported five cases of "stammering" that appeared during treatment with thyroid extract and disappeared when treatment was discontinued.

What Conditions Precede Instances of Stuttering?

One study in particular, an experimental investigation by Hill (1954), provides slight physiological evidence that is relevant to this question. Hill investigated the possibility that the initial phases of stuttering are manifestations of stimulus-response disorganization. He recorded, under threat of penalty, speech, manual responses, and muscle-action potentials for indications of generalized muscle tone. He hypothesized from earlier work on behavior disorganization (Howard, 1928; Patrick, 1934; Pavlov, 1927; Pronko & Bowles, 1951; Sears & Hovland, 1941; Young, 1928) that normal speech would be disrupted in a manner similar to stuttering by three types of conditions: (1) extremely complex stimuli, (2) ambiguous stimuli, and, the main one, (3) threat of penalty. Thirty normal speakers were trained to respond with particular hand movements to different colored light flashes and to make a new six-second statement, prepared between trials, with each presentation of a red light. The subjects were then required to respond to ambiguous stimuli (two lights flashed simultaneously) without threat of penalty and with threat of penalty.

The complex-stimuli condition produced some disorganization. The ambiguous condition without threat of penalty produced the greatest number of stops or omissions in speech but the subjects did not appear to be under stress and the muscle action-potential measures were not increased. Speech disruption under threat of penalty, however, appeared to be more compulsive and perseverative, and generalized muscle tension, as measured by EMG, was increased. Many of the disorganized speech responses Hill found were described as indistinguishable from stuttering. Although the usual interruptions were not extreme, he reports that several would have been classed as severe stuttering in any speech clinic.

Conclusion Many conditions may be capable of disrupting speech, but some normal speakers' responses to complex or ambiguous stimuli presented under threat of penalty appear to be impressively similar to what most of us describe as stuttering. Still, this is a suggestive, not a definitive, conclusion. The analogy to stuttering could be superficial. Whereas Hill's conditions seemed to disorganize normal speech in ways similar to stuttering, this is far from a conclusive demonstration that stuttering is also a manifestation of behavioral disorganization. In fact, disruptive as stuttering would obviously appear to be, and much as the pattern may change across the years, the consistency of moments of stuttering behavior from one instance to the next points to an organized learned response, however maladaptive. The majority of stimuli investigated to date that could control emission of stuttering have been psychological. Physiological stimuli may be equally important (e.g., tensions and postures of articulatory structures), but they have not yet caught the interest of researchers.

What Conditions Occur During Instances of Stuttering?

That studies of the physiology of the act of stuttering are all but nonexistent is not surprising. On the one hand, stuttering is such a transitory phenomenon that it is difficult to trap it the instant it occurs, to say nothing of the difficulty of deciding when it starts to occur. On the other hand, physiological responses, especially of the autonomic nervous system, have various latency periods that make interpretation of the stimuli that control them doubly difficult. The closest answers currently available are from innumerable physiological studies of the effects of stuttering, done mostly prior to World War II. Since Hill (1944a, 1944b) did extensive reviews of the biochemical and physiological research, we shall use his organization; we have added a category to include some work on levels of awareness that we believe is also relevant to our question in this section.

Biochemical Review Hill's review of the biochemical literature (1944a) will be summarized and two reports of more recent date will be added. We could find no other biochemical investigations of stuttering that were done after 1944. Studies of plasma and whole-blood-constituent calcium, phosphorous, potassium, globulin, protein, and sugar level (Anderson & Whealdon, 1941; Hill, 1944a; Johnson, Stearns, & Warweg, 1933; Kopp, 1933, 1934; Seeman, 1936; Steer, 1937) show stutterers within normal limits except for somewhat elevated blood calcium and phosphorous values. The increased plasma calcium, however, could directly reflect the increased muscular activity associated with stuttering. The inconsistent trend toward higher-than-normal red and white blood cell counts and hemoglobin changes (Card, 1939; Karlin & Sobel, 1940; Kopp, 1934; Trumper, 1928; Twitmeyer, 1930) were also interpreted as normal physiological responses to increased muscular activity or to affect.

Differences in salivary pH between stutterers and nonstutterers were reported (Starr, 1922, 1928), but others found no differences (Kopp, 1934), particularly when measures were made in the basal state (Hafford, 1941). Such differences as were found are similar to those reported in normal speakers and in the same individual under various circumstances (Baker & Eye, 1935; Winsor & Korchin, 1938, 1940). Increases in urinary

205

creatinine were said to accompany improvement in speech in one stutterer described as a "subbreather." These increases also accompanied deeper breathing (Stratton, 1924). The work on oxygen and carbon dioxide (Kopp, 1933; Ritzman, 1943; Starr, 1928; Trumper, 1928) showed no differences from normal in the basal state, and heightened CO_2 tension following severe stuttering. Such increases would be expected from respiratory inefficiency due to hypoventilation (Starr, 1928).

More recent research by Johnson and his group (1959) has demonstrated without much question that alveolar CO_2 partial pressure is remarkably similar for stutterers and nonstutterers and that stuttering is not associated with latent tetany. They measured alveolar CO_2 partial pressure of twenty adult male stutterers and of a similar group of nonstutterers before and after speaking and before and after hyperventilation. They reasoned that if stutterers are poised on the brink of some biochemical or neurological imbalance, then hyperventilation should precipitate more blocking. The experimental conditions produced no changes in stuttering, but, interestingly, a slight decrease in fluency of nonstutterers.

McCroskey's (1957) metabolic study of twenty adult stutterers and a matched group of nonstutterers is also relevant. The groups were similar in basal metabolic rate and in the extent of increased metabolism during the speech act. The similarity was greater, however, for stutterers who had completed therapy and, presumably, were stuttering less.

Physiological Review We will summarize Hill's integration of the physiological literature (1944b), as we did his survey of biochemical research, and will add what little work has been done since the review in 1944. He considered respiration, cardiovascular changes, muscular tone, reflexes and eye movements of stutterers in relation to the physiological reactions of normal speakers during startle.

Although consistent patterns of breathing disturbances have been reported, no individual stutterer is apt to exhibit them all (Van Riper, 1936). One of the most characteristic reactions of stutterers, though, is the sharp, rapid, initial inspiration (Fagan, 1932; Fossler, 1930; Scripture, 1923; Steer, 1935; L. E. Travis, 1927a; V. Travis, 1936) which is also a typical normal response to a startling stimulus (Berg & Beebe-Center, 1941; Blatz, 1925; Brunswick, 1924; Cannon, 1929; Darwin, 1873; Landis, 1926; Mosso, 1896; Scott, 1931; Skaggs, 1926). Another frequent reaction during a block is fixation of respiratory musculatures (Bluemel, 1928; Mills & Streit, 1942; Murray, 1932; Scripture, 1923; Steer, 1937; Stetson, 1933; L. E. Travis 1925, 1927a, 1931; V. Travis, 1936; Trumper, 1928). Similar action of the diaphragm seems to occur in normal speakers following a strong stimulus (Brunswick, 1924; Faulkner, 1941; Skaggs, 1930). Stereotyped prolonged inspiration and expiration with short respiratory movements superimposed are also typical of stutterers (Fletcher, 1914; Fossler, 1930; Steer, 1937; L. E. Travis, 1927a; V. Travis, 1936; Van Riper, 1936)—a finding supported by recent European work (Schilling, 1960)—and compare rather closely with the arrest, slowing, and rehearsal of breathing movements of normal speakers following shock (Blatz 1925; Brunswick, 1924; Landis, 1926; Mosso, 1896; Shackson, 1936; Skaggs, 1926; Steer, 1937). Vertical (thoracic) and horizontal (abdominal) incoordinations of respiratory movements have been reported frequently for stutterers (Fletcher, 1914; Henriksen, 1936; Mills & Streit, 1942; Seth, 1934; Steer, 1935, 1937; L. E. Travis, 1927a, 1934; V. Travis, 1936). The same movements have been observed, usually in less exaggerated form, in normal speakers (Mosier, 1944; Steer, 1935; Stetson, 1933; Travis, 1931). But the greater variability of respiratory movements reported in stutterers (Fossler, 1930; Hill, 1942; Mills & Streit, 1942; Murray, 1932; Seth, 1934; Steer, 1935; Strother, 1935, 1937; V. Travis, 1936) is seen in normal speakers when they are shocked (Berg & Beebe-Center, 1941; Caster, 1932; Lacey, 1941). Finally, shallow breathing and stuttering have often been related (Gordy, 1928; Murray, 1932; Starr, 1928; Trumper, 1928; Van Riper, 1936), but shallow breathing has also been related to shock (Blatz, 1925; Hill, 1942; Landis, 1926; Skaggs, 1930; Walker, 1938; Wever, 1930), psychosis (Alexander & Saul, 1940), and neurosis (Bard, 1940; Mudd, 1928), and the disappearance of shallow breathing to lessening of stuttering (Trumper, 1928). The research on breathing adaptation in stutterers by Starbuck and Steer (1954) supports this last finding.

Hill (1944b) makes the point in discussing cardiovascular changes that so many physical, chemical and reflexive factors operate as antecedents that accurate analysis of cardiac functioning is extremely complex. With this caution in mind, he presented evidence of increased and irregular heart rates for stutterers preceding and during speech, no difference during basal conditions of silence and rest, and increased rate and irregularity in normal speakers following sudden stimuli. To the extent that blood pressure changes occur during stuttering, they resemble those normally evidenced in startle (Berg & Beebe-Center, 1941; Blatz, 1925; Fletcher, 1914; Lacey, 1941; Landis, 1926; Mosso, 1896; Ritzman, 1943; Robbins, 1919, 1920; Sherman, 1941; Skaggs, 1926, 1930). The work on sinus arrhythmia, which frequently reflects disturbed respiratory patterns, has not consistently revealed differences between stutterers and nonstutterers or between sexes (Palmer & Gillett, 1938, 1939; Ritzman, 1943). Such differences as do exist seem attributable to the valsalva effect and differences in circumstances. Vasomotor reactions of normal speakers to startling stimuli are also quite similar to the responses of stutterers during speech difficulty (Fletcher, 1914; Lund, 1939; Mosso, 1896; Robbins, 1919, 1920; Travis, Tuttle, & Cowan, 1936).

The literature reviewed supports the belief that stutterers are characteristically in a state of raised muscle tone, especially before stuttering, that is considerably reduced after blocking (Brown & Shulman, 1940; Mowrer, 1940; Shackson, 1936; Travis & Fagan, 1928; Travis, Tuttle, & Bender, 1936). The work of Johnson *et al.* (1959) indicates clearly, however, that stutterers are not in a state of latent or active tetany. Hill included some European studies on oculocardiac and solar plexus reflexes (Hogewind, 1940; Sovak, 1933), and we include a more recent one (Sedlácek, 1948), that are based too much on speculation about autonomic nervous system (ANS) functioning to need more than mention in passing. The research in the 1920s on patellar and achilles reflexes, on the other hand, can be considered. It indicated heightened responses during stuttering and depression during free speech, whereas in normal speakers these reflexes increase during speech and problem solving (Travis & Fagan, 1928; Tuttle, 1924).

Additional evidence of the similarity in stuttering and startle can be seen in eye-movement and pupillary-reflex disturbances. When either stuttering or startle responses are weak, only an eye blink may be recorded, but when they are strong, the eyes are dilated and are either firmly fixated or exhibit erratic twitchings (Gardner, 1937; Jasper & Murray, 1932; Moser, 1938; Murray, 1932).

A major limitation, based on methodological considerations and recent evidence, must be emphasized about the extent to which inferences can be drawn from the earlier work, especially the biochemical, cardiovascular, and muscle-tension studies. The data reported in these types of investigation were not gathered immediately before, during, or after stuttering blocks; rather, they were gathered before, during, or after *periods* of stuttering. In other words, we do not know from them exactly what happens around the moment of stuttering.

Sheehan and Voas (1954) cast some light on the problem with electromyographic (EMG) evidence that the peak of tension in the masseter muscles during stuttering occurs toward the end of a block. This is not where we would expect to find the greatest tension if stuttering does involve a startle response. Still, electromyographic recordings reflect CNS activity directly and ANS influence only indirectly, so their data could point to efforts by the stutterer to terminate a block initiated by startle or by any other condition that may have produced it.

Taylor (1965) shed further light on the matter recently. She used a multivariate analysis of variance to interpret GSR and heartbeat-interval differences in the 14-second period before and after blocks, and a univariate analysis of heartbeat-interval variations (accurate to within less than two milliseconds) before and after blocks in periods of 3, 6, 9, 12, and 14 seconds. She found no difference in either analysis. If startle does occur or if speech is disorganized during a moment of stuttering, it is either of such short duration as to be undiscerned three seconds before a block, or else it does not involve autonomic nervous system responses of sufficient magnitude to be detected by the highly sensitive measure of heartbeat interval. Her evidence, moreover, does not support the idea that moments of stuttering represent conflict behavior; at least not if the avoidance aspect of the approach-avoidance conflict is considered to have an autonomic component of anxiety or fear.

The other physiological research on the moment of stuttering is on scattered aspects of the problem. Snidecor (1955) did a study on the loci of tension during stuttering and found them focused around the respiratory mechanism, as might be expected. Along a different line, Travis (1934) obtained muscle-action potentials from the right and left masseter muscles in 24 stutterers and 24 nonstutterers. He found the bilateral EMG data for 22 nonstutterers practically identical, whereas the action potentials for 18 of the stutterers were strikingly dissimilar. Williams (1955), in a more recent study, has shown without much doubt that all of the earlier bilateral action-potential differences (Steer, 1937; Strother, 1935; L. E. Travis, 1934; Travis, Tuttle, & Bender, 1936), for the masseter muscles at least, could be attributed to erroneous assumptions about EMG measures and to uncontrolled conditions. He found no

209

EMG differences between stutterers and nonstutterers when they performed under the same circumstances.

Level of Awareness   Hill (1944b) described the moment of stuttering vividly:

> *The chaos that occurs during the period when psychological contact with the situation is broken off is probably appreciated by but few people who do not stutter. Stuttering in this regard often becomes an unpleasant adventure in which the individual figuratively, and sometimes literally, closes his eyes and jumps into the dark. The response that is demanded by the situation is just not there. It would not be so disconcerting if orderly responses of speech merely stopped. The individual might reorient himself. But the difficulty of the stutterer is chiefly brought about by the disorganized contraction patterns, and other biological reactions, which replace the orderly progressions of speech.*

This is a description of a condition in which the stutterer presumably loses contact with external reality for a brief moment, a moment during which his conscious awareness of what he is experiencing would appear to be diminished. Various types of evidence are available that support the proposition that awareness is reduced during stuttering. Johnson and Solomon (1937), in their study of expectation, inferred that anticipation of blocking is a process involving a low level of consciousness. Herren (1931) had stutterers and nonstutterers rhythmically press bulbs attached to a recording apparatus. He reported the performance of nonstutterers as unaffected by speech and the same as that of stutterers during silence. On the other hand, during tonic blocks stutterers' hand movements ceased abruptly for as long as 22 seconds, while during clonic blocks there were skipped beats or decreases in extent of movement. Along a different line, Froechels and Rieber (1963) reported stutterers as manifesting "visual and auditory imperceptivity" during instances of stuttering. Several years earlier, Lovett-Doust and Coleman (1955) measured stutterers (although not during stuttering) and controls for the critical flicker fusion (CFF) threshold, considered to be indicative of neurological efficiency. The controls had higher thresholds than

the stutterers, thus pointing to reduced discriminatory awareness that the authors thought suggestive of a neurogenic basis
for stuttering.

Early electroencephalographic studies have provided another
type of evidence that is somewhat contradictory and ambiguous, but, overall, can be interpreted as supportive of reduced consciousness. Travis (1937) recorded brain potentials of
eight normal subjects that were correlated with periodic intro-
spective reports of the conscious state being experienced. He
concluded that the large potentials (alpha waves) are indicative
of mental blankness and abstract thinking. If his interpretation
of the alpha rhythm is valid, then Freestone's (1942) report
of more and larger alpha waves in stutterers during stuttering
is supportive of low awareness at these times. Douglass (1943),
though, found more alpha waves in nonstutterers during speech
than in stutterers during fluent or blocked speech. Not enough
is known about the conditions under which the data were
gathered in these two studies to offer an explanation for the
disagreement. The other EEG investigations do not help much
because they were mainly concerned with bilateral differences
between hemispheres. Taken as a group, however, they are suggestive of more alpha activity among stutterers and would tend
to support the major body of evidence that consciousness is
reduced during stuttering.

Conclusion Hill concluded from his biochemical survey
(1944a) that the view ". . . is practically forced that biochemical differences between stutterers and nonstutterers are coin-
cident with differences in affective and muscular activity." We
are in agreement with this conclusion, but not with the one
he reached in his physiological survey (1944b). After comparing muscle tone, reflex and eye movement irregularities, and
respiratory and cardiovascular reactions during stuttering with
similar measures from normal speakers during startle, he concluded that "the marked similarities in reaction were adjudged
sufficient evidence to warrant the interpretation that stuttering
consists of a startle contraction pattern." Granted the similarities
in the physiological responses associated with stuttering and
startle, these similarities fall far short of demonstrating that
one condition is identical with the other. If we accepted Hill's
conclusion and assumed that there is this identity, then we
could just as well conclude from the evidence that all startle
responses are acts of stuttering.

Our other conclusion, based on a variety of types of evi-

211

dence, is that stutterers probably experience a period of reduced awareness of environmental stimuli before and during the moment of blocking. Whether consciousness is reduced for all stimuli or only external stimuli, whether attention is fragmented or is so focused on how to continue speaking when stuck in a block that attention is diverted from all else, or whether level of awareness and stuttering are even casually related, cannot be determined from existing research.

What Conditions Follow Instances of Stuttering?

Only two physiological investigations, to our knowledge, have been addressed to the question what conditions follow instances of stuttering. Sheehan and Voas (1954) tested a conflict theory from which tension reduction would be predicted. They measured the time between word initiation and completion in relation to maximum masseter activity (measured electromyographically) in stutterers who served as their own controls. They found the peak of tension during stuttering just before a block is terminated; the time between this peak and completion of the word was not significantly different whether the word was stuttered or fluent. Taylor (1965), on the other hand, used a measure of heartbeat intervals that was sensitive to variations of less than two milliseconds. She compared this measure at intervals of 3, 6, 9, 12, and 14 seconds before and after moments of stuttering to determine if anxiety fluctuations could be detected. She found not even a trend toward variation.

Conclusion On the face of it, these two studies would appear contradictory. Yet, they probably are not. There is no reason to doubt the data from either study. The difference probably lies in the different measures that were used. Sheehan and Voas used an instantaneous measure of CNS action-potentials to masseter muscles. Taylor used a sensitive measure of heartbeat intervals that, nevertheless, provides a relatively slow account of ANS changes. What appears to happen, then, is that tension in the speech musculature (under CNS direction) rises as the stutterer works his way through a block and is sharply reduced following termination of the block. This tension and its reduction do not, however, appear to be associated with a visceral experience of fear.

What Conditions Perpetuate Stuttering?

One of the most perplexing questions about stuttering is why it persists when it seems so obviously maladaptive and punishing. The type of physiological research that we have included in this section is that bearing on the question whether or not stuttering reduces anxiety or varies in relation to it. Theoretically, if it does reduce anxiety, it would be reinforced and thereby perpetuated. Unfortunately, "anxiety" is but a hypothetical construct. The behavioral and physiological conditions to which it refers can only be inferred from the measures used. Heart rate, blood pressure, galvanic skin response (GSR), palmar sweat, respiration rate, electroencephalogram (EEG), and muscle tension are among the various indexes of it that have been reported. Each responds to a different pattern of autonomic and central nervous system functioning. One measure may reflect fear, another may reflect readiness to respond, but both may be employed to indicate "anxiety." Moreover, the same emotion may exhibit different physiological correlates under different conditions. As Ax (1964) observed, "It would not be surprising if the physiological patterns of fear in a person while running just ahead of a hungry lion in the jungle differ considerably from those of fearing an electric shock while reclining in the laboratory." Anxiety, then, is a term that has been used to refer to a variety of states, not all of which necessarily involve fear or apprehension. Its many possible meanings should be considered in evaluating the significance of the following reports.

A prevalent concept is that the stutterer experiences dread and apprehension before and during the moment of blocking. Brutten's work several years ago (1957, 1959, 1961, 1963), of anxiety in disfluency and expectancy adaptation, seemingly supports this idea. He found covarying adaptation of disfluency and palmar-sweat scores in his group of 33 stutterers. But Gray (1963; Gray & Brutten, 1965), reported no significant changes in palmar-sweat scores concomitant with increases or decreases in stuttering. Berlinsky (1954) also found no consistent relationship between stuttering and indexes of transient anxiety, of radial pulse rate, respiratory amplitude, rate of respiration, and changes in skin conductance. Moreover, Taylor (1965) investigated GSR and heartbeat interval immediately preceding and following stuttering blocks as well as during periods of fluent speech and found no indication at all of anxiety being associated with moments of blocking.

Hagen (1965), using a sample of eight men in an exploratory study of frequency of stuttering and open expression of aggression, included heart rate, blood pressure, GSR, EMG, and respiration-rate measures to extend the range of observed behavior of stutterers under stress. Systolic blood pressure was

213

the only statistically discriminating physiological response he found, and it may be suspect. Curiously, it showed greater reduction for those stutterers whose blocking increased when they were not allowed to retaliate after being instigated to anger than it did for those who were allowed to retaliate and whose stuttering accordingly decreased. One of the more congruent of the several possible interpretations of this finding is that stutterers experience more relief for their anger, and possible anxiety, through stuttering than through direct expressions of aggression.

The stutterer is apparently no more anxious than the non-stutterer during periods of rest. This conclusion is supported partially by the early work of Scarbrough (1943), who found no EEG differences between 20 stutterers and 20 normal speakers during minimal activity, by Douglass (1943), who reported no difference in alpha waves during silence or speech, by Correll (1956), who found no EEG differences during photic stimulation between stutterers and nonstutterers, and by Brown and Shulman (1940), who measured intramuscular pressure during rest and found their 24 stutterers no more tense than their 24 normal speakers. On the other side, Umeda's casual observations of his GSR and respiratory records (1960a) suggested to him that stutterers have a tendency to high anxiety. Similarly, Amirov (1960) characterized the motor system of one group of adolescent stutterers as having a preponderance of "excitatory process"; the EEG records following photic stimulation were interpreted for a second group, though, as typified by an "inhibitory process." Knott, Correll, and Shephard (1959) also presented some ambiguous evidence on this problem. Utilizing Ulett's EEG measures of anxiety (Ulett *et al.*, 1952), they investigated two groups of stutterers and a group of non-stutterers during silence and found only one group of stutterers "anxiety prone." All three groups differed one way or another, but the two groups of stutterers differed more extensively from each other than either differed from the non-stuttering group. One explanation offered for this puzzling result was that the experimenter with the "anxiety prone" stutterers was an attractive young woman.

Berlinsky (1954) has provided evidence that anxiety increases if the stutterer is not allowed to speak. Using changes in skin conductance as a criterion of transient anxiety, the greatest anxiety among his fourteen stutterers occurred when they were not permitted to speak. He concluded that "stuttering acts as a cathartic activity relieving the anxiety of the stutterer. The *stuttering* is inferred to be the cathartic activity and *not* the speech itself."

Conclusion Theorists searching for a functional relationship between anxiety and stuttering are destined for frustration. Tantalizing leads from one physiological study are contradicted by another. Then, too, there is the frustration of trying to specify the processes, physiological or behavioral, to which the term "anxiety" refers. At this point, none of the studies has produced definitive evidence that would require the selection of one theory over another concerning the relation of anxiety to stuttering and its preservation.

What evidence we have points consistently to the probability that the act of stuttering per se is not anxiety reducing; no one has yet produced measures of autonomic functioning that vary with the instance of stuttering. This leaves open the credible possibility that stuttering behavior is embedded in, or is perhaps an integral part of, a larger pattern of behavior that is reinforced, stuttering and all. For example, if the only way the stutterer has learned to speak under certain anxious conditions is by tensing his articulators—by stuttering when his desire to speak under these conditions is sufficient for this pattern of speech to be emitted—this is the pattern that will be reinforced and these are the conditions that will constitute discriminative stimuli for the stuttering response. Such a possibility would permit anxiety and stuttering to vary independently of each other yet remain related as functions of common variables—and would account for the apparently contradictory findings produced to date.

What Conditions Reduce Stuttering?

Several factors, ostensibly reflective of the organic condition, have been related to reductions in stuttering. These include the effects of hearing loss, auditory masking, delayed feedback, rhythm, and drugs. With the exception of drug effects, these factors appear to us to be more appropriate for behavioral than physiological discussion. All of them, though, have been interpreted by some investigators as having organic significance. We would rather err in favor of those with this predilection and include what are essentially behavioral findings than to exclude what some would believe to be legitimate evidence of a physiological basis for stuttering.

Reduced Hearing The relationship of hearing to stuttering and its reduction seems reasonably clear. When hearing is reduced 50 decibels or more by deafness, hearing loss, or auditory masking, the frequency and severity of blocking apparently decreases considerably. Backus (1938) surveyed 13,691 children in 206 schools for the deaf and found 55 stutterers, .04 percent of her population. Of these, only six had congenital hearing losses great enough to prevent normal acquisition of speech. Harms and Malone (1939a, 1939b) agree from their work that stuttering is a rarity with total loss of hearing. Maraist and Hutton (1957), studying the effects of auditory masking on stuttering, reported a sizable decrease in severity at 50 decibels of masking and close-to-normal reading at 90 decibels, which is essentially the same finding that Shane (1955) reported. Likewise, Cherry and Sayers (1956) demonstrated total inhibition of stuttering during high-intensity white noise and greater reduction from low-frequency than high-frequency noise. Sutton and Chase (1961) also found that white noise clearly improved the speech of stutterers, but they found, too, that noise only during silence preceding speech, and wearing earphones without noise, improved speech. Curlee (1964), in a pilot attempt to explore this puzzling effect of noise during silence, confounded the picture further by finding that the stuttering of four of his five subjects was not appreciably affected by 90 decibels of white noise whether it was introduced 30 seconds before, 10 seconds before, beginning with, or 10 seconds after beginning reading.

Auditory Feedback and Rate   The studies of Nessell (1958) and Lotzmann (1961) both indicate that delayed auditory feedback greatly reduces and in many cases eliminates even severe stuttering. Lotzmann, using delay times of 50 to 300 milliseconds, found an optimal delay time that varied with the individual beyond which the blocking-reduction effects of delay diminished. He also noted that the less severe stutterers often reacted to delayed feedback like normal speakers with a cluttering type of response. That there is a difference between stuttering and the disruption effect of delayed side-tone has been demonstrated by Neelley (1960). Wolf and Wolf (1959) have speculated about different types of stuttering being the effects of different discontinuities in the feedback system.

The functional relationship between delayed auditory feedback and disfluency has been demonstrated during the last several years by Goldiamond (1960, 1964) and by Perkins (1967). Working independently with more than 70 adult stutterers, they have shown that, without exception, the act and feeling of stuttering is eliminated under conditions of 250 milliseconds of auditory delay when the speaking rate is slowed to about 30 words per minute. This rate can be increased as delay time is shortened and stutter-free speech will still be preserved. If, however, a speaker, whether stutterer or non-stutterer, attempts to "beat" the delayed side-tone by accelerating the rate, his speech will be disrupted and his disfluencies will be exaggerated. The effects of auditory delay are not inherent in the stimulus but rather in whether the speaker accelerates or decelerates in his speaking response.

Rhythm Historically, speaking in rhythm to a regular beat has been one of the oldest therapies short of surgery, and one of the most effective in the reduction or elimination of stuttering. In 1837 in Europe the Isochrome was introduced. It provided a rhythmical beat for the stutterer to follow as he spoke. Essentially the same instrument appeared in the United States as an Orthophone (Beech, 1967). For various reasons the dramatic reduction in stuttering when speech is paced by rhythmic devices did not meet with professional favor in this country during the past half century. To the extent that rhythm was used, it was considered a bogus treatment. One reason for distrusting it was that its effects usually ceased when the rhythm stopped. A few years ago, Meyer and Mair (1963) revived this treatment in Britain but still could not solve the relapse problem.

No one has understood why rhythm works temporarily nor why it will not work permanently. One explanation has been that stutterers suffer a motor speech deficiency for which imposed rhythm compensates. As we saw earlier, this possibility cannot be discounted, but the supporting evidence could just as well be a consequence as a cause of stuttering. Another explanation has been that rhythm is effective because it is distracting. Barber's work (1940) did not test the concept but merely demonstrated several conditions under which it was effective. More recently, Beech (1967) and Fransella and Beech (1965) demonstrated that distraction per se does not systematically decrease stuttering, thereby disqualifying distraction as a basis for the effects of rhythm. They also demonstrated that even though slow speech rates reduce stuttering, this effect is independent of the effect produced by rhythm. The number of explanations for the success of speaking in time to a metronome has been reduced, but the discarding of alternatives does not account for the success, and the enigma remains.

Drugs A variety of drugs have been investigated in the treatment of stutterers. Published reports have dealt mainly with the use of the tranquilizer meprobamate (DiCarlo, Katz, & Batkin, 1959; Holliday, 1959; Kent & Williams, 1959; Maxwell & Patterson, 1958), although some work has been done with iodine (Serra, 1960), trifluoperazine and d-amphetamine (Fish & Bowling, 1965), haloperidol (Gattuso & Leocata, 1962), reserpine (Mitchell, 1955), prostigmin (Schaubel & Street, 1949), hydroxyzine (Yannatos, 1960), thiamine (Hale, 1951), nembutal (Love, 1955), benzedrine (Love, 1955), and lactose placebos (Love, 1955; Palasek & Curtis, 1960; Schilling, 1963a). Some unpublished research on chlorpromazine and atarax is also reported by Kent (1963).

By and large, these studies have not demonstrated a significant reduction in stuttering from drug treatment. The differences that do obtain are mostly trends that consist mainly of reported feelings of relaxation and reduced muscular tension, particularly from meprobamate, or they are speculations floating in the clouds of uncontrolled observation. For example, Fish and Bowling (1965) observed that stuttering of organically mentally retarded persons lessened with d-amphetamine. They point out in the title, however, that their results were from an uncontrolled study. Similarly, Serra (1960) casually observed that most brain-damaged stutterers he had treated with iodine therapy improved, and Gattuso and Leocata (1962) reported improvement of 80 percent of children under eight who received haloperidon but little change in the stuttering of older children. And Hale (1951), in his pilot investigation of thiamine in the reduction of tension in stuttering young children, reported 80 percent observable improvement in 2- and 3-year-olds, 50 percent in 4-year-olds, and none to speak of in children above 5. As with all of these studies, the findings could have resulted from numerous factors other than drug effect. That they could well be chance results is indicated by Penson's (1955) follow-up of Hale's pilot work by a comparison of the effects of thiamine on 32 nonfluent young children and 22 fluent control subjects. He found no differences between groups in regard to the effects on fluency before, during, or after thiamine dose.

Closely akin to drug treatment is carbon dioxide (CO_2) therapy. Reported by Meduna (1958) for the treatment of neurosis, it has been applied by physicians as a therapy for stuttering and has received a mixed reception. Smith (1953) considers it the treatment of choice over speech therapy. Arthurs *et al.* (1954) found no sustained difference between a CO_2 therapy group of 16 adult stutterers and a matched control group. Kent (1961) polled American members of the Carbon Dioxide Research Association for the use of CO_2 therapy with stutterers. Relatively few replied, but of those who did 14 reported unfavorable results and 15 were slightly favorable towards its use. Stutterers for whom onset of the problem was in adolescence or later seemed to respond better than did those with earlier onset. She concluded that the question of the usefulness of CO_2 as an adjunct therapy is open to research. We concur.

Conclusion The consistency of reports of reduced or eliminated stuttering under the two conditions of rhythmic activities and of delayed auditory feedback in conjunction with slow reading rate leaves little doubt of their effectiveness. Severe hearing loss and auditory masking also appear to be effective in reducing stuttering, but not as consistently. Our impression of drug research, on the other hand, is summarized by Burr and Mullendore's observation (1960) that "the experimentation performed to date has failed to provide the specific information necessary to predict how a specified dose of a particular tranquilizer is likely to affect a stutterer."

EVALUATION OF
PHYSIOLOGICAL APPROACHES

The net result of the physiological studies accomplished so far is not impressive. Much of the work appears to have been undertaken in an attempt to either prove or disprove the existence of a physiological variant that would distinguish stutterers from nonstutterers. Those who have sought such a variant have assumed the burden of proof for demonstrating its existence. Their evidence has not been sufficiently convincing to establish their position. On the other hand, if those who have concluded that the stutterer is physiologically no different from the nonstutterer were to assume a similar burden of proof, their position would also be tenuous. The sum of the matter is that if we address ourselves to the question whether or not the stutterer is physiologically different from the nonstutterer, we are almost as uncertain of the answer now as we were thirty years ago.

Certainly, individual stutterers who deviate radically from the norm can be isolated; the same is true for normal speakers. Common characteristics can be found among stutterers; these same characteristics are common to normal speakers. Yet, the

219

question that has been pursued most persistently, especially with physiological investigations, has been, What makes stutterers different from normal speakers? Time and again, careful research has shown this to be an unrewarding question, but the slightest clue seems to be sufficient to set a new rash of explorers scurrying after differentiating evidence. That stutterers differ from normal speakers only by virtue of stuttering (and even that difference is elusive) is apparently difficult for many to believe.

Logical Inconsistency

If the search for constitutional differences has not produced viable research leads, it has certainly yielded its share of logical inconsistencies. Those who have pursued the possibility of a constitutional predisposition to stuttering are presumably looking for a condition that could account for the onset of stuttering. Such a condition, ostensibly, need not persist once the problem took root and was flourishing on its own. To detect this condition, one would not search, logically, among older children and adults; yet, it is among these age groups that most of the investigations have been done.

One could argue that because predisposing organic conditions are unnecessary past onset of stuttering, any detectable constitutional differences at these older ages gives added weight to the probability of their contributing to the problem in the first place. Such an argument ignores the good possibility that any observed differences could be a consequence of stuttering as readily as a cause. Moreover, existing physiological differences raise the very sticky issue of how to explain fluent speech. If a constitutional defect can be found to account for stuttering, then, logically, we must reverse the problem and search for constitutional conditions that account for the stutterer's speech when he does not stutter.

Organic Versus Functional

Another logical inconsistency with which we are fond of trapping ourselves is the organic-functional dichotomy. At best, this distinction is a form of shorthand that undermines precise thinking; at worst, it is taken literally. "Organic" is a handy equivalent for "physiogenic," a term, when applied to speech pathology, that usually means the disorder is caused by a defect in the anatomy or physiology of the mechanisms regulating speech. "Functional" is equivalent to "psychogenic," a term that *connotes* that the disorder is learned, a case of diagnosis by exclusion. What "psychogenic" typically *de*notes is in-ability to find a "physiogenic" basis for the disorder, *ergo*, it must be learned (West *et al.*, 1957).

Unless we wish to conceive of learning as a mystical experi-ence, we are as obligated to explain it physiologically as we are disordered speech behavior or any other behavior. Learn-ing is as basically behavioral as anything we do. Invoking it as a "functional" explanation when no "organic" basis for causality can be found ignores the fact that learning is an operation of the organism.

New Directions

If we assume that every instance of behavior has a corre-sponding instance in each physiological system, we assume that a change in behavior requires a change in physiologic response. This assumption permits a blessed economy. It enables the in-vestigator to use behavior as a screening device for profitable physiological leads.

No evidence points convincingly to differences between the stutterer as a person and the normal speaker as a person, yet this is the trail that most physiological research has chugged along for years. Conversely, the one invariant that comes closest to being established about stuttering is what the stut-terer *does* when he stutters, but the traffic on this physiological research route has certainly created no congestion to date.

Several leads look promising. One theme concerns stress in relation to stuttering. Is the act of stuttering stressful? Does it vary with different types of stress? With different amounts of stress? Are patterns of stress in relation to stuttering the same in children as in adults? Is there a developmental se-quence? Do the patterns run in families of stutterers? Are the patterns different in boys and girls?

Another theme concerns disfluency. Are disfluencies judged as stuttering different physiologically from disfluencies judged as normal within the stutterer? Between stutterers and non-stutterers? Do clonic and tonic stuttering differ physiologically? What are the physiological correlates of severity of stuttering? What physiologic changes occur from the beginning to the end of a block? Are various types of disfluency characterized by typical physiological patterns? Within stutterers? Between stutterers and nonstutterers? Between boys and girls? Are de-velopmental changes discernible? What are the physiological bases for the effects on disfluency and stuttering of slow speak-ing rate? Of rhythm? Of singing? What are the physiological correlates of disfluency rate? In children? In adults? In boys? In girls? In families of stutterers?

Still another theme concerns the processes by which speech is regulated. Are reductions in discriminative awareness associated with stuttering physiologically demonstrable? Do they reflect reduced consciousness or shifts in attention? Do they vary with sensory modality? Are they associated with various types of disfluency? In stutterers? In normal speakers? In children? In boys? In girls? What are the discriminative stimuli in the regulation of fluency, disfluency, and stuttering? For auditory feedback? For tactual feedback? For kinesthetic feedback? For different ages? For boys? For girls? What is the physiological evidence for considering stuttering a behavioral reflection of disrupted thinking? What are the physiological correlates of thinking verbal expressions silently in comparison with speaking the same expressions aloud? What is the relation of the physiology of disfluent thinking to that of disfluent speech?

These leads are suggestive of lines of inquiry that might be productive of physiological differences. They are built around reasonably stable behavioral differences. As our fund of solid information grows, we can look forward to a reduction in the flood of theories with which we have been swamped: they flourish when hard facts are unavailable to require one answer or another. Let us remember that theories are not ecclesiastical canons to be preserved eternally. Their chief value is in pointing toward the most productive directions to follow and questions to ask that will enable us to extend our knowledge.

References

References that are listed here only by author and year of publication appear in complete form in the Bibliography.

Alexander, F., and Saul, L. J. (1940) Respiration and personality: A preliminary report. I. Description of the curves. *Psychosomatic Medicine, 2,* 110–118.

Amirov, R. Z. (1960) Further results of the study of higher nervous system in stuttering. In *Third Session* of the Institute of Defectology, Moscow: Academy Pedagological Science, pp. 152–153. In *Deafness, Speech and Hearing Abstracts, 2* (1962), 74.

Anderson, J., and Whealdon, M. L. (1941) A study of the blood group distribution among stutterers. *Journal of Speech Disorders, 6,* 23–28.

Arend, R., Handzel, L., and Weiss, B. (1962)

Arthurs, R. G. S., Cappan, D., Douglass, E., and Quarrington, B. (1954) Carbon dioxide therapy with stutterers. *Diseases of the Nervous System, 15,* 123–126.

Ax, A. (1964) Goals and method of psychophysiology. *Psychophysiology, 1,* 8–25.

Backus, O. (1938) Incidence of stuttering among the deaf. *Annals of Otology, Rhinology and Laryngology, 47,* 632–635.

Baker, K. H., and Eye, M. G. (1935) The reliability of the pH of human mixed saliva as an indicator of physiological changes accompanying behavior. *American Journal of Psychology, 47,* 222–240.

Barbara, D. A. (1946) A psychosomatic approach to the problem of stuttering in psychotics. *American Journal of Psychiatry, 103,* 188–195

Barber, V. (1940) Studies in the psychology of stuttering. XVI. Rhythm as a distraction in stuttering. *Journal of Speech Disorders, 5,* 29–42.

Bard, P., Ed. (1940) *Macleod's "Physiology in modern medicine."* St. Louis: Mosby.

Beech, H. R. (1967) Stuttering and stammering. *Psychology Today, 1,* 48–51, 61.

Berg, R. L., and Beebe-Center, J. G. (1941) Cardiac startle in man. *Journal of Experimental Psychology, 28,* 262–279.

Berlinsky, S. L. (1954)

Berman, A. B., and Train, G. J. (1940) A genetic approach to the problem of stammering. *Journal of Nervous and Mental Disease, 91,* 590–594.

Berry, M. F. (1937a) The medical history of stuttering children. Ph.D. dissertation, University of Wisconsin, Madison.

Berry, M. F. (1937b) Twinning in stuttering families. *Human Biology, 9,* 329–346.

Berry, M. F. (1938a) A common denominator in twinning and stuttering. *Journal of Speech Disorders, 3,* 51–57.

Berry, M. F. (1938b) The developmental history of stuttering children. *Journal of Pediatrics, 12,* 209–217.

Berry, M. F. (1938c) The medical history of stuttering children. *Speech Monographs, 5,* 97–114.

Bills, A. G. (1934) The relation of stuttering to mental fatigue. *Journal of Experimental Psychology, 17,* 574–584.

Bilto, E. W. (1941) A comparative study of certain physical abilities of children with speech defects and children with normal speech. *Journal of Speech Disorders, 6,* 187–203.

Blackburn, B. (1931) Voluntary movements of the organs

of speech in stutterers and non-stutterers. *Psychological Monographs, 41,* 1–13.

Blatz, W. E. (1925) The cardiac, respiratory, and electrical phenomena involved in the emotion of fear. *Journal of Experimental Psychology, 8,* 109–132.

Bluemel, C. S. (1928) Stammering and cognate defects of speech. Cited in M. Trumper, *A hemato-respiratory study of 101 consecutive cases of stammering.* Ph.D. dissertation, University of Pennsylvania, Philadelphia.

Böhme, G. (1965) The importance of brain-injury in early infancy in relation to stuttering. Congressus Otolaryngologicus Prague.

Boland, J. L., Jr. (1951)

Brown, S. F., and Shulman, E. E. (1940) Intramuscular pressure in stutterers and non-stutterers. *Speech Monographs, 7,* 63–74.

Brunswick, D. (1924) The effects of emotional stimuli on the gastro-intestinal tone. *Journal of Comparative Psychology, 4,* 19–79, 225–287.

Brutten, E. J. (1957)

Brutten, E. J. (1959) Colorimetric measurement of anxiety: A clinical and experimental procedure. *Speech Monographs, 26,* 282–287.

Brutten, E. J. (1961) Palmar sweating: A physiological index of anxiety. *Journal of the American Speech and Hearing Association, 3,* 359. Abstract.

Brutten, E. J. (1963)

Bryngelson, B. (1935) Sidedness as an etiological factor in stuttering. *Pedagogical Seminary and Journal of Genetic Psychology, 47,* 204–217.

Bryngelson, B. (1939) A study of laterality of stutterers and normal speakers. *Journal of Speech Disorders, 4,* 231–234.

Bryngelson, B. (1940) A study of laterality of stutterers and normal speakers. *Journal of Social Psychology, 11,* 151–155.

Bryngelson, B., and Clark, T. B. (1933) Left-handedness and stuttering. *Journal of Heredity, 24,* 387–390.

Bryngelson, B., and Rutherford, B. (1937) A comparative study of laterality of stutterers and non-stutterers. *Journal of Speech Disorders, 2,* 15–16.

Burdin, L. G. (1940) A survey of speech defectives in the Indianapolis primary grades. *Journal of Speech Disorders, 5,* 247–258.

Burr, H. G., and Mullendore, J. M. (1960)

Cannon, W. B. (1929) *Bodily changes in pain, hunger, fear, and rage.* New York: Appleton.

Card, R. E. (1939) A study of allergy in relation to stuttering. *Journal of Speech Disorders, 4,* 223–230.

Carroll, L. (1965) An investigation of the incidence of stuttering in the Los Angeles City Elementary Schools. Dissertation, University of Southern California, Los Angeles.

Caster, J. E. (1932) Emotional responses to strong stimuli. *Journal of Genetic Psychology, 4,* 131–153.

Cherry, C., and Sayers, B. (1956)

Cobb, S., and Cole, E. (1939) Stuttering. *Physiological Review, 19,* 49–62.

Correll, R. E. (1956)

Cross, H. M. (1936) The motor capacities of stutterers. *Archives of Speech, 1,* 112–132.

Curlee, R. F. (1964) An experimental study of the relationship between some selected temporal aspects of auditory masking and the frequency of stuttering. Research paper, University of Southern California, Los Angeles.

Curtis, J. F. (1942) A study of the effect of muscular exercise upon stuttering. *Speech Monographs, 9,* 61–74.

Daniels, E. M. (1940) An analysis of the relation between handedness and stuttering with special reference to the Orton-Travis theory of cerebral dominance. *Journal of Speech Disorders, 5,* 209–326.

Darwin, C. (1873) *The expression of the emotions in man and animals.* New York: Appleton.

Despart, J. L. (1946) Psychosomatic study of fifty stuttering children. I. Social, physical, and psychiatric findings. *American Journal of Orthopsychiatry, 16,* 100–113.

DiCarlo, L. M., Katz, J., and Batkin, S. (1959)

Douglass, L. C. (1943) A study of bilaterally recorded electroencephalograms of adult stutterers. *Journal of Experimental Psychology, 32,* 247–265.

Eisenson, J. (1937) A note on the perseverating tendency in stutterers. *Pedagogical Seminar and Journal of Genetic Psychology, 50,* 195–198.

Eisenson, J. (1958)

Eisenson, J., and Pastel, E. (1936) A study of the perseverating tendency in stutterers. *Quarterly Journal of Speech, 22,* 626–631.

Eisenson, J., and Winslow, C. N. (1938) The perseverating tendency in stutterers in a perceptual function. *Journal of Speech Disorders, 3, 195–198.*

Fagan, L. B. (1931) The relation of dextral training to the onset of stuttering: A report of cases. *Quarterly Journal of Speech, 17, 73–76.*

Fagan, L. B. (1932) Graphic stuttering. *Psychological Monographs, 43, 67–71.*

Faulkner, W. B. (1941) The effect of the emotions upon diaphragmatic function. *Psychosomatic Medicine, 3, 187–189.*

Fink, W. H., and Bryngelson, B. (1934) The relation of strabismus to right or left sidedness. *Transaction of the American Academy of Ophthalmology and Otolaryngology,* pp. 3–12.

Finkelstein, P., and Weisberger, S. E. (1954)

Fish, C. H., and Bowling, E. (1965)

Fletcher, J. M. (1914) An experimental study of stuttering. *American Journal of Psychology, 25, 201–255.*

Fossler, H. R. (1930) Disturbances in breathing during stuttering. *Psychological Monographs, 40, 1–32.*

Fox, D. R. (1965) Electroencephalographic analysis during stuttering and non-stuttering. Dissertation, University of Missouri, Columbia.

Fox, D. R. (1966)

Fransella, F., and Beech, H. R. (1965)

Freestone, N. W. (1942) A brain-wave interpretation of stuttering. *Quarterly Journal of Speech, 28, 466–468.*

Freund, H. (1934) Relationships between stuttering and cluttering. *Monatsschrift fur Ohrenheilkunde, 68, 1446–1457.*

Freund, H. (1952) Studies in the interrelationships between stutterers and clutterers. *Folia Phoniatrica, 4, 146–168.*

Freund, H. (1955) Psychosis and stuttering. *Folia Phoniatrica, 7, 133–152.*

Froeschels, E., and Rieber, R. W. (1963)

Gardner, W. H. (1937) The study of the pupillary reflex with special reference to stuttering. *Psychological Monographs, 49, 1–31.*

Gattuso, R., and Leocata, A. (1962) Haloperidol in the treatment of stuttering. *La Clinica Oto-Rino-Laringoiatrica, 14, 227–234.* In *Deafness, Speech and Hearing Abstracts, 4* (1964), 290.

Gedda, L., Branconi, L., and Bruno, G. (1960)

Glaser, E. M. (1936) Possible relationship between stuttering and endocrine malfunctioning. *Journal of Speech Disorders, 1,* 81–89.

Goda, S. (1961)

Gold, G. (1941) *A study of auditory perseveration tendencies of stutterers and normal speakers.* M. A. thesis, University of Utah, Salt Lake City.

Goldiamond, I. (1960b)

Goldiamond, I. (1964) Stuttering and fluency as manipulable operant response classes. In L. Krasner and L. P. Ulmann, Eds., *Research in behavior modification: New developments and their clinical implications.* New York: Holt, Rinehart and Winston.

Goldsand, J. (1942) Sensory perseveration in stutterers and non-stutterers. *Speech Abstracts, 4,* 140.

Gordon, M. B. (1928) Stammering produced by thyroid medication. *American Journal of Medical Science, 175,* 360–365.

Gordy, S. (1928) Cited in M. Trumper, *A hemato-respiratory study of 101 consecutive cases of stammering.* Ph.D. dissertation, University of Pennsylvania, Philadelphia.

Graf, O. I. (1955)

Gray, B. B. (1963) An investigation of the relationship between anxiety, fatigue, and the spontaneous recovery of stuttering behavior. *Dissertation Abstracts, 24,* 5606–5607.

Gray, B. B., and Brutten, E. J. (1965)

Gray, M. (1940) The X family: A clinical and laboratory study of a "stuttering" family. *Journal of Speech Disorders, 5,* 343–348.

Gregory, H. H., (1959) A study of the neurophysiological integrity of the auditory feedback system in stutterers. *Dissertation Abstracts, 20,* 3854.

Gregory, H. H. (1964)

Hafford, J. (1941) A comparative study of the salivary pH of the normal speaker and stutterer. *Journal of Speech Disorders, 6,* 173–184.

Hagen, A. C. (1965) An experimental investigation of the relationship between frequency of stuttering and open expression of aggression. Dissertation, University of Southern California, Los Angeles.

Hale, L. L. (1951)

Harms, M. A., and Malone, J. Y. (1939a) Hearing and stammering. *Annals of Otology, Rhinology and Laryngology, 48,* 658.

Harms, M. A., and Malone, J. Y. (1939b) The relationship of hearing acuity to stammering. *Journal of Speech Disorders, 4,* 363–370.

Harrison, H. S. (1947) A study of the speech of sixty institutionalized epileptics. *Speech Monographs, 14,* 210.

Heltman, H. J. (1940) Contradictory evidence in handedness and stuttering. *Journal of Speech Disorders, 5,* 327–331.

Henriksen, E. H. (1936) Simultaneously recorded breathing and vocal disturbances of stutterers. *Archives of Speech, 1,* 133–149.

Herren, R. Y. (1931) The effect of stuttering on voluntary movement. *Journal of Experimental Psychology, 14,* 289–298.

Hill, H. E. (1942) *Perseveration in normal speakers and stutterers.* M.A. thesis, University of Indiana, Bloomington.

Hill, H. E. (1944a) Stuttering. I. A critical review and evaluation of biochemical investigations. *Journal of Speech Disorders, 9,* 245–261.

Hill, H. E. (1944b) Stuttering. II. A review and integration of physiological data. *Journal of Speech Disorders, 9,* 289–324.

Hill, H. E. (1954) An experimental study of disorganization of speech and manual responses in normal subjects. *Journal of Speech and Hearing Disorders, 19,* 295–305.

Hogewind, F. (1940) Medical treatment of stuttering. *Journal of Speech Disorders, 5,* 203–208.

Holliday, A. R. (1959) Effect of meprobamate on stuttering. *Northwest Medical, 58,* 837–841.

Howard, D. T. (1928) A functional theory of emotions. In M. L. Reymert, Ed., *The Wittenberg symposium: Feelings and emotions.* Worcester, Mass.: Clark University Press.

Hunsley, Y. L. (1937) Dysintegration in the speech musculature of stutterers during the production of a non-verbal temporal pattern. *Psychological Monographs, 49,* 32–49.

Jasper, H. H., and Murray, E. (1932) A study of the eye-movements of stutterers during oral reading. *Journal of Experimental Psychology, 15,* 528–538.

Johnson, W. (1955)

Johnson, W., and Duke, L. (1935) Changes in handedness associated with onset or disappearance of stuttering: Sixteen cases. *Journal of Experimental Education, 4,* 112–132.

Johnson, W., and Duke, L (1936) The dextrality quotients of fifty six-year-olds with regard to hand usage. *Journal of Educational Psychology, 27.*

Johnson, W., and King, A. (1942) An angle board and hand usage study of stutterers and non-stutterers. *Journal of Experimental Psychology, 31,* 293–311.

Johnson, W., and Solomon, A. (1937) Studies in the psychology of stuttering. IV. A quantitative study of expectation of stuttering as a process involving a low degree of consciousness. *Journal of Speech Disorders, 2,* 95–97.

Johnson, W., Stearns, G., and Warweg, E. (1933) Chemical factors and the stuttering spasm. *Quarterly Journal of Speech, 19,* 409–415.

Johnson, W., *et al.* (1942) A study of the onset and development of stuttering. *Journal of Speech Disorders, 7,* 251–257.

Johnson, W., Young, M. A., Sahs, A. L., and Bedell, G. N. (1959)

Kantor, J. R. (1921) An attempt toward a naturalistic description of emotions. *Psychological Review, 28,* 19–42.

Karlin, I. W., and Sobel, A. E. (1940) A comparative study of the blood chemistry of stutterers and non-stutterers. *Speech Monographs, 7,* 75–84.

Kennedy, A. M., and Williams, D. A. (1938) Association of stammering and the allergic diathesis. *British Medical Journal, 24,* 1306–1309.

Kent, L. R. (1961)

Kent, L. R. (1963)

Kent, L. R., and Williams, D. E. (1959)

Kenyon, E. L. (1943) The etiology of stammering: The psychophysiologic facts which concern the production of speech sounds and of stammering. *Journal of Speech Disorders, 8,* 337–348.

King, P. T. (1953) Perseverative factors in a stuttering and non-stuttering population. *Pennsylvania State Review of Educational Research, 5,* 10–12.

King, P. T. (1961)

Knott, J. R., Correll, R. E., and Shephard, J. N. (1959)

Knott, J. R., and Tjossem, T. D. (1943) Bilateral electroencephalograms from normal speakers and stutterers. *Journal of Experimental Psychology, 32,* 357–362.

Koch, H. (1966) Hand preference and stuttering in twins. In *Twins and twin relations,* Chicago: University of Chicago Press, pp. 72–87.

Kopp, G. A. (1933) *The metabolism of the stutterer as evidenced by biochemical studies of blood, alveolar air, and urine.* Ph.D. dissertation, University of Wisconsin, Madison.

Kopp, G. A. (1934) Metabolic studies of stutterers. 1. Biochemical study of blood composition. *Speech Monographs, 1,* 117–132.

Kopp, H. G. (1943) The relationship of stuttering to motor disturbances. *The Nervous Child, 2,* 107–116.

Lacey, J. I. (1941) Changes in cardiac and respiratory activity in states of frustration. *Psychological Bulletin, 38,* 581–582.

Landis, C. (1926) Studies of emotional reactions. V. Severe emotional upset. *Journal of Comparative Psychology, 6,* 221–243.

Lightfoot, C. (1948) Serial identification of colors by stutterers. *Journal of Speech and Hearing Disorders, 13,* 193–208.

Lindsley, D. B. (1940) Bilateral differences in brain potentials from the two cerebral hemispheres in relation to laterality and stuttering. *Journal of Experimental Psychology, 26,* 211–225.

Lotzmann, G. von, (1961)

Love, W. R. (1955)

Lovett-Doust, J. W., and Coleman, L. I. M. (1955)

Lund, F. H. (1939) *Emotions.* New York: Ronald.

McCroskey, R. L., Jr. (1957) Effect of speech on metabolism: A comparison between stutterers and non-stutterers. *Journal of Speech and Hearing Disorders, 22,* 46–52.

Maraist, J., and Hutton, C. (1957)

Martin, R. (1962)

Maxwell, R. D., and Patterson, J. W. (1958)

Meduna, E., ed. (1958) *Carbon dioxide therapy.* Springfield, Ill.: Charles C Thomas.

Meyer, V., and Mair, J. M. M. (1963) A new technique to control stammering: A preliminary report. *Behavior, Research and Therapy, 1,* 251–254.

Milisen, R. (1957) The incidence of speech disorders. In L. E. Travis, ed., *Handbook of speech pathology.* New York: Appleton.

Milisen, R., and Johnson, W. (1936) A comparative study of stutterers, former stutterers, and normal speakers whose handedness has been changed. *Archives of Speech, 1,* 61–86.

Miller, M. (1926) Changes in response to electric shock

produced by varying muscular conditions. *Journal of Experimental Psychology, 9,* 26–44.

Mills, A. W., and Streit, H. (1942) Report of a speech survey, Holyoke, Massachusetts. *Journal of Speech Disorders, 7,* 161–167.

Mitchell, B. A. (1955) *An analysis of the effect of reserpine on adult stutterers.* M.A. thesis, Western Michigan University, Kalamazoo.

Moore, W. E. (1959)

Morgenstern, J. J. (1956)

Moser, H. M. (1938) A qualitative analysis of eye-movements during stuttering. *Journal of Speech Disorders, 3,* 131–139.

Mosier, K. V. (1944) *A study of the horizontal dysintegration of breathing during normal and abnormal speech for normal speakers and stutterers.* M.A. thesis, University of Indiana, Bloomington.

Mosso, A. (1896) *Fear.* New York: Longmans Green.

Mowrer, O. H. (1940) Preparatory set (expectancy): Some methods of measurement. *Psychological Monographs, 52,* No. 2.

Mudd, S. G. (1928) Observations on a variety of respiratory abnormalities. Cited in M. Trumper, *A hemato-respiratory study of 101 consecutive cases of stammering.* Ph.D. dissertation, University of Pennsylvania, Philadelphia.

Murray, E. (1932) Dysintegration of breathing and eye-movements in stutterers during silent reading and reasoning. *Psychological Monographs, 43,* 218–275.

Neelley, J. N. (1961)

Nelson, S. E. (1939a) Personal contact as a factor in the transmission of stuttering. *Human Biology, 11,* 393–401.

Nelson, S. E. (1939b) The role of heredity in stuttering. *Journal of Pediatrics, 14,* 642–654.

Nelson, S. E., Hunter, N., and Walter, M. (1945) Stuttering in twin types. *Journal of Speech Disorders, 10,* 335–343.

Nessell, E. von, (1958) Die verzögerte sprachrückkopplung (Lee-effekt) bei stotterern. *Folia Phoniatrica, 10,* 199–204.

Palasek, J. R., and Curtis, W. S. (1960)

Palmer, M. F., and Gillett, A. M. (1938) Sex differences in the cardiac rhythms of stutterers. *Journal of Speech Disorders, 3,* 3–12.

Palmer, M. F., and Gillett, A. M. (1939) Respiratory

cardiac arrhythmia in stuttering. *Journal of Speech Disorders, 4,* 133–140.

Palmer, M., and Osburn, C. (1940) A study of tongue pressures of speech defectives and normal speaking individuals. *Journal of Speech Disorders, 5,* 133–140.

Patrick, J. R. (1934) Studies in rational behavior and emotional excitement. II. The effect of emotional excitement on rational behavior in human subjects. *Journal of Comparative Psychology, 18,* 153–195.

Pavlov, I. P. (1927) *Conditioned reflexes: An investigation of the physiological activities of the cerebral cortex.* London: Oxford University Press.

Penson, E. M. (1955) A study of the effects of thiamine on children with speech non-fluency. *Dissertation Abstracts, 15,* 2600–2601.

Perkins, W. H. (1967) Rate control modification of stuttering. Final report, VRA Planning Grant RD–2180–S.

Pitrelli, F. R. (1948) Psychosomatic and Rorschach aspects of stuttering. *Psychiatric Quarterly, 23,* 175–194.

Pronko, N. H. and Bowles, I. W. Jr. (1951) *Empirical Foundations of Psychology.* New York: Holt, Rinehart and Winston.

Quinan, C. (1921) Sinistrality in relation to high blood pressure and defects of speech. *Archives of Internal Medicine, 27,* 255–261.

Rheinberger, M. B., Karlin, I. W., and Bergman, A. B. (1943) Electroencephalographic and laterality studies of stuttering and non-stuttering children. *The Nervous Child, 2,* 117–133.

Ritzman, C. H. (1943) A cardiovascular and metabolic study of stutterers and non-stutterers. *Journal of Speech Disorders, 8,* 161–182.

Robbins, S. D. (1919) A plethysmographic study of shock and stammering. *American Journal of Physiology, 48,* 285–298.

Robbins, S. D. (1920) A plethysmographic study of shock and stammering in a trephined stammerer. *American Journal of Physiology, 49,* 168–181.

Root, A. R. (1925) A survey of speech defectives in the public elementary schools of South Dakota. *Elementary School Journal, 26,* 531–541.

Ross, F. L. (1955)

Rotter, J. B. (1939) Studies in the psychology of stuttering. XI. Stuttering in relation to position in the family. *Journal of Speech Disorders, 4,* 143–148.

Rotter, J. B. (1955)

Scarbrough, H. E. (1943) A quantitative and qualitative analysis of the electroencephalograms of stutterers and non-stutterers. *Journal of Experimental Psychology, 32,* 156–167.

Schaubel, H. J., and Street, R. F. (1949) Prostigmin and the chronic stutterer. *Journal of Speech and Hearing Disorders, 14,* 143–146.

Schilling, A. von (1959)

Schilling, A. von (1960)

Schilling, A. von (1962) *Untersuchung über die Monotonie bei Stotterern.* Proceedings 4th International Congress of Phonetic Sciences, pp. 374–386.

Schilling, A. von (1963a) Drug support in the treatment of stuttering. H.N.O., *11,* 300–304. (*In DSH Abstracts,* 4 (1964), 82.

Schilling, A. von (1963b) Sprech-und sprachstörungen. Handbuchartikel, in J. Berendes, R. Link, and F. Zöllner, Eds., *Hals-Nasen-Ohren-Heilkunde.* Stuttgart: Thieme.

Schilling, A. von (1966) Speech pathology in Germany. In R. Rieber and R. Brubaker, Eds., *Speech Pathology.* Philadelphia: Lippincott.

Schilling, A. von and Biener, W. (1959) Measurement of the perception of vibration by means of an audiometer and results of this study in stutterers. *Nervenarzt, 30,* 279–281. In *Deafness, Speech and Hearing Abstracts, 1* (1960), 84.

Schilling, A. von and Krueger, W. (1960) Examination of motor proficiency of speech-disturbed children. H.N.O., *8,* 205–209. In *Deafness, Speech and Hearing Abstracts, 1* (1960), 80.

Schilling, R., and Schilling, A. von (1960)

Schlange, H. (1961)

Schonharl, E., and Bente, D. (1960) *Veranderungen im EEG bei Stotterern,* Hamburg: Gemeinschaftstg. Allg. Angew, Phonetik.

Schuell, H. (1946) Sex differences in relation to stuttering. I. *Journal of Speech Disorders, 11,* 277–298.

Scott, H. D. (1931) Hypnosis and conditioned reflex. *Journal of Genetic Psychology, 4,* 113–130.

Scripture, E. W. (1923) *Stuttering and Lisping.* New York: Macmillan.

Sears, R. R., and Hovland, C. I. (1941) Experiments on motor conflict. II. Determination of mode of resolution of comparative strengths of conflicting responses. *Journal of Experimental Psychology, 28,* 280–286.

Sedlácek, C. (1948) Reactions of the autonomic nervous system in attacks of stuttering. *Folia Phoniatrica, 1,* 97–103.

Seeman, M. (1936) Contribution to the pathogenesis of stuttering. *Review of Neurological Psychiatry, 33,* 399–404.

Serra, M. (1960) A contribution to knowledge of the pathogenesis and therapy of stuttering. *Arch. Ital. Laringol., 68,* 166–174. In *Deafness, Speech and Hearing Abstracts, 2* (1962), 180.

Seth, G. (1934) An experimental study of the control of the mechanism of speech, and in particular that of respiration of stuttering subjects. *British Journal of Psychology, 24,* 375–388.

Shackson, R. (1936) An action current study of muscle contraction latency with special reference to latent tetany in stutterers. *Archives of Speech, 1,* 86–111.

Shane, M. L. S. (1955) Effect on stuttering of alteration in auditory feedback. In W. Johnson and R. Leutenegger, Eds., *Stuttering in children and adults.* Minneapolis: University of Minnesota Press.

Shearer, W. M., and Simmons, F. B. (1965)

Sheehan, J. G., and Martyn, M. (1966)

Sheehan, J. G., and Martyn, M. (1967)

Sheehan, J. G., and Voas, R. B. (1954)

Sheets, B. (1941) *A study of the visual perseverative tendencies of stutterers and normal speakers.* M.A. thesis, University of Utah, Salt Lake City.

Sherman, M. (1941) *Basic problems of behavior.* New York: Longmans Green.

Skaggs, E. B. (1926) Changes in pulse, breathing and steadiness under conditions of startledness and excited expectancy. *Journal of Comparative Psychology, 6,* 303–318.

Skaggs, E. B. (1930) Studies in attention and emotion. *Journal of Comparative Psychology, 10,* 375–419.

Smith, A. M. (1953)

Snidecor, J. C. (1955)

Sovak, M. (1933) Measurement of sympathetic reflexes in stutterers. *Casop, lek, Cesk, 72,* 164–168.

Spadino, E. I. (1941) Writing and laterality characteristics of stuttering children. In *Columbia University Teachers College Contributions to Education.* New York: Columbia University.

Spriestersbach, D. (1940) An exploratory study of the motility of the peripheral oral structures in relation to defective and superior consonant articulation. M.A. thesis, Iowa State University, Ames.

Starbuck, H. B., and Steer, M. D.   (1954)

Starr, H. E.   (1922)   The hydrogenion concentration of the mixed saliva considered as an index of fatigue and of emotional excitation, and applied to a study of the meta-bolic etiology of stammering. *American Journal of Psy-chology, 33,* 394–418.

Starr, H. E.   (1928)   Psychological concomitants of high alveolar carbon dioxide; a psychobiochemical study of the etiology of stammering. *Psychology Clinic, 17,* 1–12.

Steer, M. D.   (1935)   A qualitative study of breathing in young stutterers. *Speech Monographs, 2,* 152–156.

Steer, M. D.   (1937)   Symptomatologies of young stutter-ers. *Journal of Speech Disorders, 2,* 3–13.

Stetson, R. H.   (1933)   Speech movements in action. *Trans-actions of American Laryngology Association, 55,* 29–42.

Stratton, L. D.   (1924)   A factor in the etiology of a sub-breathing stammerer: Metabolism as indicated by urinary creatine and creatinine. *Journal of Comparative Psychol-ogy, 4,* 325–346.

Stromsta, C. P.   (1958)   Role of bone-conducted side-tone to stuttering. Progress Report, U.S. Public Health Service Grant B–1331.

Stromsta, C. P.   (1959)

Stromsta, C. P.   (1964)   Effects of bone-conducted side-tone on stuttering. Preliminary Final Report, U. S. Public Health Service Grant NB 03541–03.

Strother, C. R.   (1935)   *A study of the extent of dyssyner-gia occurring during the stuttering spasm.* Ph.D. disserta-tion, Iowa State University, Ames.

Strother, C. R.   (1937)   A study of the extent of dyssyner-gia occurring during stuttering spasms. *Psychological Monographs, 49,* 108–128.

Strother, C. R.   (1944)   Rhythmokinesis in stutterers and non-stutterers. *Journal of Speech Disorders, 9,* 239–244.

Strother, C. R., and Kriegman, L. S.   (1943)   Diadocho-kinesis in stutterers and non-stutterers. *Journal of Speech Disorders, 8,* 323–335.

Sutton, S., and Chase, R. A.   (1961)

Taylor, M.   (1965)   *An investigation of physiological meas-ures in relation to the moment of stuttering in a group of adult males.* Dissertation, University of Southern Cali-fornia, Los Angeles.

Travis, L. E. (1925) Muscular fixation of the stutterer's voice emotion. *Science, 62,* 207–208.

Travis, L. E. (1927a) A phono-photographic study of the stutterer's voice and speech. *Psychological Monographs, 36,* 109–141.

Travis, L. E. (1927b) Studies in stuttering. I. *Archives of Neurology and Psychiatry, 18,* 673–690.

Travis, L. E. (1928) A comparative study of the performances of stutterers and normal speakers in mirror tracing. *Psychological Monographs, 39,* 45–50.

Travis, L. E. (1931) *Speech pathology.* New York: Appleton.

Travis, L. E. (1934) Dissassociation of the homologous muscle function in stuttering. *Archives of Neurology and Psychiatry, 31,* 127–133.

Travis, L. E. (1937) Brain potentials and the temporal course of consciousness. *Journal of Experimental Psychology, 21,* 302–309.

Travis, L. E., and Fagan, L. B. (1928) Studies in stuttering. III. *Neurology and Psychiatry, 19,* 1006–1013.

Travis, L. E., and Knott, J. R. (1936) Brain potentials from normal speakers and stutterers. *Journal of Psychology, 2,* 137–150.

Travis, L. E., and Knott, J. R. (1937) Bilaterally recorded brain potentials from normal speakers and stutterers. *Journal of Speech Disorders, 2,* 239–241.

Travis, L. E., Tuttle, W. W., and Bender, W. R. G. (1936) An analysis of precedence of movement in simultaneous contraction of homologous muscle groups. *Archives of Speech, 1,* 170–178.

Travis, L. E., Tuttle, W. W., and Cowan, D. W. (1936) A study of the heart rate during stuttering. *Journal of Speech Disorders, 1,* 21–26.

Travis, V. (1936) A study of the horizontal dysintegration of breathing during stuttering. *Archives of Speech, 1,* 157–169.

Trumper, M. (1928) *Hemato-respiratory study of 101 consecutive cases of stammering.* Dissertation, University of Pennsylvania, Philadelphia.

Tuttle, W. W. (1924) The effect of attention or mental activity on the patellar tendon reflex. *Journal of Experimental Psychology, 7,* 401–419.

Twitmeyer, E. B. (1930) Stammering in relation to hemorespiratory factors. *Quarterly Journal of Speech, 16,* 278–283.

Ulett, G. A., *et al.* (1952) Psychiatric screening of flying personnel. IV. An experimental investigation of development of an EEG index of anxiety tolerance by means of photic stimulation: Its validation by psychological and psychiatric criteria. U. S. Air Force School of Aviation Medicine, Project No. 21–37–002, Report No. 4 (PB 107351).

Umeda, K. (1960a) The psychophysiological study upon stutterers. *Otologica Fukuoka, 6,* 377–391. (Japanese) In *Deafness Speech and Hearing Abstracts, 2,* 266.

Umeda, K. (1960b) Electroencephalographic study of stutterers. *Otologica Fukuoka, 6,* 392–396. (Japanese In *Deafness, Speech and Hearing Abstracts, 2,* 356.

Van Dusen, C. R. (1939) A laterality study of non-stutterers and stutterers. *Journal of Speech Disorders, 4,* 261–265.

Vannier, J., Saumont, R., Labarraque, L., and Husson, R. (1954) Production experimentale de blocages synaptiques recurrentiale par des stimulations auditives homorythmiques avec dephasages reglables. Bordeaux: *Revue de Laryngologie.*

Van Riper, C. (1935) The quantitative measurement of laterality. *Journal of Experimental Psychology, 18,* 372–382.

Van Riper, C. (1936) Study of the thoracic breathing of stutterers during expectancy and occurrence of stuttering spasm. *Journal of Speech Disorders, 1,* 61–72.

Walker, E. L. (1938) A comparison of the conditioned respiratory response and the conditioned flexion response. M.A. thesis, University of Indiana, Bloomington.

Wegener, H. (1963) Untersuchungen über die motorik stotternder. In *Akustische und motorische Probleme bei der Sprach-und Stimmbehandlung,* Hamburg-Altona: Arbeitsgemeinschaft für Sprachheilpädagogik.

Weinburg, Bernd (1964)

Wepman, J. M. (1939) Familial incidence in stammering. *Journal of Speech Disorders, 4,* 199–204.

West, R. (1929) A neurological test for stutterers. *Journal of Neurology and Psychopathology, 38,* 114–123.

West, R. (1943) The pathology of stuttering. *Nervous Child, 2,* 96–106.

West, R. (1958)

West, R., Ansberry, M., and Carr, A. (1957) *The rehabilitation of speech*. New York: Harper & Row.

West, R., Nelson, S., and Berry, M. F. (1939) The heredity of stuttering. *Quarterly Journal of Speech, 25,* 23–30.

Westphal, G. (1933) An experimental study of certain motor abilities of stutterers. *University of Iowa Studies in Child Development, 4,* 214–221.

Wever, E. G. (1930) The upper limit of hearing in the cat. *Journal of Comparative Psychology, 10,* 221–233.

White House Conference on Child Health and Protection. (1931) *Special Education*. New York: Appleton.

Williams, D. E. (1955)

Winsor, A. L. and Korchin, B. (1938) The effect of different types of stimulation upon the pH of human parotid secretion. *Journal of Experimental Psychology, 23,* 62–79.

Winsor, A. L., and Korchin, B. (1940) Some observations on the effect of mental activity upon parotid secretion. *Journal of Genetic Psychology, 22,* 25–32.

Wolf, A. A., and Wolf, E. G. (1959) Feedback processes in the theory of certain speech disorders. *Speech Pathology and Therapy, 2,* 48–55. In *Deafness, Speech and Hearing Abstracts, 1* (1961), 183.

Yannatos, G. (1960) Hydroxyzine in the treatment of stuttering. *J. Francais d'Oto-Rhino-Laryngologie et Chirurgie Maxillo-Faciale, 9,* 293–296. In *Deafness, Speech and Hearing Abstracts, 3* (1963), 290.

Young, P. T. (1928) Studies in affective psychology. *American Journal of Psychology, 40,* 372–400.

About the Author PHILIP J. GLASNER, Instructor in Psychiatry and Pediatrics, Johns Hopkins School of Medicine, is in charge of Speech Therapy at Children's Psychiatric Service of Johns Hopkins Hospital. He is a contributing author to the volumes *Psychological and Psychiatric Aspects of Speech and Hearing* and *Psychotherapy of Stuttering,* and a contributor to professional journals including *American Journal of Public Health, American Journal of Diseases of Children, Journal of Pediatrics,* and the *Journal of Speech and Hearing Disorders.*

About the Chapter Utilizing a developmental and case-study approach, as well as original research, Philip Glasner focuses on the problem of stuttering in children.

6

DEVELOPMENTAL
VIEW

PHILIP J. GLASNER

6

In the past, most of the research and efforts at therapy have been directed toward the problems of the older, chronic stutterers. As in most chronic ailments, either organic or emotional, the treatment is long and difficult when the condition has been allowed to progress to a set pattern. Presumably, secondary psychological and somatic factors help to perpetuate the original condition. We would be justly critical of workers in allied fields who, before attempting treatment, would allow a progressive illness to develop until the condition reached a stage where the possibility of recovery or cure was questionable.

DIFFICULTIES IN DETERMINING
SOME FACTS ABOUT STUTTERING

Contrary to the statements made by many investigators, stuttering, with very few exceptions, does not begin after the age of six. Frequently the older stutterer dates the onset of his stuttering at a later period, but careful investigation will not substantiate his recollection. There is also a lack of agreement about what constitutes stuttering in a young child. The effort to differentiate a so-called primary stutterer from a secondary stutterer has led to much confusion. In a study relative to the diagnosis "primary stuttering" (Glasner & Dahl, 1952), certified members of the American Speech and Hearing Association responded to a question dealing with the term with definitions ranging from "normal speech" to "obvious stuttering with awareness." Among those who mentioned behavior, there was a wide range from "normal" to "an emotionally disturbed child." For a large group, the criterion for the distinction between primary and secondary stuttering was the awareness or lack of awareness on the part of the child, but none of the replies indicated techniques or criteria to determine awareness or lack of awareness. It is interesting that several of the respondents did suspect that children as young as two were anxious and aware of their stuttering speech. If awareness on the part of the child is to be a factor in the diagnosis of stuttering, it is imperative that definite criteria be established for determining awareness. No one who replied could give satisfactory techniques for making a careful differentiation between so-called primary and secondary stuttering.

There is, obviously, a regrettable lack of agreement about who is a stutterer. Experts tend to agree on the diagnosis in the older stutterer—he has been described in terms of symptomatology, physiology, emotionality, and personality. As a result, we have sufficient mutual understanding of him to discuss his problems. As to the young child, there is a wide disparity among experts not only regarding what constitutes stuttering but also regarding what the basic problem is. Many workers state that they do not feel qualified to make the diagnosis of stuttering in young children. Many believe it is normal for a child to be nonfluent in certain situations, but leave undetermined the point at which nonfluency becomes a cause for concern. And yet almost all the children who are brought to the specialist by their parents with the complaint of stuttering do manifest speech behavior that has attracted attention and has been marked as different, usually not only by the parents but by others as well. The parent, who has been observing the speech development of the child from infancy and is aware of his basic tendencies in speech, must have observed something that was unusual for him. And there was a reason for the change in speech behavior that first attracted the parents' attention. It cannot be assumed that most parents cannot and do not discriminate between the expected faltering in their child's speech and that which calls attention to itself. In many cases the unusual nonfluency was observed and noted by others in the environment as well as by the parents—this should be sufficient indication that something happened to the child to cause the reaction.

SOME ETIOLOGICAL FACTORS
IN STUTTERING

Any meaningful discussion of the etiology of stuttering must attempt to explain some of the few known facts recognized by most investigators. Why does stuttering almost always have its onset in early childhood? Why is there a higher incidence of stuttering among boys? Why is it that some children are affected by criticism and correction directed at their speech and others are not? Why do some children but not others tolerate or accept deviations from normal without apparent upheavals? Are there personality characteristics in young children and their parents that contribute to their mode of verbal communication? How and why is emotional strain reflected in one's speech? The more information we have pertaining to these questions, the better chance we have of finding a solution to the problems of the young stutterer and his stuttering. There is a lack of agreement not only on the answers to these questions, but also on the significance of the questions themselves. An attempt to discuss some of these questions from an empirical point of view may challenge others to set up research projects to study these problems more thoroughly.

Some therapists have said that it is not necessary to agree on the causes of stuttering before determining an approach for its treatment. Yet it would seem important to determine whether the stuttering is regarded as a neurological or semantogenic problem, a learned or habit phenomenon, or a reflection of an emotional or personality conflict. One cannot presume to establish a rationale for treatment before he knows, or believes he knows, what he is treating.

Too often in the past (and in the present) theories have been built upon partial observations of the problem. Speech is a reflection of the total personality; every therapist has seen persons with severe speech dysfunctions wherein the disturbance was a reflection of a personality disorder, a disorder of interpersonal relationships, or both. It is considered here that in the majority of cases, stuttering, particularly in the young child, is one of several signs of an emotionally disturbed or unwholesomely integrated personality.

McCarthy, in her excellent study "Language Disorders and Parent-Child Relationships" (1954), found that "speech defectives, when studied carefully for home adjustment, family background, and personality factors, seem to show marked abnormalities in these areas as well." Glasner, in an earlier study (1949) dealing with stuttering children under 5 years old, reported that in every case the stuttering was only one of a number of symptoms of emotional disturbance and that the children apparently had more than their share of indicative behavioral symptoms. Moncur, in a well-controlled study (1955), has since substantiated these findings.

Most investigators, in discussing the behavior of the older stutterer, are aware of his strong feelings of anxiety. However, they seem to be in disagreement whether this is characteristic of the stutterer or whether it was induced as a result of the stuttering. We are aware that everyone reacts with anxiety to certain situations, but we do not know whether the child who is prone to stuttering is overendowed with this trait. It has been the writer's experience that most young stutterers display excessive anxiety reactions prior to the onset of noticeable stuttering behavior and that the stuttering merely aggravates a problem already existing. The effects of strong anxiety feelings upon the human organism are well known. Anxiety often interferes with physiological functions and shows itself in psychosomatic disorders. Anxiety reactions are diverse, but the most common features (which the average person experiences to varying degrees) are palpitation, vasomotor flushing, and respiratory distress. It is one of the most disturbing of mental states and often arises from interpersonal experiences, feelings of insecurity, and frustrations. When a child's adjustment is such that he frequently experiences anxiety reactions in situations where the average child is not threatened, he has difficulty in functioning; a disorganization of speech pattern may be a result of this confusion. Should the emotional and physiological factors that precipitate the nonfluency continue frequently and with sufficient intensity, this pattern of response becomes reinforced and will continue until he can emancipate himself from the factors that predispose him to stuttering.

When attempts are made to explain stuttering on an emotional basis, the question is often raised why other children with apparently similar environmental, personality, and emotional conflicts do not develop stuttering. Children, as well as adults, behave in their own diverse individual ways—there are many different theories attempting to explain behavior, and there is no completely satisfactory answer. For instance, can it be proved experimentally that inhibited, disrupted, nonfluent speech is a reflection of a child's inner feelings? It is a moot question whether some children are predisposed to stuttering speech because of neurologic factors that we have not yet been able to isolate. What takes place neurologically in terms of speech pathways or the habitation of speech pattern is largely unknown, and with our present knowledge, it is impossible to produce conclusive evidence to support any theory experimentally. What most present-day investigators do agree upon is that stuttering speech in a young child clears up when noxious factors in the environment have been reduced and the child has made a good personality and emotional adjustment (Freund, 1966).

Johnson (1944) and Bullen (1945) have pointed out that stuttering is extremely rare in "primitive" societies. When these societies begin to have contact with a new culture, however, various emotional problems, including stuttering, begin to appear. It has been found that where the adult-child relationship and the cultural expectations for children are different from those of our civilization, the behavior problems that concern us are rare or nonexistent (Mead, 1947).

Similarly, recent studies support the conclusion that in our modern contemporary societies a child's emotional adjustment is determined by the child-rearing and cultural patterns to which he is exposed and lend credence to the theory that stuttering is induced by the resultant pressures and conflicts. Chamberlin's study (1965) explores the effect of parental attitudes and their relationship to the child's physical and mental health. Bloom (1958) concludes that children who stutter are reared under a regimen different from that of children who do not stutter. McCulloch and Fawcett (1964), in a study of various communities in Scotland displaying marked cultural differences, found variations in the incidence of stuttering as well as differences in the sex ratio between these groups. Goldman's study (1967) showed that the boy-to-girl ratio of stutterers in a Negro population was related to whether the child came from a matriarchal or patriarchal environent and was, in some way, related to cultural patterns. It was felt that the demands and pressures in a matriarchal society were greater on girls than on boys and resulted in a higher incidence of stuttering among girls. Goodwin's study (1966), also dealing with Negro children, found a higher girl-to-boy incidence of stutterers than is found in the white population and concluded that the difference was related to cultural factors. Most of the investigators reporting on the incidence of stuttering among Negro children found that there are twice as many Negro stutterers as white stutterers (Chamberlin, 1965; Neely, 1960; Wadle, 1934). Further anthropological studies could give us a better understanding of the forces that tend to affect our behavior in general and in particular those forces that tend to make our children prone to stuttering.

THE EFFECT OF PARENTAL DIAGNOSIS OF STUTTERING

Until very recently, the most prevalent theory regarding the etiology of stuttering has been the semantogenic theory (Johnson, 1955). The child is seen as essentially normal; the parent, however, is said to overreact to the normal nonfluencies of childhood by diagnosing them as stuttering, by becoming unduly concerned about them, and by making attention-focusing attempts at correction, thereby arousing the child's anxiety about his speech and leading him to stutter.

As a consequence of this theory, a study was conducted (Glasner, 1947) to learn something of the thinking and attitudes of parents regarding the occurrence of nonfluency in their young children, and to examine how these thoughts and attitudes are related to the conclusion that the child has stuttered or continued to stutter. In addition, answers to the following questions were thought to be meaningful: What is the incidence of parental diagnosis of stuttering among preschool children of both sexes? What criteria do parents use in their initial diagnosis of stuttering? What did parents believe to be the cause of stuttering in their child? What effect did parental treatment have on the young stuttering child? Did the child stop stuttering? Did he continue to stutter? Did correction make any difference?

In this study, parents of 996 children approaching the first-grade level were interviewed by a trained speech therapist. Of the 996 children in the sample, 551 were boys and 445 were girls.

It was found that 15.4 percent of all parents diagnosed stuttering in their children before the children had reached the age of 6. They made the diagnosis one and a half times as often for their sons as for their daughters. In 70 percent of the cases, the child diagnosed as having stuttered had displayed more than one of the recognized characteristics of stuttering. The parent evidently was more likely to make the diagnosis if the nonfluency observed was thought to be severe. The data did not indicate either undue anxiety (which was not directly investigated) or misperception in the judgment of parents. However, the majority of these parents later reversed their diagnosis, saying that their child had stopped stuttering. It does not seem judicious to suppose that in these cases the parents had simply lowered their standards of fluency. It is more reasonable to assume that observable changes in the child's nonfluency had occurred and that the parents' judgments were simply reflecting such changes.

The fact that a relatively high percentage of parents (4.8 percent of the total sample) maintained that the child was still stuttering to some degree leaves open the question whether the parents in this study were objective or were prone to diagnose stuttering where others would not. In an epidemiological study dealing with behavior characterisitcs of children between the ages of 6 and 12, Lapouse and Monk (1958) found that 4.2 percent of the mothers reported that their children were stuttering. In a subsequent recheck of the reliability of the parents' statements, they found that 98 percent of the mothers gave the same responses. An attempt was made to determined the validity of the response by special study involving the correlation of responses of mothers and children. It was thought that partial validation of the mothers' answers would be obtained if the same questions were asked of the children. Stuttering was one of the items showing the highest agreement. One of the conclusions of this study was that "mothers as shown by the reliability and correlation studies tend to agree most closely with themselves and with their children on behavior which is objective and clearly defined." The question to be asked from this information is, if over 15 percent of parents had considered their children under the age of 6 as having stuttered, and over 4 percent of the parents of children over the age of 6 were still labeling their children as stutterers, what is the relationship between diagnosis and the continuation of stuttering?

It was found that approximately 70 percent of the parents who had made the diagnosis actively sought to correct the disturbance; the other 30 percent were also concerned but did little about it. Of the 101 children who were actively corrected, only 36 were still stuttering without qualification, 17 were thought to be stuttering but only occasionally, and 48 had stopped stuttering. It was impossible to determine with any degree of accuracy which children had continued to stutter and which children had stopped from examining statements of what parents "did about" what they called stuttering. Some of the parents in this study said with conviction that it was precisely the corrective measures they employed that led to the termination of stuttering in their children. An analysis of the responses indicated that although approximately half of these parents did the very things that most speech therapists would have advised them not to do, the stuttering ceased. Although the present author would agree that active correction and calling attention to nonfluency are generally undesirable, the study indicates that the diagnosogenic theory of stuttering is an oversimplification of the problem and that in most cases the parents' diagnosis and subsequent reaction is only a part of the problem. This study was repeated by Goodwin (1966) in another community with relatively identical results.

It has been customary for speech therapists to confidently advise the parent to ignore the stuttering as a prerequisite to its discontinuation. But it is not easy for parents to observe such a symptom in their child and ignore it—as a matter of fact, the parent who remains aloof or detached could be open to criticism. All the parents in the Glasner study gave evidence of concern, some more than others, and the degree of concern seemed to reflect the parents' evaluation of the severity of the stuttering. They tended to attempt active correction of the nonfluency if its severity was thought to be greater.

SYMPTOMATOLOGY
AND PSYCHOLOGICAL REACTIONS
OF THE YOUNG STUTTERER

Studies of the older stutterer do not necessarily give an accurate picture of the stutterer as a child, when the problem had its onset.

In a study of 70 children under the age of five who were referred with the complaint of stuttering (Glasner, 1949), it was found that although on the whole the symptomatology in these cases was not as bizarre as one would expect to find in 70 random cases of adult stuttering, nevertheless their stuttering speech had all the characteristics of adult patients. Compulsive repetitions, extensive prolongations, obvious blocking with some of the advanced reactions were observed. The intensity and

249

compulsiveness of the repetitions had a great range of variability. The prolongations were often as marked and severe as those seen in many older patients. Distortions in pitch and breathing were often very apparent. Gross muscular movements in the play activity of some of these children were jerky and tense. An interesting observation is that as improvements were noticed in the speech, the play activity and general body movement became better organized and more graceful.

From the above observations one must assume that these children are aware of the unnaturalness of their inability to speak freely and easily. Many children under five who had not been previously regarded as stutterers would, after a period of excessive repetition or a block, blurt out or whisper, "I can't talk," and then begin to cry (Glasner, 1949). Others showed their frustration in other forms of behavior, such as walking away without completing what they had started to say; some placed their hands over their mouths whenever they were about to stutter. Some were known to avoid speaking for a period of time. We can safely state that children under five, when stuttering, do not exhibit the same calm unconcerned attitude characteristic of children with normal repetitions and speech inaccuracies.

The way a child reacts to his verbal nonfluency or stuttering speech is a determining factor in the progression of the behavior. If his tolerance level is high, he does not easily become frustrated, disturbed, or upset, and the faltering speech has little or no significance to him. His reaction also depends on whether the stuttering occurs frequently and whether the condition is intense or mild. It is logical to assume that he would have some reaction at the time of the difficulty, when his ability to talk is suddenly interfered with. That he has no word for it or that he cannot fully verbalize his feelings does not mean that it has no significance to him. Until we devise more refined techniques or criteria for measuring reactions, we should not suppose that the unexpected interruption of fluent speech has no effect on him. Of course, there are various degrees of awareness and levels of tolerance; a point to be considered is why some children tolerate nonfluency better than others.

PSYCHOGENIC FACTORS
IN THE YOUNG STUTTERER

When stuttering is regarded not as a semantogenic problem or an isolated speech disorder but as having a psychogenic origin, it is, of course, necessary to treat the case in terms of the precipitating factors. Too often it is assumed that the young stutterer can be treated for his speech symptoms without an investigation and a study of the child and his life history—as though it were possible to isolate stuttering from the total child. Treatment of this kind can often be more harmful than helpful. It is therefore regrettable that many speech therapists are untrained or inexperienced in the field of clinical psychology and are often at a loss how to handle the total situation. Only when the emotional pressures, environmental influences, and inner unrest are altered can speech in the young child become permanently relaxed and fluent.

The therapist's ability to determine the overall problem with its many ramifications will depend upon his ability to do a complete and meaningful examination. To be able to take a significant history is a skill that requires extensive training and experience. The art is not only in knowing what questions to ask but in knowing how to interpret the answers. In the course of the examination, which in itself can be a therapeutic experience, the parent has an opportunity to reflect on the total child from birth to the present: how the various members of the family have functioned and are functioning, and how they have related and are now relating to each other. The parents, possibly for the first time, can reflect carefully in an organized manner upon the various forces that have helped the family unit to function as it does.

Another vital part of an examination is the psychological testing of the child and an understanding of his feelings and behavior. As we have seen, stuttering is only one of a number of symptoms of a broad syndrome; unless the therapist can interpret the dynamics involved and is alert to the overall needs of the child, therapy will be hampered. Fortunately, more and more speech therapists are beginning to recognize the relationship in their patients between stuttering and emotional involvements and are becoming aware of their limited training in this area. They are increasingly aware that treatment of the young stutterer can be directed not necessarily to symptoms but to basically psychological causative factors (Freund, 1966). The training of the speech therapist, if he is to treat the stutterer effectively, should include training in a child-guidance or mental-hygiene clinic where he becomes familiar with all kinds of behavioral disturbances. In discussing the importance of psychotherapy in the treatment of the stutterer, Sheehan (1958a) states, "The speech therapist who can at the same time be a psychotherapist, or the psychotherapist who equally understands modern stuttering therapy, is best fitted to offer therapy to a stutterer." One cannot do practical and meaningful psychotherapy with a stutterer without a thorough understanding of the many emotional problems that will be encountered during the treatment process.

A careful examination of the child and the uncovering of any possible etiological factors should precede treatment. Stuttering in the young child, therefore, will not be approached as a single uniform problem of development, and the treatment will of necessity vary with the needs of the child (Glasner & Rosenthal, 1957).

The ability to evaluate the total situation in order to make a differential diagnosis is of paramount importance—if the wrong diagnosis is made and a child who is in need of treatment is passed over lightly, the examiner has possibly missed the opportunity to rehabilitate the child. A determining factor in deciding whether a young stuttering child is in need of immediate treatment is the overall personality structure that the child presents at the initial interview. For instance, when the sensitive child is criticized or corrected, he becomes unduly concerned and upset. The child who shows evidence of being inhibited and overcautious rather than outgoing and free will continue to reflect these traits in his speech. Such a child usually has a low frustration level and will have difficulty in tolerating nonfluency.

One of the cardinal characteristics of the child who stutters is his obvious hypersensitivity. In describing their child's personality at the initial visit, this is the most common trait that is referred to by parents. They may say, "His feelings are easily hurt; he becomes overly upset when he is criticized or disciplined; he reacts quickly to my moods; he cries easily; he cannot stand any disharmony between members of the family; he tries hard to please adults; he cannot tolerate rebuff from his friends; he is cautious and timid; he lacks confidence in himself; he needs a lot of reassurance"; etc.

What sort of environment do these children usually come from? In the first place, most of the mothers describe themselves as highstrung, nervous, and lacking in patience. They are found to be rigid, domineering, perfectionistic, and overprotective, and are the dominant of the two parents. The effect of parental dominance in child rearing is well known. Symonds (1939), in a controlled study dealing with parental dominance and submission, concluded: "Children dominated by their parents are sensitive, self-conscious, submissive, shy and docile.

In their inner life the dominated children feel inferior and inadequate, are confused, bewildered, and inhibited. In the case of the dominant parents, it was found that one parent is in ascendance, dominating the whole family situation with a character which is compulsively neurotic."

Parents are, of course, a vital part of the treatment program. Usually the child's improvement is directly related to the mother's ability to change her standards and treat the child as a person with rights and privileges, not as someone upon whom she can exert her authority. Since many investigators have recently concluded that the mother of the stuttering child is, as a rule, perfectionistic (Abbott, 1957; Despert, 1946; La-Follette, 1956; Moncur, 1955), a further discussion of this single trait seems appropriate. The ramifications of a perfectionist approach to child rearing are well recognized by psychiatrists—it is thought to be the source of many personality and emotional problems. This type of parent is interested in her child's activities to the extent of attempting to make all the decisions for the child. Kanner (1957) noted that the perfectionistic mother has rigid rules and regulations for the child as well as for herself. Feeding and eating in general become a source of tension and concern. Toilet training is usually started very early and with excessive pressure. As the child grows older, much attention is placed on posture, demeanor, cleanliness, obedience, language development, television programs, homework, and social activities, and choice of companions. The child cannot live up to these standards. No matter how hard he tries, his mother is never pleased—if he did well, he could have done better if he had tried harder.

Treating the young stutterer offers the therapist an exciting opportunity to correct an unwholesome situation that is damaging to healthy development. He can encourage the parent as well to regard the treatment program as an opportunity for helping the child and those in his environment to learn real mutual enjoyment. A child's future well-functioning is assured by affection, acceptance, and approval, not by questionable regimes that make both parent and child unhappy.

RATIONALE FOR EARLY TREATMENT

Recently some speech therapists have been engaged in the study and treatment of preschool-age stutterers because it was found that only at this age is the prognosis good. In most cases, not only does the stuttering itself disappear permanently, but the general functioning level of the child improves when the incapacitating and crippling elements in his environment have been corrected. It is therefore deplorable that there are many speech clinics and speech programs that will not accept stutterers for treatment until they are 8 years old. If treatment of the stuttering child is solely on a symptomatic basis regardless of environment, possible causative factors, and the child's other problems, then there may indeed be some justification for not treating a young stutterer. However, when a psychologically oriented approach is used, taking into consideration the mental hygiene of the child at all times, there is no possible danger in early treatment.

When a parent brings a young child for treatment there are usually many things going on that disturb the patient. Even where the total picture seems relatively mild, careful and thorough treatment is still indicated because it may prevent major difficulties in the near future. To those who may be concerned with the effects of treatment, it should be made clear that one cannot be too healthy emotionally. If there is a question of abundant treatment versus not enough treatment, it is better to be on the side of abundant treatment. Medicine and dentistry are now emphasizing the importance of a preventive orientation. And psychiatrists believe that most forms of mental illness can be much more successfully treated when the illness is in its primary stage and the personality and character processes are being developed. In recent years, they have been engaged in the development of programs wherein it will be possible for the patient to receive early psychiatric treatment so that his chances of recovery will be greatly improved. The writer initiated and developed a county-wide program of early treatment of stuttering which had three purposes: (1) to reduce the incidence of stuttering; (2) to prevent the condition from progressing; and (3) to shorten its duration (Glasner & Vermilyea, 1953).

A most interesting result of early treatment is that most of the former stutterers not only had no memory of having stuttered but did not know why they originally came to see the therapist. We can see from this achievement the benefits of a change in the focus of the problem. Too often the only advice given to parents is "ignore it and the child will outgrow it." More efforts devoted to the study and treatment of the very young stutterer at the time the problem has its onset and it is possible to obtain a more accurate evaluation of the causative factors can much improve the status of the therapy of stuttering. So much has been written relative to the understanding of the symptoms of speech behavior in the older stutterer and its effect upon the individual that many persons are of the impression that all of the stutterer's problems are caused by his stuttering. This is an erroneous conclusion that restricts treatment to a symptomatic level.

Those who have worked intensively with the young stutterer usually find that the term of treatment is relatively short. There are many cases on record where the stuttering symptoms were severe and yet it was possible to clear up the problem completely within a few months. Some results were even more dramatic and the changes came about within a still shorter period. There are, of course, cases where the child does not respond so quickly and the term of treatment is longer. The important fact to bear in mind is that in most cases the prognosis is favorable in the treatment of the very young stutterer.

PSYCHOTHERAPEUTIC APPROACH TO TREATMENT OF THE YOUNG STUTTERER

The therapeutic approach to be used in the treatment of the stuttering child will vary with the dynamics of the particular case. The relationship between the child and the therapist should be one in which the child feels that the presence of an adult does not mean criticism or restriction. Cooper (1966) has found that the therapist-patient relationship is an important variable in the therapeutic process. One of the goals is to create a situation where the child can release anxiety and inhibition. It is important that the child find an opportunity for free expression of feelings and thoughts that may be disliked or ridiculed at home. He should be encouraged by various devices, direct or indirect, to express his resentments and hostilities. If the child can function better in a free-play situation using play-therapy methods, this should be made available to him. If, however, as happens with some young stutterers, he desires to and is able to sit and talk with the therapist about himself, his wishes, his feelings, his playmates, parents or siblings, this should be his decision. There is no set type of psychotherapy to be followed or one that will help every child. For instance, in some cases the child does not necessarily obtain his emotional strength through his verbal or physical activities during the therapeutic sessions, but through the feeling that he is understood and taken seriously by an adult who considers

255

him worthwhile and is willing to help him with his problems. When the child is able to work out his problems and develop a feeling of self-importance, he can begin to assert himself with his contemporaries, his parents, and other adults.

Whether or not techniques are attempted on a direct or indirect basis to help the child develop a relaxed, effortless pattern of speech depends upon the individual case. Where the stuttering is so severe that the child is upset at his inability to speak freely, it is important to give the child some symptomatic relief and tell him that his manner of speaking can be corrected.

Most investigators agree that to a great extent the child is a product of his life's experiences. Parents can be helped to recognize that they are contributing agents to their child's personality and emotional problems and that if they participate in the treatment program, it will be more possible to bring about the changes necessary to free the child of his stuttering. Fortunately, many parents spontaneously remark during the initial visit that it looks as though they will have to be under treatment too. Parents should be encouraged to work out their problems, improve their attitudes toward the child, and increase their awareness of the child's needs—not only his general needs but his day-to-day concerns and problems. If the parents are alerted and prepared to cope with the child's changes in behavior as he undergoes treatment, they are not likely to sabotage and counteract the gains that are made. As the therapist becomes aware of the child's intimate feelings and needs, it is usually important that the parents be kept informed. Parents concerned with the total child can usually see the stuttering merely as a symptom and not as a condition to be necessarily treated in terms of physical manipulations and exercises. They often learn that they do not know their child as well as they had thought and are frequently surprised at the feelings and attitudes that are uncovered. Unfortunately, there are cases where the family constellation is such that it is very difficult to help the family make the changes necessary for the improvement of the child. Some parents are under the impression that it is possible for the therapist to help the child without involving them in the treatment process. Occasionally, parents themselves are so disturbed that it is necessary to refer them for intensive psychiatric help if the child is to have an opportunity to develop in a wholesome manner.

Group therapy for parents is often useful as an additional approach to helping parents understand themselves and their child. At these sessions, the therapist is not too active a participant but allows the parents to examine their attitudes and behavior toward one another as well as the personal material they themselves present. Some parents are able to derive support from understanding others with similar problems. They find that they can reflect upon their own behavior by observing similar behavior in others. Group therapy is becoming an accepted form of psychotherapy when utilized by trained therapists.

Where it is found that the child is basically healthy, that he is adjusting reasonably well, and that his stuttering symptoms are relatively mild, the parents are informed of the findings with the assurance that the prognosis should be favorable. Although the condition is not considered serious in this type of case, the specific factors that may be upsetting the child are discussed at length with the parents with the expectation that they will take the necessary steps to clear up the conditions that could be interfering with smooth, free speech. They are, however, given an appointment to return within a month but are informed to consult the examiner if the condition should take a turn for the worse. If the nonfluency continues and shows any sign of tension or compulsion, even though mild, the problem is discussed further with the parents and they are asked to return in two weeks. At this time, if the stuttering still continues, the child is taken on for treatment.

Treatment is a complex process, and nothing can be taken for granted. The child and the parent are seen regularly, and only after the stuttering disappears can the frequency of the visits be reduced. If the patient remains symptom-free on the reduced schedule, he is still not discharged but asked to return at infrequent periods for a check-up. Only when the necessary personality and emotional adjustments, as well as fluent speech, have become an integral part of the child's makeup can he be considered ready to be discharged.

Therapy that has as its goal not merely an amelioration of or an adjustment to stuttering but the complete removal of the symptoms as well as the factors that precipitated the disturbance will focus is efforts on the early diagnosis and treatment of stuttering. The self-perpetuating nature of stuttering with its somatic and psychological involvements creates a situation that does not usually lend itself to efficient results in the older stutterer. That the disturbing conditions which created the problem are often no longer in existence does not make the problem accessible to a favorable prognosis. We are concerned with the stutterer because of what stuttering represents and the effect it has on his future adjustment. Modern medicine has made its outstanding achievements in the field of prevention. It is to be hoped that this approach will also prevail in the future treatment of stuttering.

References

References that are listed here only by author and year of publication appear in complete form in the Bibliography.

Abbott, T. B. (1957)

Bloom, J. (1958)

Bullen, A. K. (1945) A cross-cultural approach to the problem of stuttering. *Child Development, 35,* 1–88.

Carson, C., Kantner, C. (1945) The incidence of stuttering among white and colored school children. *Southern Speech Journal, 10.*

Chamberlin, R. R., Jr. (1965) Approaches to child rearing. *Clinical Pediatrics, 4,* 150–159.

Cooper, E. B. (1966)

Despert, J. L. (1946) Psychosomatic study of fifty stuttering children: I. Social, physical and psychiatric findings. *American Journal of Orthopsychiatry, 16,* 100–113.

Freund, H. (1966)

Glasner, P. J. (1947, Nature and treatment of stuttering. *American Journal of Diseases of Children, 74,* 218–225.

Glasner, P. J. (1949) Personality characteristics and emotional problems in stutterers under age of five. *Journal of Speech and Hearing Disorders, 14,* 135–138.

Glasner, P. J., and Dahl, M. F. (1952) Stuttering: A prophylactic program for its control. *American Journal of Public Health, 42,* 1111–1115.

Glasner, P. J., and Rosenthal, D. (1957)

Glasner, P. J., and Vermilyea, F. D. (1953)

Goldman, R. (1967)

Goodwin, S. M. (1966) A comparison between the incidence of parental diagnosis of stuttering in young Negro children and young white children. M.A. thesis, Pennsylvania State University, University Park.

Johnson, W. (1955)

Johnson, W. (1944) The Indians have no word for it. I. Stuttering in children. *Quarterly Journal of Speech, 30* 330–337.

Kanner, L. (1957) *Child psychiatry.* Springfield, Ill.: Charles C Thomas.

LaFollette, A. C. (1956)

Lapouse, R., and Monk, M. A. (1958) An epidemiologic study of behavior characteristics in children. *American Journal of Public Health, 48,* 1134–1144.

McCarthy, D. (1954) Language disorders and parent-child relationships. *Journal of Speech and Hearing Disorders, 19,* 514–523.

McCulloch, J. W., and Fawcett, P. G. (1964)

Mead, M. (1947) The concept of culture and the psycho-somatic approach. *Psychiatry, Journal of Biology and Pathology of Interpersonal Relations, 10,* 54–76.

Moncur, J. P. (1952)

Moncur, J. P. (1955)

Neely, M. McC. (1960) An investigation of the incidence of stuttering among elementary school children. M.A. thesis, Tulane University, New Orleans.

Sheehan, J. G. (1958a)

Symonds, P. M. (1939) A study of parental dominance and submission. *Psychological Bulletin, 36,* 540–541.

Wadle, E. (1934) A comparison of speech defects of colored and white children. M.A. thesis, University of Iowa, Iowa City.

About the Author DR. SHEEHAN is identified at the beginning of Chapter 1.

About the Chapter This chapter essays an integration of role-theory concepts with other currents of knowledge on stuttering, and presents a fresh approach to treatment. It grows out of Dr. Sheehan's continuing, active role as a working therapist. Presented here are clinical principles, basic concepts and guidelines in treatment, with specific goals and practical procedures in achieving behavior modification and role change. Routes leading to success and routes leading to failure are indicated for the clinician.

7

ROLE
THERAPY

JOSEPH G. SHEEHAN

7

Stuttering is not a unitary disorder but a cluster of disorders of varying degrees of complexity and relatedness. Stuttering is a bog one can enter from many different pathways, and from which one may find a variety of exits. Many roads lead to Rome and to and from stuttering. Psychological subtypes appear to exist, not only as to origins, but as to behavior styles and patterns of recovery (Sheehan, 1958b, 1960; Martyn & Sheehan, 1968; Sheehan & Martyn, 1970). Varying treatment is indicated for varied stutterers, yet certain underlying principles must apply to all.

The handicap of stuttering is traditionally defined in terms of the blockings, repetitions, mouth posturings, and grimaces that the stutterer goes through in trying to utter a word, but it is much more than that.

A stutterer is one who does not know where his next word is coming from. Moreover, he does not know when the next situation will arise in which he will need that word. Even his fluency may give him little more than a feeling of thin ice. The to-be-or-not-to-be, to-speak-or-not-to-speak is always with the stutterer, and from this gnawing pervasive uncertainty springs the major portion of his handicap. The symptoms we see make up only the top of the iceberg; far greater, and more dangerous and destructive, are those that lie underneath.

The average person who meets a stutterer is similarly divided in his choices. Should he watch the debacle, or avert his gaze? Should he help the stutterer with a painfully obvious word, or let him flounder? Should he give some friendly recognition to the difficulty, or help the stutterer pretend it is not there? Knowing little about it, he gets his cue from the stutterer himself. And as a result, he usually concludes that stuttering is something very shameful.

The blockings seem to come in waves, and those waves hit hardest when the stutterer has to say something important to someone important. Yet it is not always so, and the stutterer can sometimes surprise everyone, including himself, by speaking fluently in a crisis. Such breaks are seldom really lucky for the stutterer; people may grow more intolerant, saying, "Well, that shows he can talk if he really wants to." And that same fluency may be experienced by the stutterer as a buildup of pressure for the future.

The partial predictability of stuttering, the anticipations of stuttering as a probability but not as a certainty, add a gambling aspect to the handicap. Should the stutterer enter the situation or not? Can he say the word or not? This is part of the under-the-surface, iceberg aspect of the experience of stuttering. Ironically, the most severe stutterers are most optimistic in their hopes for success and fluency, if level-of-aspiration-for-fluency may be taken as a measure. Once the stutterer commits himself to speak fluently, he increases the probability that he will stutter. Such sequential or dependent probability estimates comprise a significant portion of the stutterer's emotional burden (Sheehan, 1963).

Classification of theoretical and therapeutic approaches to stuttering, always a hazardous task for any writer, has sometimes taken strange turns. Simplifying and broadening a threefold classification proposed by Bloodstein (1958), we might group theories under three general headings: (1) constitutional or dysphemic; (2) psychoanalytic or neurotic; (3) conditioning or learning. The first is not represented here, for constitutional theories have fared badly under scientific examination, and do not lead anywhere in terms of treatment. Significantly, even the dwindling few who still hold constitutional theories propose treatment programs primarily psychological in nature and essentially unrelated to the theory. The second and third are potentially compatible in at least some respects, for neuroses are learned behaviors too.

The approach-avoidance conflict model, which has furnished our prime theoretical base for a systematic explanation of the complexities of stuttering, is sufficiently broad to include both learning theory and psychoanalytic theory, at least in some of the mutations of each. Comprehension of this breadth has been most clearly evident in the writings of Ainsworth (1957), Andrews and Harris (1964), Brutten and Shoemaker (1967), Beech and Fransella (1968), and Gregory (1968).

In a brief contribution to the Gregory book just cited, we combined a role theory approach with the conflict model (Sheehan, 1968). In the present chapter, we propose to spell out more thoroughly some of the implications for treatment. As a basic concept, we view the field of psychotherapy as moving increasingly toward specialization in the development of particular techniques for particular problems.

A ROLE-SPECIFIC APPROACH
TO TREATMENT

When stuttering is viewed as a false-role disorder—a role-specific conflict involving approach and avoidance, involving attitudinal and motoric aspects—the major directions of treatment begin to converge.

Role theory may be utilized in two distinct ways in the treatment of stuttering: (1) recognition of the overt behavior as resulting from a conglomeration of false roles; (2) recognition that the pathway out involves assigned roles, successive experiencing of role enactments, with both motoric and attitudinal changes resulting from actions, from change through doing, and that changes in the self result from successful role enactment.

To elaborate the first point, stuttering may be said to be a false-role disorder in that the observable behavior consists largely of behavioral residues of the tricks, crutches and devices originally employed as disguises.

Every stutterer becomes in time a "walking museum," or perhaps a "talking museum," of those crutches, devices or mannerisms he has employed to conceal his stuttering. The history of the stuttering pattern of any one individual is clustered in what he does each time he stutters. In the adult, unraveling the tangle of false behaviors is a major goal of therapy.

Stuttering is typically reported as having a gradual onset, in spite of a widespread tendency to search for some dramatic event. Any emotional shock or illness may be blamed, or any other luckless stutterer within artillery range is therefore assumed to have been an imitative model. Despite this search, few stutterers or their parents are able to pin down the onset of stuttering as either dramatic or sudden. (Johnson *et al*, 1967). Spontaneous recoveries also appear to be gradual (Sheehan & Martyn, 1966, 1970; Martyn & Sheehan, 1968)—which seems to be true of recovery processes in general. (Sheehan *et al*, 1957; Wingate, 1964; Shearer & Williams, 1965). In its incipient stages, stuttering behavior itself appears as simple repetitions and hesitations, though in some instances complete blocks and struggle behavior are reported to be present from first observation. Stuttering patterns usually begin simply, and snowball in complexity as the stutterer continues to search for devices and distractions.

The acquisition of new responses in stuttering patterns has been described by the author in learning theory terms as follows:

> In attempting to say a difficult word the stutterer finds that employing a novel response, such as a sudden intake of breath, releases the word more quickly due to the disinhibiting effect of response-produced stimuli. With continued use the device loses its disinhibitory properties and becomes incorporated into the characteristic pattern of the stuttering. The response loses its voluntary characteristics along with its effectiveness, and the stutterer soon finds himself gasping automatically with every stuttered word. This cycle is repeated as he seeks relief in other novel responses (Sheehan, 1951).

In this way, every stutterer carries with him the vestigial remains of devices he has used to conceal stuttering and in this sense becomes a "walking museum."

By observing a stutterer we can guess with accuracy what has been suggested to him in the past. For example, a stutterer who gasps or who takes too deep a breath and then wastes it has probably been told "how to breathe." In many respects stuttering is a conscious, compensatory interference with an automatic process. (For an early version of this concept, see James Hunt, 1863.)

265

Just as walking would be awkward if we tried to direct our feet consciously, so talking becomes awkward for the stutterer when he has to overcome fear and an avoidance tendency and force himself consciously to speak—and not just to speak, but to speak as perfectly as possible. Under the same set, even a superior speaker with no history of stuttering would tend to break down in fluency. To this we could add the time pressure set which the stutterer has learned to internalize and impose upon himself (Sheehan, 1958a; Stunden, 1965).

Faltering during speech often carries with it social penalties just as dramatic as faltering during walking. Moreover, the process of speaking is a sensitive barometer of emotional upset. In *The Psychopathology of Everyday Life* (1914), Freud noted the sensitivity of speech in these words:

> *There is no doubt that the disturbances of the speech functions occur more easily and make less demand on the disturbing forces than other psychic acts.*

The case of the stutterer is compounded by the learned effort to avoid the social penalties associated with faltering or blocking in speech. The parallel to walking is furthered by the plank-walking analogy:

> *If a child is learning to walk, you don't expect to make him stumble less by telling him to stop stumbling. Stuttering is a result of trying to avoid stumbles or bobbles in speech. Therefore warnings to watch his speech only make the child try to avoid little slips and the stuttering increases. Children should not have to speak under pressure. It's like walking a four-inch plank—you could do it easily flat on the floor, but not so easily if it were placed across a chasm (Sheehan, 1950).*

Concentrated in the act of stuttering are many potentially disruptive sets: (1) the set to conceal and to avoid any overt manifestation of difficulty; (2) the set to go forward in a conscious effort to overcome avoidance, producing forcing, heightened muscle tension, and wrong postures and sounds; (3) the set to speak as perfectly as possible, to inhibit any potential "stuttering"; (4) the internalized time pressure set; (5) the set to interrupt oneself, to come to a dead stop the moment any stuttering behavior surfaces; (6) the set to go to lengths to portray a false role to the listener, to keep up the sham that nothing is happening, even after stuttering has become painfully evident to all.

THE FICTION OF NORMALITY

The psychology of everyday stuttering is characterized by the flimsy pretense on the part of both speaker and listener that the stutterer has no defect and is speaking like everyone else. We may call this the fiction of normality or perhaps the "baby hippopotamus effect."

Though moments of grimacing and blocking on the part of the stutterer intrude very conspicuously into the conversational situation, the stutterer engages the listener in a kind of implicit understanding that the difficulty will not be mentioned. The listener is drawn into the magical defense that what we refuse to see is not there. It is as though somebody put a baby hippopotamus on the table in plain view, and everybody pretended there was nothing there at all. An Emperor's Clothes effect in reverse! Perhaps more simply, a perceptual defense, an example of cognitive shift due to dissonance.

Paradoxically when a stutterer attempts to cast himself in a more fluent role when speaking as himself, he is more likely to stutter. When he accepts more easily the probability of stuttering, recognizes the hippopotamus on the table, and does not try to pretend or to enact false roles, he is able to be a more fluent speaker. Therapy for stutterers is largely a matter of dispelling fictions so that the roles become more appropriate—and of enacting roles so that the fictions are further diminished.

CYCLIC VARIATION AND
THE FLUENCY CARRYOVER ILLUSION

Most stutterers have spent the bulk of their lives with the mistaken impression that experience in speaking fluently will carry over, that they can suppress their stuttering in this way. We may call this the "Fluency Carryover Illusion." In the belief that he may make his occasional or artificially induced fluency extend, the stutterer is constantly reinforced by prestige suggestion of all kinds. Not only do friends, neighbors and family frequently encourage belief in the fluency illusion, but the history of the treatment of stuttering is shot through with it.

What is a common illusion for the stutterer has become an

unstated premise for too many experimenters and therapists. For example, those attempting to apply operant conditioning principles seem easily excited by intervals of fluency experimentally induced through such techniques as masking noise or delayed auditory feedback. Necessarily, they depend upon a premise that such fluency can be made to carry over. None has shown any convincing scientific evidence that such carryover is possible, yet the premise of fluency carryover is implicit in their procedures: a premise, we hereby state explicitly, that is highly questionable.

After all, every stutterer has spent most of his life speaking fluently—for the vast majority of words spoken by stutterers are spoken fluently (Johnson *et al*, 1967). Wavelike variation is characteristic of stuttering, as has been observed clinically for years, and as Quarrington's studies (1956) have shown.

Recently Taylor and Taylor (1967) challenged the evidence for cyclic variation and the Fear Reduction Hypothesis and related hypotheses suggested by Sheehan (1958a) and Quarrington (1956). One source of disagreement seems to have been that in our original exposition of conflict theory (1953, 1958a) the order of duration of the waves was not sufficiently spelled out. There are large waves, ripples, and ripples within large waves. The crests and troughs may vary widely from one person to another, and within the same person at different times. But the cyclic characteristic of stuttering is not confined to a narrow time segment. The pattern of variation may include second-to-second, minute-to-minute, hour-to-hour, day-to-day, week-to-week, month-to-month, and even year-to-year. Stuttering may also vary according to the life stage of the individual stutterer (Sheehan, 1969).

Thus, important individual differences exist among stutterers in cyclic variation and on other dimensions. Some stutterers show minimal variation, others maximal. In speaking of wavelike variations in stuttering frequencies on a group basis, it is important to recognize that stutterers do not all follow a common pattern and that some show much less cyclic phenomena than others. Among stutterers, even variation is not invariable.

But whether or not an orderly cyclic variation in stuttering can be shown, the evidence is ample from studies of the frequency of stuttering in relation to the adaptation and consistency effects that most stutterers speak most of their words fluently (Johnson, 1955).

Fluency does not beget more fluency. Rather it appears that episodes of fluency lead to episodes of stuttering (Sheehan,

1958a; Quarrington, 1965; Conway & Quarrington, 1963). If true, these statements are strong evidence that mere experience in speaking fluently will not lead anywhere in terms of a permanent solution to the problem of stuttering.

PARTIAL IRREVERSIBILITY
AND PROVISION FOR FEAR

From the principle of partial irreversibility of punishment-based learning (Solomon & Wynne, 1954) it is difficult to see how anyone can believe that the stutterer will not ever again experience the fear-eliciting cues that have become so strongly conditioned to the act of speaking. Through extinction and counterconditioning, one may make the fluent response temporarily ascendent in the hierarchy. But what of the future? Will fear never return? If the stutterer does experience fear again, what is he to do? From the curve of forgetting, the future probability of reinforcement of competing responses, leading to return of the suppressed stuttering behavior, is almost inevitable. Unless there is some provision for fear and future failures, the therapy itself will fail.

Therefore, the stutterer must learn how to cope with moments of fear and anxiety and panic. What is he to do when he stutters? Perfect fluency is the biggest illusion of all, and the stutterer has learned an intolerance of bobbles and disfluencies in his own speech. Severe stutterers especially seem to have developed high and unrealistic levels of aspiration for fluency (Sheehan, 1963a).

The stutterer does not need to be taught how to be fluent; he is able to be fluent part of the time anyway without such teachings. Rather, he needs to be taught how to respond when fear is signaling. Among other things he needs to learn how to stutter. Part of every stutterer's difficulty is that he doesn't know how to stutter. But he can learn! He can learn how to stutter openly and easily, something he has never experienced, rather than how to speak fluently, something he has experienced many times without permanent effect.

THE PRIMARY LOSS
VERSUS THE SECONDARY GAIN

If stuttering is a defense, as it appears to be in certain cases, it is a most punishing kind of defense. Cannot the process of symptom choice do better? Is there no better way to escape competition, achievement pressure, or other role-expectation?

Two assertions frequent in the literature are that stuttering is attention-getting behavior (especially as it first appears in childhood), and that stuttering is perpetuated by the sympathy it arouses (see for example, Wischner, 1950, 1952b). Interestingly, neither assertion appears prominently in the writings of those who have gone through the experience of stuttering. Those who stutter report clinically that overprotection is the hardest to bear of all audience reactions, that it is experienced by them as a rejection, and that other forms of rejection are at least as frequent as sympathy. As for the thesis that stuttering is a negative bid for attention, why then doesn't the stutterer display his symptoms more freely and easily? Avoidance is characteristic of even the young child stutterer who develops the slightest awareness. Moreover, attention-getting is not typically confined to a single behavior mode such as speech. The child or adult demanding attention diversifies his effort—he wants to be noticed in all sorts of ways—manner of dress, making loud noises, and other intrusive activity of all kinds.

Stuttering involves a primary loss—a defeat of the ability to communicate. Whatever "gains" accrue to this loss are secondary indeed. We have a strong clinical impression that intellectual achievement pressure is a frequent contributor to the onset of stuttering, so that stuttering may in that sense be an ego-protective conflict. But we still hold that with the onset of the problem called stuttering, the primary loss far outweighs anything that may later be rationalized as a secondary gain. An amputee veteran may experience some sympathy (most of it unwelcome) along with a multitude of frustrating social reactions. But does the gain exceed the loss? Would he trade back, given the opportunity? These are the questions that must be asked of the stutterer. In considering secondary gain as a "reinforcer" for stuttering, why overlook the primary loss? Consider how eagerly the stutterer has grasped for every straw of distraction that yielded quick fluency and the temporary illusion of cure. The residues of such follies are part and parcel of the stuttering pattern—the "walking museum" discussed elsewhere in this chapter.

To summarize this section, we conclude that: (a) while stuttering may serve as an ego-protective device in some cases, the primary loss of ability to communicate fluently vastly exceeds the secondary gains from peoples' reaction to the loss; (b) stuttering is not easily understood as a negative bid for attention, for related attention-getting behaviors are wanting in the stuttering child and even the occasions for speaking are rapidly subjected to avoidance learning; (c) since rejection of all kinds is frequently experienced by the stutterer, and since sympathy itself is frequently experienced as a rejection, the notion that sympathy is a positive reinforcer appears poorly suited to explain the perpetuation of stuttering.

For adequate explanation of the reinforcement of stuttering, we have to look elsewhere. Why does reinforcement fail in four out of five cases (Sheehan & Martyn, 1966; Martyn & Sheehan, 1968)? Why do not all stutterers follow the same patterns of reinforcement (Sheehan, Cortese, & Hadley, 1962)? Why do some stutter more under punishment and others more under reward (Frederick, 1955)?

ROLE CHANGE AND RESISTANCE

All of us resist change, and the stutterer in therapy is no exception. Most stutterers have learned to be wary of efforts to help them, for so many useless suggestions are freely offered by anyone. Although such initial resistance is virtually a part of the presenting problem, the really substantial resistance is likely to come following a certain amount of progress. The stutterer who moves easily at one stage in therapy becomes unaccountably bogged down at another. Apparently, improvement and recovery in themselves involve role changes calling for difficult adjustments. The stutterer may become disappointed in the results of his new partial fluency, due to the loss of protective functions and secondary gains. He finds that he is not a "giant in chains" but an ordinary mortal who has many other limitations which had been obscured by his stuttering along with some of his capabilities. He discovers that there are two ways to be disappointed in life. One way is not to get what you wish for. The other way is to get it.

Though every therapist needs to be aware of the possibility of resistance, for he will experience it, the concept is dangerous in that it may easily make the therapist cynical. You have to have hope yourself in order to kindle hope in a stutterer, and so many stutterers have had their hope responses extinguished. At the very least, the stutterer should not have to overcome the resistance of the therapist concerning his own potentialities. Faith in the integrity of the individual and in his ability to move toward positive change is a therapist *sine qua non*. If there are cardinal virtues for therapists, then hope, faith and empathy must rank at the top.

271

As an example of the "will toward health' and self-corrective potential, stutterers often come to feel guilty and wrong about their tricks and crutches—guilty about fooling people, guilty about representing themselves falsely. Given an orientation that stuttering is a conflict and a false-role disorder, they readily sense what is true self-portrayal and what is false. When they play false roles and conceal their stuttering behavior, they sense that their actions are wrong.

The stutterer who resists therapy may be hanging on to his symptomatic behavior and protecting his "secondary gains," but this tenuous concept does not automatically apply to all resistance. Some resistances are quite appropriate, and as Rank pointed out many years ago (Rank, 1936) the will of the patient to resist the therapist may be one of his most important assets. More simply in the case of stuttering therapy, often the stutterer is wise in rejecting therapy suggestions that have so often failed for him in the past. Every stutterer is shaped through previous nonreinforcement to resist certain kinds of suggestions, like the constant refrain, "Now relax, think what you have to say, and take a deep breath!" One of the first tasks for any therapist should be to dissociate himself from such aborted efforts of the past.

During the course of even the most enlightened therapy, the stutterer may reject an idea or a technique because it is really not suited to his needs. A stutterer undergoing therapy should always be entitled to consideration of the possibility that he is right and the therapist is wrong. Within the smorgasbord of therapy techniques, there may be valid reasons for an individual's rejection of certain dishes. Not everybody has to do everything—that is not therapy but regimentation.

CRITERIA FOR
' NEW" THERAPY TECHNIQUES

Under the banner of behavioral approaches, especially, recent years have seen a burgeoning of "new" therapy techniques. Many of these echo back to the sorry early history of the treatment of stuttering (Cf. Van Riper, Chapter 2, this book). Techniques employing masking noise or delayed auditory feedback, or "time out" postponement devices, or experimental manipulation of punishment contingencies, all have their forebears—the not very illustrious genealogy of the quacks. Often the distraction they are based upon is less sophisticated than the devices stutterers themselves show upon initial interview in the clinic.

The trouble with stuttering, as always, is that everything works—immediately—and for a time afterward.

In a journal of the American Speech and Hearing Association, of all places, commercial ads have begun to appear offering mechanical devices for treating stuttering. They are billed as representing a "new behavioral approach." Yet nothing is "new" except the improved technology that renders the devices portable; while a gadget is not behavioral at all. Nor does it represent what can fairly or properly be called a behavior therapy. The attempt to suppress and avoid moments of stuttering by such a means reflects old-fashioned symptomatic therapy at its worst. Commercial exploiters of mechanical devices have attempted to clothe the discarded methods of a sorry past with the raiment of modern experimental psychology. They are quacks in Wundt's clothing. The hands are presented like the hands of Skinner or Wolpe, but the voice is the voice of Bogue.

Despite a number of continuing theoretical puzzles, we do know enough about the factors surrounding stuttering to treat the majority of cases successfully. The price is courage on the part of the stutterer and skill on the part of the clinician. Any stutterer who goes thoroughly through the Role Therapy program presented in this chapter will shed a substantial portion of his handicap. Recent pioneering studies on the outcome of stuttering therapies including our own demonstrate this very clearly (Gregory, 1969).

What guidelines are available by which to judge a proposed "new" therapy technique? How is the practicing therapist to evaluate various procedures now appearing in the literature under imposing experimental auspices? From our view of stuttering as a multilevel approach-avoidance conflict, as a self-role conflict and a false-role disorder, we propose the following criteria:

1. Does the technique lead to approach behavior or to avoidance behavior?
2. Is the technique true to the self or does it represent a false role? Based on honesty or falsity?
3. Does it allow for future fear and fluency failure? Does it provide a means for dealing with the inevitable?
4. Does it call for behavior expression or behavior suppression?

273

5. Does it call for 'control" of something that really isn't there?
6. Does it create dependence upon itself or provide eventual freedom?
7. Does it produce fluency directly or indirectly? Does it hinge upon the spread of artificially induced fluency?
8. Are the results lasting and permanent, or logically only temporary? For example, are basic attitudinal changes toward self and others facilitated?
9. Does the therapy offer the stutterer eventual independence of the therapist?
10. Is the technique systematically related to a comprehensive theory of stuttering and supported with scientific evidence?

Subjected to such scrutiny, many frequently advocated and widely used techniques nominate themselves for the discard pile. Yet stutterers are still exhorted to forget the problem, to relax, to take a deep breath, to take a pill, to get hypnotized, or to walk around with a portable noise generator.[1] Each of these violates nearly all of the listed criteria.

For example, speaking with a noise-producing modified hearing aid produces immediate, temporary, and very false fluency. Rather than leading to independence, it fosters dependence on both gadget and therapist. It is clearly suppressive, calls for vigilance and control, is premised upon successful avoidance of stuttering, and is designed upon the fantastic hope that falsely created fluency can be stretched to cover all occasions.

CRITERIA FOR SUCCESS
AND FAILURE IN THERAPY

What are the distinguishing features of success in stuttering therapy, and what are the hallmarks of failure? What are the therapeutic end-products like? What would be considered a success?

Every therapist has worked with a number of stutterers he might place on either side of the ledger, as well as those who might be more clearly considered as a success or a failure. For

[1]For an hilarious satire on the operant approach to stuttering by means of distraction, see "The Operant Control of Stuttering Through Arm Swinging" by "Benjamin Q. Buque" in the *WMU Journal of Speech Therapy*, Vol. 6, No. 2, May 1969, Editor, C. Van Riper, Western Michigan University.

the dichotomy of success and failure, we all recognize, doesn't really hold in any simple fashion.

Seldom is it success with a capital "S" or failure with a capital "F", for there are gradations. Moreover, there are dimensions of speech improvement and psychotherapeutic improvement.

The time at which the assessment is made enormously affects the categorization of success and failure. Some who go forth having completed therapy with apparent success later bog down and become failures. Others show a delay in the factor of readiness for change, yet during therapy pick up an approach they later put into practice successfully. A few seem unable to accept help from a therapist and do not really begin to move until they become self-directed, until they become their own therapists (Sheehan, 1963b).

Yet we know that the determinants for success do not lie within the stutterer only, nor the therapist only. The interaction and the relationship are of crucial importance—what Stunden (1966) has called the client-clinician match. One man's failure could have been another man's success!

Despite the foregoing complexities, let us attempt a set of criteria for success and for failure. To be either, a case would not have to have all of the distinguishing marks, but a predominance of them would put him in the category.

Therapy can be considered a success: If the stutterer can speak fluently much of the time; if he has "fluency capacity" so that he is not constantly forced to exercise vigilance and control; if the way he speaks does not intrude conspicuously into the situation; if he has reasonable freedom from anxiety over possible stuttering; if he has a reasonably positive and well-integrated self-concept; if he is capable of handling most speech challenges; if he is able to get what he wants through speech without strain and anxiety in the process; if he is able to say what he wants to say when he wants to say it; if he can cope with major crises in his life without major relapse.

The stutterer should not have to go on "working on his speech" the rest of his life. The goal for a success should not be therapy interminable, but a growth beyond therapy. A good therapist should enable the stutterer to become independent of him, just as a good parent works to help his child become independent of him.

Therapy can be considered a failure: If the stutterer continues to avoid words, dodge speaking situations, and to use tricks or cover-up; if his stuttering conspicuously comes between him and his listener; if he is still addicted to crutch phrases or exhibits great tension in initiating words; if he is not rising to normal challenges of possible speaking situations; if he has to devote major energy to the process by which he speaks; if he goes on to further therapy after alleged completion of the first therapy; if he has to speak in an artificial manner or if he has to carry with him some kind of device such as a portable masking noise generator or an electrolarynx. Again, the term "failure" implies a category from which no one ever escapes. Yet today's failure may be tomorrow's success, and conversely, today's success may become tomorrow's failure—hence the need for follow-up data. In any case, the foregoing are some of the most readily observable distinguishing features of success and failure in stuttering therapy.

ROUTES THAT LEAD SOMEWHERE; BASIC CONCEPTS

From the view of stuttering as a self-role conflict involving approach and avoidance tendencies, principles of treatment logically follow. Perhaps the clearest way of presenting these is in the form of a "clinical philosophy," as it might be stated to the stutterer.

Designed primarily for adults, the following is useful with adolescents and older children, provided that the parents and other significant figures are dealt with first or simultaneously. Before these are presented to children, the usual precautions should be observed, *viz.*, (1) recognition of members of the family as members of the problem; (2) strong clinical effort to identify and to remove pressures on the child; (3) clear evidence that the child is long into the secondary stage, that he shows extreme forcing and struggle and has a vivid conception of himself as a stutterer; (4) reasonable clinical assurance that initiation of direct dealing with stuttering will not have adverse effects.

Although there may be danger in dealing with young stutterers too directly or too soon, a typically greater hazard is perpetuating a false mystery. Once the child has a clear conception of himself as a stutterer it is healthier to be open about it, otherwise the pointed omission of any reference to his stuttering behavior is interpreted as a taboo. Parents and clinicians frequently underestimate the child's ability to be open and honest; they unwittingly push more of the iceberg beneath the surface.

Moreover, the ideas presented below have been found to be essentially supportive for any stutterer.

1. Stuttering is a false-role disorder. You will remain a stutterer so long as you continue to pretend not to be one.

2. Just as you have stuttered most of your life up to now, you will stutter somewhat the rest of your life.

3. You have a choice as to *how* you stutter. You do not have a choice as to *whether* you stutter.

4. What you call your stuttering consists mostly of the tricks, the crutches you use to cover up.

5. Your stuttering is like an iceberg—most of the handicap you keep concealed beneath the surface. Get more of it up above the surface, and you will get rid of it more easily.

6. Your stuttering is *something you do*, not something that happens to you. It is your behavior, not a condition. Not a defect nor an illness, but a series of mistakes you continue to make. Mistakes you can correct with a little self-study and courage.

7. Working on your stuttering can be fun—to attack and conquer situations from which you have always retreated.

8. Role therapy is not something interminable. You have learned a set of attitudes, feelings and habits. You can learn a new set of attitudes, feelings and habits.

9. It is far better to stutter openly and honestly than it is to use a trick, especially if temporarily successful.

10. Your stuttering won't hurt you and your fluency won't help you.

11. In accepting yourself as a stutterer, you choose the route to becoming a more honest, relaxed speaker.

12. You have a choice—you can exercise a choice to stutter openly and smoothly.

13. The more you run away from your stuttering, the more you will stutter. The more you are open and courageous, the more you will develop solid fluency.

ROUTES THAT LEAD NOWHERE; COMMON FALLACIES

Though the therapy outlined in the foregoing may be linked historically to Dunlap and his idea of negative practice, and to variant forms of this idea in the writings of Van Riper,

Bryngelson and Johnson, the therapy itself is radically different from many concepts common in "stuttering therapy."

So many temptations for short-cut and quick, magical "cure" beset the stutterer, offering the glittering promise of immediate though temporary fluency, that some "don'ts" need to be offered along with the "do's."

In contrast to the above principles, here are some notions that you should reject, for they increase "holding back:"

1. "Control." If you try to "control" stuttering, you are likely to be suppressing it, covering up, and this aggravates the problem. For it is the direct opposite of the basic goal of being open.

2. "Block," neurological or otherwise. There is no block to keep you from going ahead, only your own crutches and effort to avoid.

3. "Symptom." Your stuttering is your own behavior, something you have learned, something you can unlearn. It is not a "symptom" of an illness or of some deep personality disturbance. It is neither an entity nor something that happens to you, but the result of your effort to cover up.

4. Distractions, tricks, and crutches of all kinds. This includes portable noise generators and delayed feedback gadgetry. You need courage, not apparatus. No machine will ever cure you.

5. "Faking." Pretending to stutter or "faking" won't help you, though honest voluntary stuttering can. You "fake" too many things already. This is part of the problem. Far better to work for open stuttering, to share with your listener what you are doing by letting him see and hear your stuttering.

6. "Guilt over fear." You must expect during therapy to experience fear, for it is only that way you can progress. A block is not a failure; a fear is not a failure. They are the raw materials of stuttering therapy.

7. "Relaxation." Like fluency, relaxation should come as a by-product of open display of stuttering. You cannot always be relaxed and you should not count on rituals to reduce tension. You can learn to stutter in a more relaxed way, and you will begin to lose your forcing when you have become sufficiently open.

8. Direct effort for fluency. You do not need to learn how to speak fluently, for you do that already when you do not try to cover up and get in your own way. When

you have gotten rid of the last island of avoidance in your own behavior, you will find that you have become fluent within normal limits.

COMMON SOURCES OF
DISCOURAGEMENT
IN STUTTERING THERAPY

A role-taking psychotherapy, or behaviorally oriented speech therapy, such as we have evolved for stuttering, carries unique disadvantages along with its equally unique advantages. Among some of the disadvantages, which can lead to transitory motivational problems and feelings of discouragement in the stutterer, are these:

1. A feeling of guilt building up during therapy over not doing well enough.
2. A feeling of hopelessness, that he can't really change his style of stuttering.
3. A feeling that he must spend the rest of his life trying to "control" something, that eternal vigilance is the price of fluency.
4. A misguided perception that therapy must be a process interminable, rather than realization that when he accepts himself fully as a stutterer and relinquishes his struggles to cover up, he will be able to speak naturally and easily.
5. "Slumps" or little relapses resulting from the operation of Jost's Law of Habits and the Law of Forgetting. Since recently acquired attitudes or habits inevitably fall off faster than the old, he must keep the initiative for a sustained period.
6. Unintentional inviting of relapses by letting speech go in "easy" situations, and concentrating only on the "hard" situations. When the stutterer does this, he lets the Hullian learning principle, $sEr = D \times H$, work to his disadvantage. With frequent repetition of the wrong response (H), then any slight buildup in anxiety or fear (D) multiplies the tendency for the response to occur (sEr, or Excitatory Potential). Accepting the role of stutterer openly and easily in simpler situations, or stuttering openly, smoothly and easily in these situations, will increase the probability of success in situations in which fear and avoidance are present.

279

WHO SHOULD BE THE THERAPIST?

Broadly speaking, all treatment of the stutterer is to be regarded as a species of psychotherapy. A unique feature of stuttering therapy is that so many specialized therapy techniques have been developed, especially for the adult. This development stems from the circumstance that by far the bulk of the handicap consists of secondary features. On the side of what Brutten and Shoemaker (1967) call "conditioned negative emotionality" are such feelings as guilt, shame, tension, and dejection (Sheehan, Cortese, & Hadley, 1962). On the motor side are such instrumentally acquired behaviors as struggling, grimacing, timing movements, running starts, fluent asides, etc. etc. Except for primary guilt and shame, these are secondary behaviors, extensively catalogued as such by Van Riper (1937a, 1937b) and more recently by Johnson, Darley, and Spriestersbach (1962).

A psychiatrist colleague, Dr. Samuel Futterman, once raised the intriguing question, "Are there any other problems or neuroses in which so large a proportion of the treatment effort is directed at the secondary features?" Within the framework of analytically oriented psychotherapy, we could think of none. The treatment effort to which we referred was a therapy for stuttering viewed as a multilevel approach-avoidance conflict (Sheehan, 1953, 1958), which we would today describe as a role-taking psychotherapy and an early form of behavioral therapy.

If the treatment of stuttering is a specialized form of psychotherapy, then who is best fitted to offer this therapy? Two central requirements are knowledge and clinical expertise in psychotherapy as broadly defined, together with knowledge and clinical expertise in the specific problem called stuttering. Just being a psychiatrist, or a clinical psychologist, or a speech therapist, or a psychiatric social worker is not enough. The disorder of stuttering is a peculiar tangle with many special features; it has been heavily researched and has a rich literature. Any stutterer seeking treatment is entitled to an assurance that his therapist has at least read the literature sufficiently to acquaint himself with major findings, and particularly with the many specialized techniques which have been developed to cope with this problem. Yet the stutterer's trust is constantly abused, typically on the convenient and lazy assumption that stuttering must be just an outward symptom of deeper maladjustment, to be treated by "ignoring the symptom" and getting back to the source through psychotherapy.

The search for "the source" of the symptom in adults often turns out frustratingly for both patient and therapist. In a general sense, the source of stuttering is unknown and unknowable. The insight model, which was so well suited to treatment of Viennese hysterics at the turn of the century, does little for any but the most repressed stutterer. Moreover, the most important insights are not obscured in the mists of the past, but are readily available in the present.

For example, the stutterer needs to know what he is doing, and he typically does not. He can readily learn that avoidance is harmful and that eye contact helps. With effective techniques easily at hand, why let the stutterer flounder for an indefinite and seemingly interminable period while searching for buried complexes? When a stutterer who has had three years of analysis cannot look you in the eye, the inescapable conclusion is that something was lacking in the therapy. The same is true for any therapy, including operant conditioning.

Some of the most prominent practitioners of operant methods are equally guilty of failure to heed the literature, and appear to have little more going for their methods than the ancient and fickle principle of distraction. (For evidence on this point, see Biggs & Sheehan, 1969.) They have resurrected direct-fluency methods long discarded by speech pathology, and have vested them with the trappings of modern experimental psychology. Yet they have provided no convincing evidence that laboratory fluency can be carried into life.

When their methods fail, the stutterer is left with nothing at all. In fairness to the overassuming analyst criticized earlier, at least the stutterer has some possibility of deriving general benefits from the therapy even if the observable speech behavior does not change much.

Here is a summary of the qualifications of the clinician:

> *Any therapist who works with stutterers has a basic obligation to inform himself about the many special features of the disorder. If the therapist is to fulfill his ethical obligation to any child who entrusts himself for treatment, he needs to know the problem. For example, he needs to know that much of what we see as stuttering behavior is learned, that stutterers do not require psychotherapy merely because they are stutterers, that they are essentially like non-stutterers in most respects. The therapist who would work with stutterers has the duty of*

281

reading the literature that has accumulated on the problem. Usually, supervised clinical experience in working with the problem of stuttering, with at least one course which deals specifically or substantially with stuttering therapy, and with child therapy, is advisable. But even those who possess qualifications as speech therapists should study stuttering, observe and interact with stutterers, and perhaps assume the role of a stutterer in sufficient speaking situations to experience and understand some of the social rejection and frustration the disorder brings. In addition to this knowledge and experience, the therapist should know that while there are different approaches, there is a substantial core of agreement among those who specialize in therapy for stutterers (Speech Foundation of America, 1964).

Speech pathologists and students in training frequently slight role-taking experiences for themselves. Learning the pattern and enacting the role of the stutterer you have in therapy, not just in the clinic but in the hard outside world, has no parallel as a means of understanding the psychology of stuttering.

An issue frequently raised with respect to the qualifications of the therapist is whether a stutterer should become a therapist for other stutterers. Some training program directors will not let stutterers become therapists unless they become very fluent speakers first. We would exactly reverse that stipulation; normal speakers should not become therapists until they have first become stutterers. We refer, of course, to extensive and intensive experience in taking the role of the stutterer. The fluency needed by the therapist is not in speech but in understanding.

THE STUTTERING EQUIVALENT

Since stuttering is a problem of the social presentation of the self, nearly everyone has an equivalent problem. A long nose, freckles, a scar, runt-like stature, obesity—all these are fairly obvious. In his heavily autobiographical novel, *Of Human Bondage*, Somerset Maugham symbolized his stuttering by giving his hero a club-foot. His descriptions of the morbidly curious behavior of the children on the playground make familiar reading for any stutterer.

Life is full of parallels for the social handicap of stuttering.

The fascination that stuttering holds for many people is explainable on this basis. From the equivalents of stuttering come an opportunity for understanding by the clinician. If he is to help the stutterer in openness and role acceptance, he must accomplish a similar feat within his own personality.

Along with taking the role of a stutterer, the clinician needs to identify, accept and openly display his own stuttering equivalent. Since every therapist builds his therapeutic style around his own personality, this is a feature that he can share with the stutterer—provided that he demonstrates in action for the stutterer his acceptance of his own stuttering equivalent. He who would preach the objective attitude must also show it within his own identity problems, not once but many times.

TAKING THE ROLE OF THE STUTTERER

The role experiences of a stutterer have a certain uniqueness, which can only be tapped by role-taking. Speech clinicians who would qualify themselves to work with the stutterer could best begin by entering the role, not once as a gesture but many times.

Instead of merely "faking" stuttering to a few people as a part of an introductory speech pathology course, or superficially during his clinical training, the clinician should have shared the stuttering experience over a significant period of time. If he has not done so, he is depriving himself and his stutterers.

Taking the role of a stutterer, finding out what it is the stutterer experiences, is the principal way the clinician can overcome the handicap of being a normal speaker. In order to help the stutterer, a *doing* kind of therapy is needed; a behavior-oriented therapy. As we pointed out in Chapter 1 and elsewhere, the stutterer is changed by what he *does*.

Too many direct their energies into intellectualizing. They are quite receptive to traditional insight-oriented psychotherapy because this is so often a kind of intellectualizing once-removed. To talk about feelings is very easy. To talk about the literature on stuttering is even easier. To be yourself without pose of sham or pretense, to be yourself openly, here is the fundamental personal challenge. For a stutterer this means accepting openly the role of a stutterer and displaying openly those blocks he would experience from previous conditioning. The Achilles' heel of most normal speaking therapists who try to work with stutterers is simply that they are not willing to do what they ask their stutterers to do and what is necessary for both to do.

To go through the experiences of a stutterer is enormously sensitizing. To a therapist we might say: "Go into a store and stutter very severely to the clerk. In anticipation what do you do? You rehearse the experience. You visualize it beforehand just as the stutterer does. You sidle up to a counter and you notice some people nearby, so you wait until they go away because you don't want bystanders around. Then, when you do try to stutter, you chicken out and become more fluent than you thought you were going to be."

Perhaps the greatest value of the foregoing assignment stems from the resistance the clinician typically feels. When he has overcome his reluctance and gone through the experience, he will never be cavalier about telling the stutterer to be objective; will never again act as though there's nothing to it.

The clinician may find himself sabotaging the assignment, and will thereby learn how easy and tempting this route is. He goes into a store and starts out boldly enough: "G-g-g-g-give—, g-give—ah, ah, ah—me a p . . . package of Smith Bros. Bla—Bla—Black C—C-C-Cough Drops." So far, so courageous. Then he notices a bystander viewing him warily, and suddenly undergoes a remarkable improvement: "Thank you very much. They're my favorite brand. I've relied on them for years."

This is exactly what a stutterer is tempted to do in any assignment involving open identification of himself as a stutterer. The clinician who has felt the temptation to step out of role and gotten rid of it—perhaps by succumbing—will be alert to this possibility when he plans the situation with stutterers. A negative suggestion that the stutterer will probably "chicken out" the first time in this manner is often facilitating toward success or at least permissive toward initial failure.

PSYCHOTHERAPY THROUGH ACTION

Role-taking psychotherapy is not merely a verbal therapy depending upon recollection of past events. Rather, it is an action-oriented therapy in which the stutterer is changed, not by what he thinks about, nor by what he talks about, but changed by what he does.

Insight-oriented psychotherapy may facilitate change when it is a *supplement* to action; insight retards change whenever it serves as a *substitute* for action.

Feedback upon the self results from successful role enactment. There may be tremendous psychotherapeutic effects of such enactment. The status gap is not changed merely by bandying words under conditions of psychotherapeutic isolation. We have evolved a therapy in which the stutterer is encouraged to go forth into the real world and to experience.

Psychotherapy itself is becoming more experiential—you are changed by experience; you are molded by experience. The therapist who can share the process of going out and meeting the social rejection that the stutterer sometimes meets is much more in tune with the stutterer. He will have deeper empathy and understanding.

Here are three cardinal elements in therapy:

1. Empathy—some feeling of emotional rapport, an emotional inter-reflection. Therapeutic communication does not always have to be verbal, but empathy is the first element.

2. Hope—it is necessary that the therapist offers some hope for the stutterer to give him a chance, perhaps, to face in a new direction—to try things he's never had an opportunity to try before.

3. Challenge—which puts him more on his own and gives him responsibility for doing what he wishes to do— what he had been unable to do—and some kind of positive social consequence. This is very much like the Hullian, Dollard and Miller principle of drive, cue, response and reward as conditions necessary for learning. That is, in order to improve, in order to go through this arduous learning process we call therapy, the stutterer has to want something. He has to see something, perceive something, do something and get something, and he is going to be changed as a result of what he does. In learning theory terms, these are: Drive, Cue, Response, and Reward, and are fundamental to all new response acquisition.

Psychotherapy by action and by role-taking is more demanding of the therapist. The process requires clinical sensitivity and clinical judgment, but the results are worth it.

On the other hand, discussion of feelings is a widespread therapist's crutch. The clinician can easily—too easily—respond to anything with, "How do *you* feel about it?" Yet what most people in trouble need is not a wallowing in visceral response, but a plan of action. To talk about feelings is fairly easy; to do something in response to feelings is what is difficult.

Role-taking is the royal road to insight into another, and action is the royal road to psychotherapeutic change.

THE DEMAND-SUPPORT RATIO

With any parental relationship, or any therapeutic relationship, the following two questions are crucial:

1. How much is demanded of the individual?
2. How much emotional support is offered to meet these demands?

First let us consider the parent-child relationship. What is demanded of the child? What role expectations are set up for him? What are his duties and the constraints on his time? In what sense is he not permitted to be a child but required to meet adult needs? Is the child showing the behavior patterns of a child or those of a little adult?

To the other side of the coin: how much love and support does the child receive? Some parents who are relatively demanding provide abundant interpersonal help in meeting the demands. Similarly, some children are neglected to the point where they receive little of either demand or support.

The most favorable situation is one of low demand and high support; from such a situation can come initiative, responsibility, and self-realization. Probably the least favorable is that with high demand and low support to meet the demands. In our clinical experience, the latter constellation is more frequently found in stuttering than the others. Although personality assessment of parents of stutterers has not shown impressive differences (see Chapter 3), no measure has yet been devised for the Demand-Support Ratio.

In an action-oriented, role-taking, *doing* therapy, such as we developed for stutterers, the relationship of emotional support to role expectation becomes particularly critical. Just as every parent should be evaluated in terms of the Demand-Support Ratio, so should every therapist. How much does he demand of the stutterer? And how much support does the therapist provide to help meet these demands? It is in this context that the relationship between the stutterer and the clinician must remain essentially psychotherapeutic. Therapists who merely hand out a set of techniques in an offhand or authoritarian way are dooming their cases and themselves to failure. Assignments tend to fail when they are too vague, carelessly given, impossible of recording, not attuned to the factor of readiness for change, or when the clinician is insufficiently supportive. The Demand-Support Ratio is a principle or criterion to be applied broadly to any psychotherapy or to any behavior modification therapy.

CLINICAL PRINCIPLES

In spelling out the operations of therapy, one may easily be accused of a cookbook approach. So much clinical avoidance of this accusation is evident in our literature that it is amazingly difficult to find any description of the operational aspect of therapy anywhere. The student searching for straightforward answers to his straightforward questions on techniques in therapy rapidly finds himself in a verbal maze. When he asks, "What do you do in therapy?" the fog rolls in.

We have tried to meet both the clinician's need for specific procedures and the profession's need to avoid regimen in two ways. First, we do give examples of procedures that may usually be followed with benefit, and second, we embed these in a context of clinical principles:

1. In role therapy with stutterers there is a cumulative or snowballing effect. The role assignments of early therapy are to be continued and should become an habituated part of the stutterer's daily style. For instance, emphasis on establishing eye contact before speaking and maintaining it during moments of stuttering begins early in the therapy but continues throughout.

2. New procedures are best introduced *one at a time*, so that the stutterer attains some mastery before meeting the next challenge.

3. Since the activities of stuttering therapy overlap, more than one assignment may be directed toward a particular goal.

4. In a particular situation, it is usually advisable for the stutterer to work on one subgoal at a time. For example, if his goal is entering a highly feared situation and he does enter it, this counts as a success no matter how miserably he may have done in the situation. From the standpoint of casual listener esthetics, he may have blocked horribly. No matter! He moved forward in the face of fear—something he must do many times to succeed in therapy.

5. Innovations of technique by the inexperienced therapist are to be avoided. There is always much room and need for innovation and creativity in planning with the stutterer *how* therapeutic goals are to be accomplished.

6. Since the introduction of a new technique is motivat-

ing, therapists are constantly tempted to introduce them prematurely, as a means of keeping the stutterer going. The result is a piling up of halfheartedly acquired methods, none of which the stutterer is able to use with any degree of command.

7. No procedure, however meritorious in itself, should be used indiscriminately with every case. The needs of the individual must always be considered.

8. Specific methods or techniques are tools which may be used well or badly, though none suggested here are particularly dangerous.

9. Timing is crucial in all clinical work. Activity appropriate at one point may be inappropriate at another. Similarly, a particular method may accomplish different goals at different stages in therapy.

10. The success-failure ratio must be kept in balance on the success side. If the stutterer is failing, then the goals and subgoals need to be reexamined.

11. Every method used with a stutterer should meet the basic criteria of facilitating honestly rather than posing, and approach rather than avoidance.

12. Most assignment failures are the fault of the clinician, not the stutterer. An assignment should always contain enough challenge to help the stutterer move forward but not so much as to be overwhelming. In an action-oriented approach, therapeutically induced guilt over non-fulfillment of roles can be a major problem. The clinician should do all he can to keep this guilt to a minimum.

13. All therapy should include continuous evaluation of the effects it is currently producing. Changes associated with improvement may in themselves produce problems which the therapist must be prepared to cope with.

14. The procedures of therapy are designed to help the stutterer break out of the vicious circle of self-reinforcing avoidance. When a stutterer continually resists or sabotages his own improvement, he cries out his need for deeper or more broadly based psychotherapy.

15. The therapist role has many similarities to the parental relationship. Effective therapy must always be based upon an essentially psychotherapeutic and facilitative relationship between clinician and stutterer. Whether

a technique succeeds or fails, or should be introduced at all, may hinge upon the quality of the therapeutic relationship.

16. Every therapist, like every parent, must recognize that his progeny will become independent of him. He should do all he can to facilitate that process and to help the stutterer become his own clinician, or perhaps better, his own clinical resource.

BASIC THERAPY PROCEDURES

In this section we list, with brief explanations where necessary, a number of practical methods in therapy. Developed originally for adults, with modifications appropriate to age level and with due sensitivity to the roles of family members in the ongoing problem, these methods apply to any stutterer who must be worked with directly. For an adolescent or older child stutterer irretrievably into the secondary stage, these are a few of the differences which must be considered: (a) The child is often dragged or drafted into therapy, so that his motivation differs. What starts out as the parents' project must become his own if he is to succeed. (b) His level of conceptualization differs and the rationales for the techniques must be simplified. Usually, it is better to get a stutterer involved in action-taking without heavy preliminary explanation. Reasons for procedures seldom have to be explained to those who have performed them. (c) In the child the stuttering is much more likely to be serving a protective function.

Before undertaking one of the following procedures, the clinician needs to have assimilated thoroughly the Clinical Principles of the preceding section. Though the order of listing forms an approximate sequence in which the techniques are introduced in group or individual therapy, various modifications may be undertaken by the clinician in the light of his sensitivity and judgment.

The following procedures are phrased as they might be directly to the stutterer:

1. **Eye Contact** Interpersonal communication is nearly always facilitated by eye contact, and that between speaker and listener is particularly important. You soon learn that you shape the audience response depending on the attitude you display. If you avert your eyes when you stutter, you increase the shame and the

mystery, and you lose touch with your audience. Four points are particularly worth noting:

(a) Establish eye contact *before* you begin to speak. Two or three seconds of quiet eye contact can get you off to a better start.

(b) Some people will look away no matter how much you try to keep contact. To succeed, it is sufficient that *you* look at them.

(c) At first you may find yourself staring people down, but don't worry about it. You can over-correct a little and then let the pendulum swing back. No stutterer ever had a sustained problem of too much eye contact.

(d) Later on you may occasionally look away from your listener, which is natural. But be sure you don't look down or away just at the moment of stuttering.

2. **Discussing Stuttering** You can begin accepting your role as a stutterer by discussing freely the problem of stuttering and the fact that you've begun therapy. You might do a "Gallup-type" poll with a sample of strangers and find out what their attitudes are. Let all your friends hear you talk about stuttering so there's no taboo and they also feel free to discuss it.

3. **Exploring Your Stuttering** We want to explore your stuttering, and we invite you to do the same. Oddly enough you probably do not know what you do when you "stutter." Because it is unpleasant, you have probably covered it up from yourself as well as others. Let us discover all the tricks and crutches you use now or ever have used. When you have explored your stuttering pattern, you will not have so much fear of the unknown.

4. **Learning the Language of Responsibility** Your stuttering is not something that happens to you, but something that you do. See if you can observe and describe your stuttering in language that recognizes that you have a part in it, that it is your own behavior. You are doing the doing. You have responsibility and you have choice. Read Dean Williams' article (1957) and learn what he means by the "it," or animism in stuttering.

5. **Monitoring** Your first job is to observe continuously what you do, a process we call monitoring. If you

really monitor well, you will begin to drop many of your crutches automatically. You can make faster progress by alert monitoring than by consciously trying to prevent your crutches.

6. **Initiative and Fear-Seeking** You will progress much farther and speak much better if you keep seeking out feared words and situations instead of just letting them happen to you. The "initiative set" is incompatible with the "avoidance set" for each new speaking situation. In stuttering therapy you never stand still. Unless you are pushing back the frontiers of fear and difficulty, you are lapsing into retreat.

7. **Exposing the Iceberg** Get as much of your stuttering above the surface as you can. And after studying the iceberg diagram (Chapter 1, figure 2) draw your own "iceberg of shame and guilt" in different situations during the day.

8. **Counting Successes and Failures** Keep expanding your successes, and your failures will dwindle. For example, count it as a success if you stutter openly and get more of your iceberg above the surface or if you are able to make your stuttering more overt.

9. **Stuttering Openly and Easily** Make your stuttering a public event. Let your listener know exactly the kind of trouble you are having through an open display of your stuttering.

10. **Resisting Time Pressure** Record instances of how you react to time pressure, and create several such situations for yourself. How much of the pressure you felt was due to the other person's behavior and how much was your own internalized time pressure set? Note words and situations in which you hurry yourself when there is no need for it.

11. **Pausing and Phrasing: Use of Silence** One of the most conditionable of responses, breathing is notoriously associated with fear states. Lapsing into silence is a natural defensive biological reaction all the way up and down the phyletic scale.

    Part of your built-in time pressure system as a stutterer is that you never pause for breath except in the "dead stops" before feared words. You need to learn to phrase and pause normally so that you do not begin speech on residual air. Much of your problem of forcing results from your failure to pause, with initiation of long sentences on residual air, and almost inevitable hanging up even *before* your first feared word. At that point you may be long out of breath, but your intolerance of silence is such that you dare not pause. If you do, you may feel obligated to go back for a running start on the phrase, and you may actually get stuck at an earlier point. No wonder that your speech may seem hopelessly entangled in a thicket of everbranching phrasing changes!

12. **Reducing Struggle**   You struggle because you try to avoid and conceal and deny your stuttering. This is a principal source of your muscle tension. Monitor closely and observe carefully several blocks. After each ask yourself, "Why did I force so much? What was I trying to cover up?" It is much better to ask yourself, "Why force?" than it is to tell yourself to relax, for that only becomes a source of more tension. Though it is folly to try to relax as a means of avoiding stuttering, it is a perfectly good idea to explore how relaxedly you can stutter, provided you are open about it.

13. **Voluntary Stuttering**   The principle of negative practice stated that you can eliminate bad habits by practicing them consciously. Research has shown that the most effective form of voluntary stuttering is a smooth syllable prolongation or "slide" on non-feared words. You should slide, or stutter voluntarily, principally on non-feared words. You may also find it useful to slide as an alternative method of stuttering on feared words. However, unless you keep safety margin as suggested below, this can easily become a crutch.

14. **Nonreinforcement**   You will find that there is a motor or instrumental side to your stuttering, as well as the emotional or attitude side. So far we have concentrated on attitude and openness, because that is of first importance. However, for eventually smoother speech, you must begin to do something about the vicious circle of self-reinforcement of your tricks. Whenever you use a trick to get the word out, you are strengthen-

iny your habit of using that crutch, and you will be more likely to use it next time. Monitor well enough to sense what is the *moment of release*, the point at which the fear seems to have subsided sufficiently so you feel you can say the word. This is your main point of reinforcement. Here are three examples of ways to weaken the reinforcement of your stuttering pattern. (1) See whether you can stutter smoothly and openly beyond release. By making your "block" longer you can make it easier. (2) If you find you have used a jerky release anyway, or have used a trick, say the word a second time stuttering more smoothly and openly. (3) Say the word over and over again until you have said it at least once fluently. Be public about it. You thereby bring about reinforcement of a newer and smoother style of stuttering—and eventually of speech.

15. **Safety Margin and Tolerance for Disfluency**   Most stutterers keep themselves under tension by trying to speak as perfectly as possible. Oversatisfy the fear or do a little more stuttering voluntarily than you would otherwise have to do in each situation. Then you do not have to strain to be as fluent as possible. When you oversatisfy the fear and develop an acceptance of your natural disfluencies and bobbles, you will have developed a "safety margin." As a healthy byproduct of safety margin, you will become much more fluent.

16. **Direct Natural Speech Attempts**   Early in therapy we discouraged direct attempts at fluency and helped you learn to scoff at "false fluency." When you have become more open and have dropped your crutches you may be ready for a next important step: direct attempts on feared words. There is nothing wrong with consciously directed fluency provided no tricks are being used. At this point you can also begin to work on better phrase emphasis and inflection, more effective use of silences and pauses and other features of effective speaking.

17. **Adjusting to Fluency**   You may be astonished that fluency is anything to which you would have to adjust. Yet it is a central problem in the consolidation of im-

provement. Just as in the early phases of therapy, you had to accept your role as a stutterer, so in the later phases, you have to accept your role as a more normal speaker. The second adjustment is sometimes bigger than the first one. You have to overcome the feeling that all fluency is false and undeserved. You may even need to accept the responsibility and disappointment that results when you learn that your conquest of stuttering does not magically solve every other problem in life.

THE SMORGASBORD
OF STUTTERING THERAPY

Therapies for stuttering often take the form of a mixed bag, a variety of techniques. Within the same therapy we may find elements which motivate the stutterer toward approach, toward avoidance, or toward both at the same time.

In the smorgasbord of stuttering therapy, a variety of techniques is made available, and the client tastes, rejects or accepts based on his individual inclinations. One man's favorite dish is anathema to another, though all methods must meet the basic criteria of facilitating approach rather than avoidance, fostering self-acceptance and openness.

It is fascinating to observe the individual reactions to the "same" therapy program as presented in our beginning group. Assuming in Rankian fashion the presence of a growth impulse, a will to health, an underlying drive toward positive personality change, this self-selection of therapy methods appears highly desirable.

Just as infants in the classical Davis "free-feeding" experiments tended to choose for themselves the diet their bodies needed, so stutterers in therapy, when properly oriented toward the elimination of posing and false role-playing, tend to choose role assignments they need. They may grasp for role enactments beyond their reach, but that is another problem.

As an example of the mixed ingredients of therapy, let us take the author's personal experience as a clinic stutterer during 1939–41. Avowedly, the therapy was a shotgun approach (Van Riper, 1943, 1958). Stuttering was seen as evidence of insufficient cerebral dominance, which the therapy in part aimed to correct. This portion of the therapy, which made up the majority of the activities within the clinic, consisted of: simultaneous talking and writing; vertical board writing; rhythm practice with jaw bite, tongue protrusion, and panting; abandonment of two-handed activities such as typing and piano-playing, and use of the preferred hand wherever possible in order to improve one's margin of cerebral dominance.

Since I was already as thoroughly right-handed as it is possible for anyone to be, and since the activities were tedious and monotonous as well as logically irrelevant, I reached an early satiation point and refused to carry out that part of the therapy. I could not learn to throw myself into a "real block," nor learn to experience and react to the experience of what were supposed to be my neurological blocks.

Though I must have seemed a resistant "black sheep," I could not commit myself to exercises that made no sense in relation to stuttering as I had experienced it all my life. Alone in my room, I seemed to have plenty of cerebral dominance, for I could talk perfectly well. Why should my cerebral dominance vanish when I went to see the personnel manager of Kellogg's about a job? That was like facing up against a sheer cliff towering over me—the element that we have since researched as the role of authority in stuttering (Sheehan, Hadley, & Gould, 1967). Why should I bite my jaws or tap my fingers or pant my breath in unison with a rhythm pattern on a record disc in the speech laboratory? To be sure, I had read Travis's systematic formulation of the theory, expressed with brilliance and clarity in *Speech Pathology* (Travis, 1931). The experimental evidence amassed up to that time seemed overwhelming, but I could not seriously believe that it really applied to my case.

And I was right. In the light of today's evidence, my skepticism was sound. In pointing this out I lay no claim to sixth-sense infallibility, but rather wish to illustrate the principle that the stutterer often knows and senses what is good for him, if given a chance by the therapist.

One man's poison is another man's meat, and there were stutterers in the same clinic who seemed to gain some measure of security and fluency from the regimen just described. Whether this was due to cumulative suggestion or to the Hawthorne effect is anybody's backward guess. But I did observe it, though the improvement may have derived from other aspects of what was a fairly complex therapy program. Maybe they belonged to a different subtype, another subspecies. The "same" therapy may be experienced in entirely different ways by different stutterers. Yet to me the margin of dominance that needed strengthening was not cerebral but interpersonal.

Illustrating further the principle that therapy is often experienced as a mixture, other elements in Van Riper therapy circa 1940 provided me crucial experiences and turning points. For example, for the first time I had an alternative to the old panicky feeling of approaching difficulty. I could stutter in a different way. I could stutter voluntarily, and in time was able to do so without so much wincing, grimacing, and hatred. I learned that the trick I used at the moment of release, or point at which I could complete the word, soon became incorporated into my habitual pattern. When I thrust open my mouth or bobbed my head and successfully brought the word out, these behaviors were strengthened. The probability of their occurrence next time was increased. Easily recognizable today as the reinforcement principle, this was one of the most important ideas in Van Riper's therapy. He held the concept and taught it to me in the early 1940s, long before it appeared in the literature. The experimental modification of stuttering through nonreinforcement, which I carried out as a doctoral study at Michigan during 1948–1949, derived from his technique of "cancellation" (Sheehan, 1951).

To return to my experiences in the clinic, through advertising my stuttering I lost some of the fear of discovery. Through study of the literature, stuttering lost some of its mystery —though ample remained and still does. Through contact with other stutterers, I discovered that I was not alone, but a member of a rather large fraternity, and that Van Riper himself was a stutterer unashamed. And a conspicuously successful one. Though even when I left to become a chemist in 1941, I had not learned "control" and still stuttered severely, I had improved sufficiently to see a ray of light at the end of the tunnel.

Working on my own, I set about to eliminate every last trace of avoidance. Control? Forget it! Control means suppression, and there's nothing there to control, nothing but yourself. By the time I had succeeded in reducing every last vestige of avoidance of words or situations, I was stuttering smoothly with ever decreasing frequency and speaking with a constantly expanding fluency.

That, at least in part, was my route to recovery. I suppose I did what every stutterer needs to do, that is, pick and choose (though not just on the basis of what's easy) and adapt the therapy to himself, to make it his own project. In this respect our stuttering therapy is and perhaps should be a smorgasbord.

What a therapist offers a stutterer is much like the teaching a parent offers a child—part of it will be lost, and part may have great impact, but you cannot foresee which part will be which.

THE GROUP AS THERAPIST

Since stuttering is an interpersonal self-presentation disorder and occurs in a social context, group therapy is a natural choice for adults. In combination with varying degrees of subgroup and individual therapy, we have worked out a fairly unique structure unifying stuttering therapy with major aspects of psychotherapy.

Stutterers can do things for each other in groups that no individual therapist can accomplish. Social isolation, at least in the lonesome sense of feeling like a probable freak—or an improbable one—is a core feeling in stuttering. Against this background, the discovery that you are not alone, that your experiences are shared and sharable with others like you, can be in itself enormously therapeutic. Particularly is this true if the group is used as a springboard for action.

Groups are always to some extent at the mercy of their composition, and group members can be destructive as well as supportive. As Travis once pointed out, in a group you are exposed not only to the support of other egos, but the criticism of other superegos (Travis, 1953). How can the therapist keep the group moving toward legitimate therapeutic goals, yet still let the members feel that it is their group and that they are doing the moving? This is one of the major challenges for any group therapist, particularly in the action-oriented, role-taking therapy needed by most stutterers.

The group therapist working with stutterers needs to be active and influential without becoming such a dominant force that the members are too dependent on him. He needs to be highly permissive on the feeling level, without being completely permissive or casual on the doing level. What the stutterer does in response to his feelings is of greatest importance —it is at the very heart of stuttering therapy.

On this point, we might say to a stutterer something like this:

> *Catharsis is great for the soul, but if you are*
> *going to change, you have to get into action, to*
> *do something. You are changed by what you do,*

297

> *not by what you think about, read about, talk about, write about, intellectualize about, or emote about. Ventilation may help you feel better about your failings but unless you change your reinforcement pattern you are going to continue them.*

Clinical sensitivity and interpersonal judgment, essential requisites for any group psychotherapy, are constantly demanded in working with stutterers. The beginner may lead too much or too little—and so may the experienced therapist on a bad day. Though the dangers of being too domineering are readily perceived, unless some leadership and challenge is exercised the group may drift toward avoidance.

For example, in the early 1950s we fostered the development of a stutterer's club known as Stutterers Unanimous. The membership was open to those who had passed through the clinic for at least a semester, and was visualized as having a kind of maintenance function. The members might help each other as Alcoholics Anonymous does, but without divine guidance or invocation.

In an effort to be democratic, we kept a hands-off policy and didn't provide secular guidance either. Unhappily for this venture into clinical democracy in action, the experiment went sour. Leaderless at first, the club was soon taken over by a few clubbily-motivated "officers" and their wives, with by-laws, minutes, treasurer's reports and other officious procedures. The meetings became massively boring to all those who still wanted to do something about their stuttering problem, and these better members soon departed, leaving for those who remained a well-geared vehicle for social withdrawal from the world of those who did not stutter. At some meetings they even swapped new distraction devices, and hunted the pink pill! The counterfeit currency and the real could not coexist, and the real disappeared.

The group alloy is a function of the mettle of its members.

Fortunately, not every group turns out as did Stutterers Unanimous. Since that experience, we have utilized many advanced stutterers who have been through our therapy program as auxiliary clinicians. They merge into the clinic staff, providing a mix of normal speakers and stutterers. Perhaps the mix helps to prevent the social withdrawal that for stutterers' clubs is always an available tangent.

Outstanding examples are Leonard, formerly a very severe

stutterer whose case is reported in the Speech Foundation of America (1968) booklet, *Stuttering: Successes and Failures in Therapy;* and Thomas, who described his path toward recovery at the 1968 meetings of the American Speech and Hearing Association in Denver. Both appear in the educational film, *The Iceberg of Stuttering,*[2] where their interactions with others may be observed. In each case, the acquisition of a new role as an auxiliary member of the clinic staff solidified the virtually complete recovery each has already achieved.

The Council of Adult Stutterers, led by Gene Walle and Michael Heffron of Catholic University in Washington, D.C., has developed a large, successful, and enthusiastic society of stutterers. Significantly, they identify themselves publicly as stutterers through publications and television programs. With or without formal enrollment in therapy, such public identification and group role acceptance tends to have major therapeutic effects.

FOOTBALL HUDDLE THERAPY

The structure of the adult stutterer's group may be likened to that of a football huddle. Although the analogy is crude, it does convey picturesquely the reciprocal roles of clinician and group member. We may begin something like this:

> *This group is like a football huddle. It is not the whole game, but an analysis and planning session. You're going to get a chance to play with a new system—an S-Formation—a How-You-Stutter formation. We're going to show you a new way to play this game. We are your coaches. We can teach you the system. We can give you new plays and some ways of hitting a line. But you have to carry the ball. You have to do the blocking—if we may be forgiven a very bad pun. Most of all, you have to carry the ball into the game to score a victory, and only you can do it. We can show you a new way of tackling this problem. But we're on the side-lines. Taking the ball and running with it for a touchdown is up to you. How much do you*

[2]Available from Academic Communication Facility, University of California, Los Angeles.

> *want to win this game? How much are you*
> *willing to do?*

"Football huddle therapy" dramatizes the fundamental point that therapy is a center for role analysis and action-planning. The game is won or lost in the real world outside the clinic. The reiterated weekly or daily challenge is, "In terms of what your own observation tells you, what do you *need to do?* What *will you do* between now and next time?"

As in every game of life, there are players who choose to remain on the bench. Others sound great in the huddle but shirk the playing; their role perceptions are fine but their self-concepts do not permit enactment of the roles. Still others have potential but lack available readiness for change. For these some form of psychotherapy is indicated, be it insight-oriented or merely supportive. Many others could be outstanding but never get a chance to be on the team.

An important advantage of the football huddle structure is that it permits the clinician to shatter the magic-wand expectations that are twin residents with despair in the psychology of stuttering. The analogy of the coach sitting on the sidelines, while the game is really played by the man on the field, is a useful model of the stutterer-clinician relationship.

FEATURES OF GROUP
AND INDIVIDUAL THERAPY

Following are some of the special reasons for employing group therapy in the treatment of adolescent and adult stutterers:

1. Since stuttering is a social relations disorder, and occurs in an interpersonal context, it is naturally treated in a social setting.
2. The damaging and limiting self-perceptions of the stutterer have been created through successive reinforcements from the opinions of others. Change can best come about through "significant others" (Mead, 1934) as the members of the stutterer's group typically become.
3. Since the therapy itself is an action-oriented, role-taking psychotherapy, and requires courage in facing situations from which the stutterer has always retreated, group support and sharing of the adventure

of tackling feared situations is often needed to carry the stutterer through.

4. For the adolescent, peer relationships are especially important—moreover, mixing adolescent and adult stutterers for a portion of the group or subgroup meetings facilitates positive opinion change.

5. Part of therapy consists in "Discovering your own stuttering patterns and underlying attitudes in relation to those of others. Sharing opens up the process. You find that you are not alone, that your experiences and feelings are not unique, that you are not a freak who belongs in a closet."

6. Stuttering behaviors, tricks and crutches, and avoidances of all kinds may likewise be compared and contrasted. "Look around you. There are many different ways to stutter. What is so good about your particular stuttering pattern? You have a choice. You can go on your old way or learn a new way. You do not have a choice about whether you stutter, but you do have a choice about *how.*"

7. "Responsibility for your own behavior, for the fact that you are doing the doing, is of great importance. In a group you can learn this in interaction with other stutterers as you observe their descriptions of their stuttering as something happening to them, or as a condition, rather than as something they are actually doing."

8. Initiative may be originated or inspired in a group experience.

9. A stutterer who has authority problems with an individual therapist may be more comfortable in a group.

10. Discussions in a group may facilitate insight, and there are some who may talk about things close to themselves more freely in a group than in face-to-face individual therapy.

11. Finally, in a group therapeutic dependency may be diluted.

On the other hand, certain advantages accrue from individual contact:

1. Each person feels that he needs to have some individual contact with his therapist. Groups may be the main healing medium, but client expectations call for individual conference.

2. Obviously, certain aspects of case history may be more efficiently covered in individual sessions. We have found the Recovery Interview useful (Sheehan & Martyn, 1966), as well as the Sentence Completion Test for Stutterers (Sheehan, 1956; Griffith, 1969) and the Lanyon Severity Scale (Lanyon, 1967).

3. Since members of the family are always members of the problem, some contact with them is desirable, particularly with adolescents or stutterers still living in the parental home. In a single family interaction, the clinician may glimpse interpersonal dynamics that might take months to appear or might never surface at all.

CONFLICT LEVELS
AND THERAPY SEQUENCE

The view of stuttering as a self-presentation disorder and a self-role conflict in its probable origins, as a speaker-listener status gap problem in its most important manifestation, points to certain logical directions in therapy. First, the self-esteem and security of the stutterer needs to be built up, especially in the speaker role. Second, the awesomeness of the listener needs to be decreased through better interpersonal relationships. These are similar to common prescriptions for any psychotherapy.

Psychotherapy and speech therapy for stutterers, or what has come to be called stuttering therapy, are similarly in concert in the goal of reducing "holding back" or avoidance behaviors of all kinds. Stuttering is a double approach-avoidance conflict, with self and role conflicts representing deeper levels. Other conflict levels include: word, situation, feelings, and relationship.

> *The blocking in speech may reflect a conflict between speaking or not speaking a feared word, meeting or avoiding a threatening situation, expressing or inhibiting unacceptable feelings, accepting or rejecting certain social roles or interpersonal relationships, and entering into or retreating from certain lifelong endeavors, aspired roles, and other competitive callings (Sheehan, 1954a).*

For the adult, it is usually advisable to offer speech therapy first, and let the person's reactions to speech therapy serve as an index of his need for psychotherapy. That is, with the adult, we begin with word and speech situation fears, which are of most immediate concern to him anyway, offering the experiences typically afforded by "stuttering therapy," in reality a specialized psychotherapy, a form of behavior therapy.

A useful feature of the differentiation of the conflict levels is that for the child the sequence is typically the reverse of that for the adult.

For the Adult	For the Child
1. word	5. self-role (ego protective)
2. situation	4. relationship
3. feeling	3. feeling
4. relationship	2. situation
5. self-role (ego-protective)	1. word

FOR THE CHILD:

FAMILY-CENTERED THERAPY

Let us avoid for a moment the semantic problem of whether the child is to be called a stutterer, or whether he is primary, transitional, secondary (à la Van Riper, 1963b), or in one of Bloodstein's developmental stages (Bloodstein, 1960a; 1960b). With a young child still living in the parental environment, still caught in the matrix out of which his stuttering emerged, such tortured exercises in taxonomy are largely academic. The major directions of therapy are clear and specifiable in any case.

With a young child still in the family circle, direct speech therapy should more often be a last resort rather than a starting point. In our studies of spontaneous recovery from stuttering, at least some of the discouraging results of public school therapy appeared to stem from offering direct speech therapy to a child too early, without any substantial relief of the background pressures. Small wonder for this sorry condition. Working with the family is enormously difficult, and often the system does not provide incentives for it. Working with the stuttering child is usually much easier, and the system does reward this with daily attendance records. What is the beleaguered therapist to do? Parents are often hard to budge, even for skilled, experienced and authoritative clinicians.

What are the "clear and specifiable directions" of therapy for the child? First, a recognition that the problem does not reside inside the skin of the child. Members of the family are members of the problem (Johnson, 1961). The stuttering child is the parents' symptom (Travis, 1957). He is a statement about them—and they are quite correct in regarding it as unflattering. Yet they may in fact not be dramatically different or worse in their handling of their child than other parents whose offspring did not respond with a symptomatic reproach. Putting pressure on a child is like driving across a railroad crossing without looking. Most of the time you can get away with it. But the gain is not worth the risk. The parents of stutterers were probably not behaving conspicuously worse than others. They just got caught at it.

With the child, we ask first, What are the defensive needs of this stutterer? What are the competitive pressures? What are the functions that stuttering as a symptom is serving? We examine the relationships that the young stutterer has with his parents, siblings and school associates. We explore his feelings in areas not particularly pertaining to speech, and use his stuttering as a guide to problem areas. A psychotherapeutic approach necessarily involves consideration of all the significant others, all the important figures in the child's life.

Frequently we explore the family pressures and other environmental factors eliciting onset stuttering behaviors in young children with assignments for the parents. These assignments should be given in writing and should call for a simple but thorough written report.

During the next week observe five situations in which your child had a particularly great amount of difficulty. For each situation observe carefully and answer thoughtfully the following:

1. To whom was he speaking?
2. What was he trying to say?
3. What form did his difficulty take? What did he actually do?
4. To what observable pressures in the situation was the stuttering a response?
5. How did he react to his own difficulty? How much awareness did he show? What did he do to cover up or otherwise struggle with the difficulty?
6. How did his listeners react? What did they do and say?
7. How did he react to their reactions?

8. In your own words, what is causing him to continue to have difficulty?

Write down each answer immediately or as soon as possible after you observe, so you do not have to depend too much on recall.

For the five situations in which he is most fluent or speaks most easily or successfully, observe and answer thoughtfully these questions.

1. To whom is he speaking?
2. What was he trying to say?
3. How fluent was he? Did he have little bobbles or disfluencies that he seemed to ignore or react to easily?
4. What was there about this situation that made speaking easier?
5. Did he seem aware that he was speaking better than usual? Did he go on and on?
6. How did those listening react to his relative fluency? Did they show surprise? Did anyone praise his fluency or tell him that he was improving?[3]
7. How did he react to any listener reactions he may have received?
8. In your own words, why was he able to speak better in the situation you observed?

Data provided the clinician by the foregoing assignment, and others like it, are of two kinds:

First, the answers themselves point significantly to certain interpersonal and situational factors. For example, if the child has his worst moments in situations where a younger brother or sister is competing for attention, this is an obvious lead. Did the best speech occur in a quiet one-to-one relationship with a playmate? With mother, but not with father? With father, but not with mother? Is somebody a constant source of interruption threat? What situation seems to provide the most security, as reflected in speech? These are the raw data of parent counseling with young stutterers.

Second, and equally significant is the evidence contained in

---

[3]In the typical situation of the young stutterer neither one of these comments is advisable since they may easily have destructive effects. The comment "that was fine, you didn't stutter at all" is well intended but misguided. Even a very young child easily concludes that if he is good when he speaks fluently, he must be bad when he stutters. Much experimentation shows that for most stutterers, increasing the penalty has the predominant effect of increasing the frequency of stuttering.

the parent's response to the assignment. When a mother brings in shoddy notes carelessly scrawled on the back of an old envelope, as we have experienced in actual cases, she gainsays her glib statement that she is willing to do anything for her child. The parent who reports that he did not have opportunity to make the observations, or did not have time, is bringing in the most important data of all. Such examples could be multiplied many times. Dealing with the parent and the problem at this point is a challenge to the general clinical and psychotherapeutic skills of the clinician.

We cannot emphasize too strongly that the foregoing assignment is intended primarily as a guide to interpersonal factors —not just how the child is doing on his speech. Too often we find therapists balancing delicate semantics with parents over labels to describe speech behavior, shrinking in the process from dealing more with significant relationships within the family. Many parents indulge in a search for a mechanism, or hope for some simple physical cause. Organic theories of stuttering may have flunked the test of scientific survival, but they still have great appeal to the parent who is offended by any suggestion that he may have been responsible and ought to change.

Where the young stutterer must be worked with directly, it is often desirable to have a second clinician deal exclusively with the parents. In this way the stutterer feels that he is getting the attention of a parent figure who is not reporting everything back to the parents. Many general techniques of family therapy (Satir, 1964) may be applicable here.

For older and more severe stutterers we sometimes add an optional assignment for parents: to learn their child's stuttering pattern well enough so that they can imitate it, to learn to enact his role in outside situations enough to experience directly some of the social reactions the stutterer must experience. Though difficult, if they can be cajoled or challenged into doing it, the resultant motivation toward reducing pressures can be dramatic.

Unhappily, parental incorrigibility is a frequent problem in stuttering. Those who resist the assignment most are likely to be most in need of acquiring a better empathy with their stuttering offspring. And those who created the symptom by putting on pressures fail to heed even the most earnest clinical pleas to ease up, after having failed in the first place to be deterred by the emergence of stuttering behaviors.

If the parents cannot rally to a clinical appeal and the pressures continue, then we have no choice but to try to teach the child how to cope with his stuttering. With other avenues of appeal exhausted, we offer the child a miniaturized and child-adapted model of what we might do for an adult. However, such direct therapy for a child living with his parents offers many complexities beyond those already present in adult therapy. For example, we sometimes undertake the clinically risky enterprise of helping the young stutterer learn how to cope with his parents.

Unless the child has a sharply developed awareness of himself as a stutterer, and is actively struggling to keep his stuttering hidden, we should not deal with his word or situation fears in specific terms. Even for children who seem to be thoroughly into the secondary stage of stuttering, the level of awareness may not be at all comparable to that seen in the adult secondary stutterer. An indirect approach is advisable in the beginning even though the child shows a great many secondary characteristics. With young secondary stutterers, it is probably better to try first a program aimed at relieving the conflict at role and relationship levels and to use speech therapy only after indirect measures have failed. Leave the child alone, and treat the parents! This is a great motto in speech pathology, but it is broken more often than the Ten Commandments.

The adult stutterer remains an adult stutterer because he will not accept his role as stutterer and will not give up his avoidances. Examine clinically the situation behaviors of any stutterer who is not making progress, and you will find many "Islands of Avoidance," or areas of reservation of the old concealment behavior.

The child stutterer remains a stutterer because his parents will not permit their pressures on him to subside. A child who continues to stutter is a child whose parents put on too much pressure in the first place and then refuse to relent. In every sense he is his parents' symptom.

Since stuttering can and does become self-perpetuating to some extent, even the removal of the pressures may require some time for a noticeable diminution of the stuttering. As noted in Chapter 8, recoveries involve fundamental changes in the self-concept and take time.

SUMMARY

Stuttering is a role-specific disorder that can include many different personalities, and is not a unitary phenomenon. As a false-role disorder and a disorder of the social presentation of the self, stuttering is amenable to a role-specific therapy. Therapy should not aim at immediate fluency, but at the reduction of fear, avoidance, and false-role mannerisms. Therapy methods may be evaluated according to whether they lead to approach behavior or to avoidance behavior, and whether they lead to authentic or to false-role enactment. Criteria for success or failure in therapy are specified. Stuttering involves a primary loss as well as secondary gain. Psychotherapy may be seen as a process of role-taking, and "stuttering therapy," a special example, is a pioneering form of behavior therapy. Every stutterer selects from the smorgasbord of therapy those experiences most significant for him. "Control" is a fallacy in therapy because it leads to suppression. Responsibility, choice and initiative are key elements in adult therapy. With young stutterers some form of family therapy is essential. Since stuttering is a social milieu problem and a self-presentation problem, it is best treated in a social context.

References

References that are listed here only by author and year of publication appear in complete form in the Bibliography.

Ainsworth, S. (1957)

Andrews, G., and Harris, M. (1964)

Beech, H. R., and Fransella, F. (1968)

Biggs, B. E., and Sheehan, J. G. (1969)

Bloodstein, O. N. (1958)

Bloodstein, O. N. (1960a)

Bloodstein, O. N. (1960b)

Brutten, E. J., and Shoemaker, D. J. (1967)

Conway, J. K., and Quarrington, B. (1963)

Dollard, J., and Miller, N. E. (1950) *Personality and psychotherapy.* New York: McGraw-Hill.

Dunlap, K. (1932) *Habits: Their making and unmaking.* New York: Liveright.

Frederick, C. J., III (1955) An investigation of learning theory and reinforcement as related to stuttering behavior. Ph.D. thesis, University of California, Los Angeles.

Freud, S. (1914) *The psychopathology of everyday life.* New York: Modern Library.

Gregory, H. H. (1968)

Griffith, F. A. (1969)

Hunt, J. (1863) *Stammering and stuttering, their nature and treatment.* London: Longmans, Green.

Johnson, W. (1955)

Johnson, W., *et al.* (1961a)

Johnson, W., *et al.* (1962)

Johnson, W., *et al.* (1967)

Lanyon, R. I. (1967)

Martyn, M. M., and Sheehan, J. G. (1968)

Quarrington, B. (1956)

Rank, O. (1936) *Will therapy.* New York: Knopf.

Sarbin, T. R. (1964) Role theoretical interpretation of psychological change. In P. Worchel and D. Byrne, Eds., *Personality change.* New York: Wiley.

Sarbin, T. R. (1954) Role theory. In G. Lindzey, Ed., *Handbook of social psychology.* Reading, Mass.: Addison-Wesley.

Satir, V. M. (1964) *Conjoint family therapy.* Palo Alto, Calif.: Science & Behavior Books.

Shearer, W. M., and Williams, J. D. (1965)

Sheehan, J. G. (1950) The fight to speak. University Explorer broadcast, University of California, Berkeley. Columbia Broadcasting System, May 27.

Sheehan, J. G. (1951)

Sheehan, J. G. (1954a)

Sheehan, J. G. (1958a)

Sheehan, J. G. (1958b)

Sheehan, J. G. (1960) Research frontiers in stuttering. Psychology Speech Clinic, UCLA (mimeographed).

Sheehan, J. G. (1963a) The effect of role commitment on stuttering. Paper read at Ninth World Congress of the International Society for Rehabilitation of the Disabled, Copenhagen, Denmark, June 23–29.

Sheehan, J. G. (1963b) Successes and failures in stuttering therapy. Symposium, American Speech and Hearing Association, Chicago, November 5.

Sheehan, J. G. (1968)

Sheehan, J. G. (1969)

Sheehan, J. G., and Martyn, M. M. (1966)

Sheehan, J. G., and Martyn, M. M. (1970) Stuttering and its disappearance. *Journal of Speech and Hearing Research,* *13,* No. 2. Reprinted on E. P. Trapp, and P. Himelstein, *Readings on the exceptional child: Research and theory* (Revised). New York: Appleton, 1970.

Sheehan, J. G., and Voas, R. B. (1957)

Sheehan, J. G., Cortese, P., and Hadley, R. G. (1962)

Sheehan, J. G., Hadley, R. G., and Gould, E. (1967)

Sheehan, J. G., *et al.* (1957) A symposium of recovered stutterers. American Speech and Hearing Association, Cincinnati, November 18.

Skinner, B. F. (1957a) The experimental analysis of behavior. *American Scientist, 45,* 343–371.

Skinner, B. F. (1957b) *Verbal behavior.* New York: Appleton.

Solomon, R. L., and Wynne, L. C. (1954) Traumatic avoidance learning: The principle of anxiety conservation and partial irreversibility. *Psychological Review, 61,* 353–385.

Speech Foundation of America (1960) *On stuttering and its treatment.* Memphis, Tenn.: M. Fraser.

Speech Foundation of America (1964) *Treatment of the young stutterer in the school.* Memphis, Tenn.: Fraser.

Stunden, A. A. (1965)

Stunden, A. A. (1966) Computer simulation of therapy: The client-therapist match. *Journal of the American Speech and Hearing Association, 8,* 100–104.

Taylor, I. K., and Taylor, M. M. (1967)

Travis, L. E. (1931) *Speech pathology.* New York: Appleton.

Travis, L. E. (1953) Talk before the Western Speech Association, Tucson, Arizona, October 15.

Van Riper, C. (1937a) The growth of the stuttering spasm. *Quarterly Journal of Speech, 23,* 70–73.

Van Riper, C. (1937b) The effect of devices for minimizing stuttering on the creation of symptoms. *Journal of Abnormal and Social Psychology, 32,* 185–192.

Van Riper, C. (1943) In E. Hahn, *Stuttering: Significant theories and therapies.* Stanford, Calif.: Stanford University Press.

Van Riper, C. (1958)

Van Riper, C. (1963b)

Williams, D. E. (1957)

Wingate, M. E. (1964)

Wischner, G. J. (1950)

Wischner, G. J. (1952b)

About the Author Dr. Sheehan is identified at the beginning of Chapter 1.

About the Chapter Progress towards the conquest of stuttering can only be as solid as our research on the disorder. If we are to move ahead we must constantly find better ways—we must discard unserviceable, unworkable ideas and test out promising new concepts. In a closing chapter entitled "Research Frontiers," the author delineates common methodological pitfalls and offers principles for future scientific exploration of the problem called stuttering.

8

RESEARCH
FRONTIERS

JOSEPH G. SHEEHAN

8

THE KNOWN AND THE UNKNOWN

The known facts on stuttering are outnumbered by its mysteries. We do not know a precise cause of stuttering, nor whether a single precise cause exists. The treatments for stuttering, and the conditions under which it appears and disappears, are extremely diverse. Although vast research effort has gone into various attacks on the problem of stuttering, many basic features about the disorder remain puzzling.

The clinical phenomena are fairly well recognized and have been extensively described and catalogued in terms of primary symptoms, secondary symptoms, and symptoms transitional between these two pages (Van Riper, 1963). In this country the term "stuttering" is employed by those who have done most of the scientific work on the problem as a generic term including both the repetitive patterns more common in children and the blocking, grimacing behavior characteristic of the adult. At one time the term "stammering" was widely used, either as a euphemism or in an abortive effort to break the disorder into two subclasses, those of stuttering (repetition) and stammering (silent blocking). However, the attempted distinction has been abandoned, for (1) too many cases starting out with repetitive symptoms have developed blocking symptoms, and (2) repetition appears to be a symptom common to all those formerly classed as either stutterers or stammerers.[1]

Whether what we classify as stuttering is really a single disorder or whether we deal with a group of disorders is still open to question. Research is needed on possible subtypes within the stuttering group. If subtypes exist, it is unlikely that we shall find a single therapeutic approach suitable for all stutterers. Doctoral researches, such as those of Berlin at Northwestern University (1954) and Frederick at the University of California in Los Angeles (1955), explored possible subtypes. Berlin sought through systematized history data to discover physiological groupings. Finding that some stuttered more with the prospect of reward while others stuttered more with the threat of punishment, Frederick attempted to distinguish these groups in terms of their Minnesota Multiphasic Personality Inventory (MMPI) profiles.

Severe stutterers differ in some rather special ways from mild and moderate stutterers. The spontaneous recovery rate is higher for those who were never severe. The severe were more likely to have received public school therapy (Sheehan & Martyn, 1970). They were more likely to have begun with complete blockings, rather than syllable repetitions. Mild, moderate, and severe stutterers differed from one another in recovery from and continuation in the category of stuttering. Moreover, mild stutterers and severe stutterers differed in their levels of aspiration.

The puzzling lack of personality pattern characteristic of stuttering might be explained if stable subgroupings could be determined.[2] Such a discovery might well lead to the development of principles that would prevent an inappropriate approach in certain cases. If it can be confirmed by replication or cross-validation that, as Frederick suggests, reward serves as a reinforcing mechanism for some stutterers and punishment serves as a reinforcing mechanism for others, then it becomes highly important for success in treatment that the therapist understand with which type he is dealing.

The probability that stuttering is not a unitary disorder grows as we delve further into the issues of the reinforcement

---

[1] A clinical observation pointed out by Froeschels and by Van Riper and corroborated by a phonetic analysis of stuttering phenomena (Sheehan, 1946).

[2] Even if such subgroups could be isolated, however, the process of therapy would by no means be identical within each subgroup.

of stuttering, the puzzle of its continuation despite its apparent unserviceability. The study by Sheehan, Hadley, and Cortese (1962) explored dimensions of guilt, shame, tension, and dejection in graphic portrayals of stutterers' behavior before, during, and after the moment of stuttering. Marked differences in the patterns for individual stutterers suggested that varying patterns of possible reinforcement may occur in different stutterers and that the nature of reinforcement did not appear to be the same for every stutterer. Some appeared to operate on a reward basis, others on a frustration basis.

Further support for the view that stutterers differ markedly as individuals appears in the varied ways in which they recover spontaneously, and in the finding that more than three-fourths of those who develop stuttering as a problem recover spontaneously (Sheehan & Martyn, 1966; Martyn & Sheehan, 1968; Sheehan & Martyn, 1970).

Sometimes stuttering as a disorder of the rhythm of speech is found associated with cluttering,[3] although this association is too rare to throw much light on the problem of stuttering. Bloodstein (1958), Freund (1966), and Weiss (1950) have extensively considered the possible relationship of stuttering and cluttering. We feel that perhaps the most significant commonality is that time pressure is a striking feature of each. In a recent doctoral study at UCLA, Stunden found that stutterers differed from nonstutterers on a word-association task administered under time pressure. As a part of his role conflict, the stutterer develops a built-in, internalized time pressure system, and this appears to be true of the clutterer.

Our knowledge of stuttering is founded upon exploratory studies, survey research, experimental studies, and the consensus provided by repeated clinical observation. Oddly, many of the findings based upon research studies are less widely accepted than are a number of those based upon clinical observation. Perhaps certain clinical observations are so striking or meet such social agreement that no one is motivated to do a study to check on them, while experiments by their nature are usually devoted to resolving areas of question or controversy.

Our task in this chapter is to summarize what is known of

---

[3]Perhaps the best definition of cluttering, like stuttering a disorder of the rhythm of speech, is still that of John Wyllie (1894): ". . . a torrent of half-articulated words, running after one another like peas in a spout."

stuttering, what is partially known, and what is yet largely unknown. As we move through this task, we will try to indicate the underpinnings of fact or belief. It may be well to relate some of the common clinical observations first. They provide some of the best introduction to the disorder and give important clues to its probable nature. So much is known clinically about stuttering that the list is necessarily incomplete and touches only what are generally regarded as major features of the disorder.

WHAT WE KNOW ABOUT STUTTERING

1. Distribution Throughout World

Stuttering has been known for centuries and is today to be found among practically all peoples all over the globe. Cultural variability appears to have some influence upon incidence figures, with possibly fewer stutterers among, for example, North American Plains Indians (Johnson, 1959; Lemert, Chapter 4; Sapir, 1915; Stewart, 1960), but more stutterers among the Moslem Indians of Durban, South Africa (Sheehan, 1960), and among the detribalized Bantu of Johannesburg (Aron, 1960, 1962). Most peoples of the world appear to have well-recognized words for stuttering, many of them onomatopoeic in character (Aron, 1960, 1962; Sheehan, 1960). For example, the Kikuyu word for stuttering is "kuhindahinda" which literally means "stuck in the tongue."

2. Incidence in United States

The incidence of stuttering in the United States is somewhat less than 1 percent of the population (American Speech and Hearing Association, 1957).

3. Age of Onset

The age of onset of stuttering falls principally between 2 and 7, with apparent peaks at 3 and 5.

4. Spontaneous Recovery

Of those children who ever develop a definite problem of stuttering, as judged by themselves and others, approximately four-fifths recover spontaneously (Sheehan & Martyn, 1966, 1970; Martyn & Sheehan, 1968).

This result is depicted graphically in Figure 1. The ratio is lower for severe stutterers, and higher for the mild. For stut-

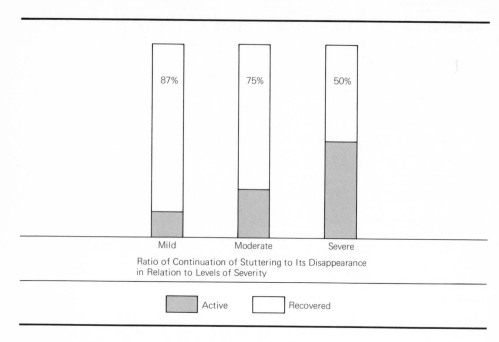

Figure 1 *Disappearance and Continuation of Stuttering in Relation to Severity*

terers who were ever severe, only about one-half recover spontaneously, while for those who were never worse than mild, about seven-eighths recover without treatment.[4]

Recovery tended significantly to occur in early adolescence and early adulthood. As with onset, recovery appears to be a gradual process.

5. Sex Ratio

A striking feature of the disorder is the sex ratio. For reasons that have remained mysterious, about four to five times as many males stutter as females, (American Speech and Hearing Association, 1957; Andrews & Harris, 1964; Johnson *et al.*, 1959; Schuell, 1946).

[4]No wonder medical practitioners so often counsel parents that the child will outgrow stuttering! On how many other disorders are their predictions right 80 percent of the time? Yet nothing in this happy predictive state mitigates harm to the unlucky child who is denied help when he needs it.

6. Familial Incidence Pattern

Repeated studies have shown that stuttering runs in families. While early investigators took this as evidence of a genetic causation, most modern investigators (e.g., Johnson, 1959, and Johnson *et al.*, 1967) have attributed familial incidence to cultural factors. Reported familial incidence may be spuriously high due to what we have called *differential preliminary search*:

> *Stutterers and their families who come into clinics are likely to have searched out the possibility that some relative stutterers, especially since it is supposed to run in families. Each spouse will have scanned the family tree of the other in an effort to discover a stutterer roosting there. Control group families will not have made a comparable intensive search for a stutterer, for they came in for a different problem, or no problem at all* (Sheehan & Martyn, 1967).

7. Physiology

Stuttering has been reported to be related to shift of handedness, but contradictory findings have cast doubts on this observation. No undisputed relationship between stuttering and handedness can be said to exist (Johnson, Darley, & Spriestersbach, 1962; Johnson *et al.*, 1967). Stuttering has not been shown to be related to other problems, either neurological biochemical, or physiological (see Perkins, Chapter 5 in this book).

8. Personality

Stutterers do not show any typical or characteristic personality pattern. Moreover, stutterers do not differ from nonstutterers on any established and measurable dimensions of personality (Goodstein, 1958; Johnson, 1959; Sheehan, 1958b; Sheehan, Chapter 3 in this book).

9. Distraction and Suggestion

Many stutterers relate that they can sing without stuttering; sometimes they can whisper without stuttering. Both of these examples—and there are exceptions to each—seem to involve another key element in stuttering, that of distraction. Any novel stimulus, procedure, or ritual seems to be capable of distracting the stutterer so that the behavior suddenly diminishes. Some stutterers are known to speak more fluently temporarily under strong suggestion or hypnosis.

Bloodstein (1950a) cited distraction effects as one of the two conditions responsible for almost "all of the reductions in stuttering recorded in this study." Biggs and Sheehan (1969) have shown that a famous study, claiming to show operant conditioning in stuttering (Flanagan, Goldiamond, & Azrin, 1958), involved nothing more substantial than the old principle of distraction.

10. Variation with Speaker-listener Relationship

When speaking alone, stutterers tend to be fluent—a significant feature of the disorder. The stutterer is like anyone else except when he talks—an ancient joke that tells us something. Talking involves the speaker and a listener, a relationship between two persons, and it is in the context of the speaker-listener relationship that the stutterer has his difficulty. Telephone and bystander situations involve special threats due to reduced feedback; they are face-to-face situations once removed. Interestingly, a few stutterers experience just the opposite effect and find the telephone their easiest situation. A bystander may evoke more stuttering, when direct speech to the listener is relatively easy. A few stutterers report difficulty when reading aloud to themselves, but it seems they project an audience even when alone. Stuttering, then, has an interpersonal character; it occurs primarily in the context of attempting expression of meaning and feeling in a face-to-face relationship. The problem stems in some degree from the feelings of the stutterer about himself as a person and as a speaker and his feelings about the listeners to whom he must relate via speech (Sheehan, 1953, 1968).

TOWARD A SCIENCE OF COMMUNICATION DISORDERS

1. Verifiability

Verifiability is the ultimate criterion of science. A finding on the relationship between stuttering and handedness, for example, should hold up on replication (repetition of the experiment with a fresh sample of subjects) or cross-validation (checking the validity of predictions from one study to another). From this criterion the science of speech pathology is in a rather sad state. All too few experiments have been subjected to repetition, and those that have been repeated by experimenters with a different theoretical bias have tended to turn up contrary findings.

From the standpoint of methodology, the problems of research in stuttering are not basically different from those in other branches of science. The literature on stuttering has suffered, as it has also frequently benefited, from the circumstance that a large number of highly motivated persons with little knowledge in other fields have sought to make contributions. Many have themselves been stutterers, and they have tried to advance our knowledge in what they felt to be a neglected area. Until recently, relatively few of those best equipped in statistical and experimental knowledge have troubled themselves with the stutterer. Greater attention to the problem of stuttering is needed, particularly from those with backgrounds in anthropology, linguistics, sociology, psychiatry, social psychology, and group dynamics.

Despite the essential unity of scientific approach with stuttering and with other problems, so many methodological traps have beset research workers on stuttering that it may be well to point out some of the more avoidable dangers and present a few suggestions and rules.

Many speech clinicians are dubious of experimentation and see no value in it. Perhaps we should focus a moment on this attitude.

Why test at all? Why carry out studies?

Because though we can discover much through our clinical impressions, we cannot verify and cross-check except by formalizing our propositions and controlling our observations. When we do this adequately, we have an experiment. Figuratively speaking, an experiment is a way of taking an idea that we may have been carrying around for some time and throwing it back to the subjects themselves, then letting them tell us by their response whether or not it is true.

Unfortunately, experimental training all too often brainwashes a developing worker in the field to such an extent that (1) he avoids all research; or, (2) he confines himself to trivia that are easy to test. Perhaps along with knowing our methodology we should also encourage greater flexibility in daring to undertake exploratory or case studies where indicated.

2. Rigor and the Need for Replication

Two kinds of rigor, both necessary for clean-cut experimental investigation, should be distinguished: (1) *statistical rigor*, pertaining to choice and utilization of techniques of data analysis; (2) *procedural rigor*, pertaining to substantive aspects of the data. Even the simplest statistical tools can be utilized to accomplish a great amount of work. More sophisticated statistical methods may often increase the efficiency of the work without necessarily involving greater rigor. Good experimental procedure, on the other hand, results largely from knowledge of the substantive content of the field. For procedural rigor, it is essential that we know stutterers and their contrariness as experimental animals, and that we possess enough clinical or experimental experience with stuttering to know what variables to control. In nearly any study this process can be materially faciliated by carrying out a pilot study before the procedure and design become frozen. Many experimenters, too eager to stop and invest hours or days running a few subjects and completing a pilot study, embark on their first investigation and unwittingly invest months or even years in gathering the wrong data under the wrong conditions utilizing a faulty procedure. Where procedural rigor is lacking, as in an unwanted confounding of variables, no statistical techniques can salvage the study.

Because of better knowledge of the variables, replication work tends to be more rigorous but less exciting, for it merely confirms the previous work or casts doubts upon it. While such work is sorely needed by the field, it lacks personal appeal to the young research worker who is naturally more desirous of producing something "original." The cumulative result is often a schizophrenic proliferation of "findings" which are seldom coupled together in any thoughtful way, and which often cannot be reconciled when they are placed side by side. Personality comparisons of stutterers and nonstutterers, summarized by the author (see Chapter 3) and others, may be cited as something of a horrible example in this regard. A similar statement could be made for biochemical and physiological comparisons (see Perkins, Chapter 5).

3. Need for Truly Random Sample in Observational Study

In some respects the obtaining of a truly random sample of the population is more important in a purely observational study than it is in an experimental study.

There is a distinction between observation and experiment which is important even if not always clear-cut. In the simplest experiment, we take some handy samples of subjects, randomly assign them to one or the other of two groups, and run the experiment. Because of the random assignment, we may use standard statistical tools to determine if the observed difference between the two groups after treatment is real or to be attributed to chance. If we obtain a significant result, then we may conclude statistically that our two treatments had different effects for this particular ready sample of subjects. Generalization to other subjects must be made on the basis of scientific or extrastatistical judgment. Such generalization will be more or less tenuous, but it does have one solid statistical finding upon which to proceed.

By contrast, in an observational investigation we simply set out to see what occurs naturally. In such circumstances, a truly random sample becomes highly important, more so than in the handy sample that could suffice for an experiment proper. For if we set out primarily to describe certain characteristics of the sample, we need to be able to generalize the description as being characteristic of the population, i.e., stutterers as a group.

METHODOLOGICAL HAZARDS
IN RESEARCH ON STUTTERING

1. Limitations of the Clinic Sample

Naturally enough, what we know about stuttering is based largely upon those who seek help and treatment, or who can be led to come for treatment. Those who recover by themselves and those who remain stutterers but do not come into our clinics probably differ in some important ways from the clinic stutterers, but we have not been able to study these groups enough to know what the differences are. Other stutterers experience a remission lasting several years and then under some stress, such as military combat, become more severe stutterers than they had ever been before. Still others become so discouraged with early abortive attempts at treatment that they abandon hope. Those we get in our clinics as adults tend to be a persistent breed. Practical necessities provide our research population. Stutterers who refuse to seek treatment or who recover spontaneously do not pose a clinical problem but they do pose a scientific problem (Sheehan & Martyn, 1966; Sheehan & Martyn, 1967). Stutterers who come for treatment differ from stutterers who do not, and this limitation of the population from which the sample is drawn does restrict our ability to generalize toward a broader understanding of stuttering as a disorder.

How are we to overcome this deficiency? One of the primary

ways would be to gather a large-scale national sample of the population which would automatically capture within it many recovered stutterers, relapsed stutterers, stutterers who seek treatment, and stutterers who do not seek treatment. Such a sample would permit a systematic comparison of these subgroups as well as studies of the properties of the total group ever classified as stutterers. The foregoing should not be construed to mean that nothing short of a nationwide random sample is worth anything. Much in the way of experimentation and considerable in the way of observation may be carried out on a local scale. The results may be less generalizable, but a big survey may be wasted until enough local information is built up to conduct it efficiently and incisively.

2. Bias from Self-selection to Certain Clinics

While geography is probably the most important single determiner of what stutterers go to which clinics, there is another selective factor that cannot be ignored in planning research. Certain stutterers tend to be drawn more to clinics that offer approaches in line with their needs. Those who are particularly attracted by Freudian doctrines are likely to go into analysis; those who prefer operant conditioning are likely to go to Minnesota; those intrigued by semantic approaches are likely to go to Iowa. In this way, every clinician known for a particular approach tends to get stutterers who reinforce his position. The people who go to faith healers probably differ in some important ways from the people who go to analysts.

Pending the collection of the idyllic "national sample," some correction for this bias can be achieved by including in the study stutterers from other clinics, particularly clinics that differ in treatment approach and in reference population.

3. Bias from the Experimenter

Research is largely a labor of love, and to be motivated toward undertaking a particular study, the researcher often has strong beliefs, hopes, or theoretical commitments about the expected outcome. He needs to protect his experiment from himself. Where there are observations to be made comparing or judging conditions, as in an adaptation study or in rating hostility in projective protocols of stutterers and nonstutterers, it is essential that the judgment be made without the observer's knowing which condition is being judged. Where feasible, experiments should be designed to provide against the possible influence of motivation upon perception. Most of the studies now in the literature on stuttering do not contain adequate insurance against experimenter bias—a principal source of our bewildering array of conflicting reports.

Rosenthal has shown that experimenter bias may operate in subtle ways. For example, students running "stupid" rats compared to "smart" rats in a learning task reported that the "smart" rats did significantly better. In fact, the rats did not differ at all, but were litter mates randomly assigned to the two groups (Rosenthal, 1966).

4. Bias from the Sophisticated Guinea Pig

Where it is at all possible, studies should be planned in such a manner as to ensure naive subjects. Since most studies are drawn from clinic populations, this would mean running the subjects before or near the beginning of therapy. Too often, research populations suffer from sophistication. Two examples may be used to illustrate this problem. Stutterers who run repeatedly through studies of the adaptation effect tend to become knowledgeable in certain ways. This may have been a strong factor in determining the outcome of an experiment which reported that the invariable feeling of stutterers in the moment after the block was one of relief and tension-reduction. Many of the subjects had been lectured to on the anxiety-reduction theory they were later used to verify! An expanded replication of this study with a larger, naive sample showed many other patterns.

In another study, sophisticated stutterers, who had run through many adaptation studies and could draw a curve better than most graduate students elsewhere, were used to demonstrate "adaptation of anticipation." They were asked to anticipate stuttering frequency while merely pretending to read the passages repeatedly. Not too strangely, their reported anticipations followed their previous adaptation curves. Also not strangely, a replication using unsophisticated subjects showed no such effect.

Many other such examples could be cited. The stutterer is a mean experimental animal at best. Let's not give him a head start on us!

5. Need for a Control Series

Inclusion of a control series is as necessary in speech pathology research as in other branches of behavior study. In summarizing the maze of conflicting findings on studies comparing stutterers and nonstutterers on Rorschach, Thematic Appercep-

TABLE 1	STUDIES OF RECOVERY FROM STUTTERING
Investigators	Wingate, 1964
Subjects	50 recovered stutterers.
Source	Speech pathologists and students in the field; parents and near relatives of clinic patients; friends and acquaintances of colleagues and students. Data obtained by questionnaire.
Controls	None.
Significance Tests	None.
Conclusions	Reported percentages in the sample as findings. Recovery attributed to change in attitude, direct attack on the problem.

tion, Picture-Frustration, and other projective instruments, we stated:

> The findings are not particularly consistent with each other, and some studies are not consistent internally. When inflation of probabilities, capricious interpretations, experimenter bias, and conclusions based on nonsignificant differences are eliminated, very little is left to show that stutterers are different from anyone else ... The search for personality differences between stutterers and nonstutterers may be intriguing enough so that it will be continued, but the trail does not look promising at this point. (Sheehan, 1958b)

The need for controls in speech and personality studies has similarly been emphasized by Goodstein (1958).

Shearer and Williams, 1965	Sheehan and Martyn, 1966
58 recovered stutterers.	32 recovered stutterers; 32 active stutterers.
University students personally interviewed by the investigators.	University students personally interviewed by the investigators.
None.	32 active stutterers; 366 normal speakers.
None.	Chi-square.
Sample data reported. Recovery attributed to development of adequacy and self-confidence, relaxation, greater understanding of the problem.	Four of five stutterers recover. School speech therapy negatively related to recovery. Active stuttering and stuttering as part of self-concept are related. Recovery attributed to role acceptance as a stutterer, growing self-esteem.

Some investigators, for example both Madison and Norman (1952) and Quarrington (1953), using the Rosenzweig Picture-Frustration test, have used established norms as controls. By economy of effort, this procedure probably makes possible many studies which otherwise would not be carried out. However, there are important benefits from the collection of the control group by the same investigators. Whatever the quirks of the local cultural or geographical scene in providing subjects, these are roughly equated when the same investigators collect both the experimental and control groups. The influence of unwanted variables is thereby held to a minimum.

The use of control groups is a feature lacking in many reports on stuttering. The lack has been particularly marked in studies of the efficacy of therapy techniques, in which the "before" and "after" status of a group receiving a particular treatment is given without reference to "what might have happened anyway." A control group answers this question.

TABLE 1	(continued)
Investigators	Martyn and Sheehan, 1968
Subjects	48 recovered stutterers.
Source	University students personally interviewed by the investigators.
Controls	37 active stutterers, 549 normal speakers.
Significance Tests	Chi-square
Conclusions	Expansion and replication of 1966 Sheehan and Martyn study.

1. Recovered stutterers differed in symptoms at onset, showing syllable repetitions rather than complete blockings, but not in time of onset.

2. Familial incidence distinguished stutterers from normal-speaking controls, but not active stutterers from recovered stutterers.

3. Recovery was negatively related both to severity and to receiving public school speech therapy.

4. Active stutterers in university-clinic therapy felt it had helped them improve and recommended it for others. None attributed improvement to public school therapy, or recommended it.

5. Active stutterers were more likely to have incorporated stuttering into their self-concepts.

6. Recovered stutterers differed from active stutterers in methods used to cope with the problem.

Failure to employ a control group or to restrict conclusions in the absence of one has recently appeared in a study by Wingate (1964). Using simple percentages with no significance tests, he presented sample characteristics as though they were established universe characteristics. He reported "sinistrality"

Dickson, 1968	Sheehan and Martyn, 1970
From parent reports, 196 spontaneous "remission of symptoms."	116 recovered stutterers
Parents of stutterers in the public schools.	5,138 University of California students screened during student health examinations. Ages: 17–56, Mean: 24.
From parent reports, 168 "retention of symptoms."	31 active stutterers. Ages: 17–32, Mean: 23.
t-test for proportions.	Chi-square.
Initial symptoms for remission group contained more syllable repetitions. Those who remained active showed more blocking at onset. Actives showed more severity at onset. Parents of actives did more admonishing, e.g., "start over; think before speaking; relax; take it easy." Parents of actives more often sought the help of a speech specialist, teacher, pediatrician. Parental confirmation of findings Sheehan and Martyn obtained from the stutterers themselves, *viz.*, onset in actives was severe and began with blocking, wheras onset in recovered was mild and began with repetitions.	Recovery ratio 4:1, i.e., 80% recover spontaneously. Severity and public school therapy negatively related to recovery. Familial incidence in stuttering but not in recovery from it. Agrees with Johnson (1959) on age of onset. Agrees with Dickson (1968) and with Martyn and Sheehan (1968) that recovereds had shown syllable repetitions at onset whereas actives had begun with blocking. Agrees with Wingate (1964) and Shearer and Williams (1965) that recovery is a gradual process.

in stutterers based on percentages in a group of recovered stutterers with no controls, either active stutterers or normal speakers. Table 1 presents a summary comparison of Wingate's study with those of Shearer and Williams (1965), Sheehan and Martyn (1967), Martyn and Sheehan (1968), Dickson

TABLE 2	"PREDISPOSING" FACTORS: VERBALLY REPORTED LEFT-HANDEDNESS IN THE STUTTERER AND IN HIS FAMILY
Investigators	Wingate, 1964
Subjects	50 recovered stutterers.
Controls	None.
Tests	None.
Conclusions	Under heading "Sinistrality," reports percentages in sample.

(1968), and Sheehan and Martyn (1970). Wingate's paper also illustrates unwarranted inference. From a simple questionnaire item on hand preference, he reports "sinistrality." Two inference jumps are unwarranted here: the leap from verbally reported hand usage as meaning handedness, and the further extension of handedness to include all of sidedness. When controls were used, as in the study by Sheehan and Martyn (1967), no significant difference appeared on handedness. This result is shown in Table 2.

In three evaluations of personality studies of stuttering (Sheehan, 1958, Chapter 3 in this book; Goodstein, 1958) the findings were that the better controlled the study, the less likelihood of obtaining a positive result. In fact, the most authoritatively stated positive results purporting to distinguish stutterers from nonstutterers on personality variables were those having no control groups at all.

6. Sample Size

When research studies are criticized, it is usually said with considerable piety that samples should be larger. While probably too many speech studies have been carried out with samples of

Sheehan and Martyn, 1967
64 recovered and active stutterers.
366 normal speakers.
Chi-square.
1. Active stutterers and recovered stutterers not different in reported handedness. 2. Neither stutterer group different from normal controls. 3. Parallel lack of significance for reported handedness in the family.

ten or less, there are implications to this recommendation that are not often recognized. In a review of methodology in speech and personality research, Goodstein (1958) criticized studies in speech pathology because sample sizes seldom exceeded thirty-five. Goodstein did not specify any particular sample size as being optimum for all the different problems that may be investigated in speech pathology, but rather contented himself with the recommendation that "sample size should be large enough to insure the chance of getting a significant result." While it is hard to quarrel with the essential virtue of this statement, it should not be uncritically inferred that doubling sample sizes or demanding samples of over 50 or 100 for all problems is necessarily going to do the cause of research in speech pathology a service. Quite obviously, a number of studies that are now undertaken as masters' or doctors' theses would simply never be carried out if this limitation were imposed upon them as a condition of acceptability. To this writer, it appears that it would be much better to struggle along with N's of 24 or 36 and to be sure that the studies really are completed. Replication or cross-validation of findings on studies of moderate sample size is a more efficient utilization of overall research effort.

In fact, it can be argued that sample size should not be too large. Psychologically important factors should not require a large number of cases in order to show statistical significance. The attained probability level has the same meaning regardless of the number of cases in the sample, but if it is necessary to build up the cases to one or two hundred in order to show statistical significance, then the difference in question is not as important in the psychology of stuttering as a difference that reveals itself readily on smaller samples.

7. Inflation of Probabilities

As Cronbach (1949) has pointed out, significance tests are like greenbacks; the more that are put in circulation, the less each one is worth. In studies that include a large number of significance tests, some should be expected to turn up "significant" by chance alone. All too often this factor is not taken into account either in the planning of studies or in the interpretation of results once obtained, and statistical comparisons may be undertaken that capitalize on chance features of the sample. So many studies already in the literature have reported "significant" results from inflated probabilities that many published findings need to be replicated on fresh samples.

8. Inappropriate Statistical Techniques

Especially critical here is the factor of inadequate attention to assumptions. Speech pathology as well as related fields has suffered its share from the use of F, *t*, and other normal-curve techniques when the requirements of trait normality and homogeneity of variance are not met. The results of the Norton study (1953), as reported by Lindquist, are somewhat reassuring as to the effect of violation of the assumptions of trait normality and homogeneity of variance within reasonable limits. Nevertheless, in instances where assumptions of trait normality and homogeneity of variance are untenable, and where the data come naturally in rank order or numbered form, consideration should be given to the use of nonparametric statistics such as the sign test or chi-square techniques. The book by Tate and Clelland is one of the most usable and reliable sources for nonparametric techniques (1957). These tests have the disadvantage of less sensitivity, i.e., they do not use all the information in the data. The choice of statistical techniques is up to the researcher; it should be met with sensitivity to the problems involved in the choices, and with knowledge of whatever limitations may be imposed upon the interpretation of the results.

For example, it should be remembered that direct comparison

of magnitudes of two significant levels is not permissible. When one dimension is found significant and one nonsignificant, the finding does not establish a significant difference between the two variables.

9. Treatment of Sample Characteristics as Probable Universe Characteristics

It is very easy to forget, when analyzing data from a sample, that one is not dealing with the entire universe, but only with one particular sample from the universe. Successive random samples from the same population will differ from each other in important ways. If we treat a sample as though it were representative of the universe, we trap ourselves into false conclusions.

Let us suppose, for example, that we have gathered a sample of fifty stutterers and fifty nonstutterers with the idea of comparing their handedness. We happen to observe something we had not planned to investigate, namely, that a striking number of the stutterers in our sample appear to be redheaded (or shy, or hostile, or withdrawn). We might be tempted to run a significance test on this difference and it might turn out to be "significant." Yet we would not be justified either in conducting this significance test or in concluding from it that stutterers were significantly more redheaded than nonstutterers. We would simply have capitalized on one chance occurrence, on one of many, many possible dimensions that could have come to our attention in the same way. We would only have an hypothesis to be stated before experimental test upon a fresh sample. Undoubtedly many of the false differences between the stutterer and the nonstutterer that were reported in the literature, especially during the 1930s, were derived because sample characteristics were treated as universe characteristics. Our sample will nearly always differ from our universe in some important ways, and any sample of stutterers is likely to exhibit some atypical features on some dimensions if subjected to enough scrutiny after the deed of gathering the sample is done.

METHODOLOGICAL PROBLEMS IN
STUTTERING RESEARCH

Despite their efforts at concealment, which are fundamental to so many of their problems, stutterers may be both seen and heard. Because of the overt characteristics of their behavior, stutterers provide an almost ideal population for behavior modification research—a fact long known to speech pathologists and recently the focus of more systematic attention by psychologists and other students of behavior.

Three general kinds of research in stuttering may be distinguished: the survey or *ex post facto* study, the cross-cultural studies, and the experimental studies. In examining research on stuttering, it appears that the primary difficulties lie in methodological problems inherent within the study of stuttering itself. To cope with these problems and to proceed with scientific rigor, it is essential that we know stutterers and have enough experience clinically to know what variables exist. We also need to become aware of our problems and the limitations they place upon us and the generalizations we make. No amount of statistical rigor or choice in techniques of analyzing results can overcome poor data collection. The importance of careful sample selection and choice of control groups is basic— and has been most frequently mishandled or overlooked.

In observational or survey studies, a truly random sample of the population of stutterers may be even more important than in experimental studies, for in the observational study there is a more direct line of inference from sample characteristics to those of the population. For instance, if we were restricted (for sampling purposes) to a population of redheaded stutterers, we would not be entitled to any generalizations about stutterers as a group if we were merely gathering the survey type of data. However, even such a severe restriction would not prevent our gathering in an experimental procedure much useful data on learning, reinforcement, or adaptation curve characteristics under an experimental condition such as time pressure. The absence of such a restriction as "redheads only" would be desirable, for it would permit generalization beyond the particular sample studied. But the observational study would still be most vulnerable, most sensitive to sample selection.

If we wish, as in a survey, to describe stutterers as a group, we must select a sample reflective of the whole population. Why should this be so difficult?

Perhaps it is a problem in definition of the class "stutterer." Everyone is inclined to believe he "knows" what stuttering is— but how do we determine who is a stutterer?

First, whom do we include? On the continuum of disfluency-fluency, where does stuttering begin? Should the implicit stutterer be included in our sample? The mild stutterer? The severe stutterer? The spontaneously recovered stutterer? Is stuttering a unitary disorder? (Sheehan, 1958b, 1968; St. Onge, 1963.) In most studies, the implicit stutterers (those who view themselves as stutterers but show little overt stuttering behavior) are not considered; the mild stutterers are passed over in laboratory manipulation of stuttering behavior; the very severe are sometimes excluded; the spontaneously recovered have been largely omitted, and here alone four-fifths of those who have ever had the problem called stuttering are left out (Sheehan & Martyn, 1966, 1970; Martyn & Sheehan, 1968).

Second, who determines the diagnosis? Should we depend on self-diagnosis, on self-identification, to establish the category? Parental diagnosis? Observer identification? "Sophisticated" clinical diagnosis in order to select subjects for research? Though it is true that stuttering has a certain "social visibility" (Lemert, 1951), the stutterer expends much effort in hiding the problem. Paradoxically, much of what is called stuttering behavior is made up of efforts to hide precisely what the observer then identifies as stuttering behavior. However, many of the stutterer's concealment efforts are successful, either partially or temporarily (Sheehan, 1958a). Even experienced clinicians are often fooled by the stutterer.

This aspect of the psychology of stuttering introduces special problems with reference to cultural and anthropological studies. In an investigation of a primitive society, neither the informant nor the interviewer is likely to be fully aware of how readily much of what is called stuttering can be concealed, and a precise criterion for the classification "stutterer" is lacking. The reports may be based mostly on stutterers with relatively high social visibility (see Lemert, Chapter 4 in this book).

Even cultural studies in "civilized" societies suffer from a sampling problem difficult to control because of the sample source. These studies have been directed toward such variables as socioeconomic status, class structure, upward mobility, and other status-level factors in stuttering. Though it appears that the problem of stuttering is not markedly different in primitive societies than in our own, the findings of many cultural studies are inconclusive and often contradictory.

Though there are many inherent difficulties in conducting research on the problem of stuttering, in many instances the quest for new knowledge has been needlessly complicated by the violation of simple rules of design and inference, particularly as they relate to sample selection and the use of control groups. An awareness of these problems—especially as they relate to getting an adequate sampling of the stutterer population—and an attempt to handle them should result in new leads and in more verifiable research on the problem of stuttering.

METHODOLOGICAL ISSUES
IN BEHAVIOR MODIFICATION

The recent proliferation of behavior modification experiments, especially those conceived and reported in the Skinnerese language of operant conditioning, has posed a number of methodological issues worthy of special mention.

Behavior modification is a broad term, under which "stuttering therapy" as set forth in this book and elsewhere would be included. Learning theory approaches such as those of Brutten and Shoemaker (1967), Gregory (1968), Luper (1968), Beech and Fransella (1968), Williams (1968), plus the varied offerings in the book edited by Gray and England (1969), are all recent examples of behavior modification applications. Earlier examples are Dunlap's (1932) "negative practice," which gave rise to voluntary stuttering techniques, and the speech therapies for stuttering devised by Johnson and by Van Riper. Semantic reorientation is a form of behavior modification, and so is desensitization. In his recent book, *Principles of Behavior Modification*, Bandura (1969) reviewed our experiment on the modification of stuttering through nonreinforcement as a promising early example of behavior modification (Sheehan, 1951). As pointed out in Chapter 7, the experimental procedure derived from Van Riper's speech therapy technique of "cancellation." Other examples could be cited to show that stuttering therapy has been a pioneering form of behavior modification.

Most of the work just cited has been conducted within the traditions of experimental psychology, entailing use of a generous sample of subjects, design controls on observer reliability and experimenter bias, and significance tests to filter out sample differences most reasonably attributed to chance. Stuttering is a disorder of sufficient complexity so that research endeavors require all of these safeguards.

Behavior modification in its broadest sense also includes operant conditioning, which has developed from B. F. Skinner's term for instrumental conditioning (Hilgard & Marquis, 1940) into something of a social phenomenon. In part, the form is newer than the substance; in other respects, the claims and methodologies of the operant conditioners are sufficiently unique to compel special discussion. As a starter, Skinner (1953, 1957a, 1957b) rejects learning theory as such in favor of a strictly descriptive approach, the "experimental analysis of behavior." Behavior is reinforced by its consequences. Constructs are unneeded and unwanted: inferred entities such as drive and anxiety are junked. Studies with a few subjects whose individual curves are reported with no statistics of sampling are a hallmark of the operant approach. A common method involves running one subject until a baseline of some behavior is established, introducing an independent variable, usually a positive or negative reinforcer, then measuring the presumably resulting behaviors against the baseline.

The operant approach retains the experimental method, involving a restricted set of observations within a contrived or "laboratory" procedure. Also retained is the longitudinal aspect of the case study approach, calling for repeated observations over a long period of time. A disadvantage of the experimental approach is that it tends to favor relatively trivial variables which may be readily manipulated in the laboratory; another is the restriction of the scope of observation and the possible introduction of artifacts. On the other hand, the case study approach is limited by the intrusion of unseen events and uncontrolled variables. In choosing to experiment with just a few subjects over a long period of time, operant conditioning manages to combine into one package both the disadvantages of the experimental method and those of the case study approach —without preserving the advantages of either.

Moreover, operant conditioners tend to restrict what they choose to observe, and to report findings as though there were nothing else that could be observed. For example, interpersonal processes may be just as crucial in the outcome of an experiment as they are in therapy. The work of Rosenthal (1966) and others has shown that the outcome of an experiment is heavily affected by the expectations of the experimenter.

As we have pointed out in this book and elsewhere, the disorder of stuttering is not a unitary disorder. Subtypes with discernible differences in pattern of onset and development, and in other respects, appear to exist. Not all stutterers come from a thoroughly homogenized sample of interchangeable "subjects" that can be manipulated by the experimenter without regard to their divergent proclivities. Stutterers are not empty organisms, but individuals who differ importantly among themselves.

Subject variability does not disappear just because an experimenter has assumed implicitly that it does not exist.

Since stutterers vary, how is the operant experimenter to know what kind of subject he happens to have before him? Were he more in the tradition of psychological experimentation, running 20 or 30 subjects—using sampling theory, the question would not be so critical. Presumably a good-sized sample would pick up most of the important varieties of stutterer, if indeed varieties exist. But when the operant experimenter picks only a few subjects, then the question of subject variability becomes a critical issue. The fact that operant conditioners withhold diplomatic recognition from the question does not mean that it is not highly relevant to their results.

Just because traditional safeguards on observer reliability which have characterized the development of psychological experimentation are abandoned does not mean that the experiments are not prone to historic fallacies. Just because learning theory is rejected by the Skinnerians in favor of a descriptive approach does not mean that nothing of theoretical significance is happening. Just because operant conditioners choose not to use significance tests does not mean that some of their results are not easily attributable to chance. And statistics have been an essential safeguard against reporting as "findings" results due to chance alone.

For the naive experimenter who does not know the disorder and its literature, stuttering is an attractively camouflaged trap. So amenable is the disorder temporarily to the principle of distraction—the reduced frequency of stuttering due to the introduction into the environment of a novel stimulus—that initially everything and anything seems to work.

The contingent reinforcement of the experimenter, as well as the subject, must be considered. The distraction principle is so pervasive in stuttering that anyone who experiments with the disorder is immediately reinforced by a tempting schedule. Everything new or novel works in reducing stuttering behavior simply because it is new and novel. Simply stated, this is the distraction principle. Therefore, whatever the operant conditioner chooses to impose as his experimental technique on stutterers, provided it aims directly for fluency, is bound to work just because it is novel and new. Many experimenters employ masking noise or delayed side-tone and treat the immediately resulting fluency as evidence that the stutterer can continue this improvement indefinitely. Masking noise and delayed side-tone have similar effects in bringing about quick fluency, since delayed side-tone tends to serve as a masking noise. However, there is persuasive evidence that the occurrence of fluency does not automatically lead to more fluency.

Fluency should be an indirect goal in the treatment of stuttering, not a direct goal. As we indicated in Chapter 7, this is a fundamental concept in the treatment of stuttering. Fluency should come about through the reduction of the avoidance, the holding back, the false behavior that is characteristic of stuttering.

Using a mechanical gadget to get a stutterer to speak a word or to read pages from books fluently has no effect on future probability of stuttering, as we have noted in Chapter 1. The variability of stuttering is such that the experimenter is bound to get a lot of reinforcement whatever he does. Surely this is all the more reason for following traditional methodological safeguards in researching this complex disorder. But many operant conditioners start out rejecting these safeguards, and end up with results that fail the scientific test of repeatability.

For example, we recently followed our own recommendations in this chapter and undertook the replication of a widely reprinted experiment on "operant stuttering" by Flanagan, Goldiamond, and Azrin (1958). After reviewing conflicting evidence on the effects of experimental reward and punishment on stuttering, Biggs and Sheehan (1969) noted that stutterers appeared to show varied reactions as individuals. We employed double the number of subjects of the original study and added something the original study did not have, a noncontingent control condition. Six male stutterers who enrolled in the Psychology Speech Clinic of the University of California, Los Angeles, were tested during successive readings of a given passage. Three experimental conditions were employed utilizing a 4000 cps tone at an intensity of 108 db, ISO hearing level, to determine the effect of this stimulus upon stuttering behavior: (1) an aversive condition in which the presentation of the tone was contingent upon stuttering; (2) an escape condition in which cessation of the tone was contingent upon stuttering; and (3) a random condition in which the tone was presented independent of the subjects' disfluencies.

The findings, contrary to those of Flanagan *et al.*, were that stuttering decreased in all conditions. The results are most readily explained as being due to distraction effects. Since noise reduced stuttering whether contingent or not, the reverent mention typically accorded operant research in stuttering appears far from justified. There is a real need to conduct further ex-

339

perimental checks on the claims and the methodologies of those who report highly dramatic results, as well as a general scientific need for the replication of frequently cited experiments.

Subjects in our replication rated the noise as not really punishing but somewhat distracting. If punishing at all, the supposedly noxious sound involved a fairly mild penalty. The experience of stuttering itself, which the allegedly "aversive" stimulus was supposed to control, was rated as still more punishing than the noise. Since the noise showed the functional properties of a distractor, it worked whether contingent or not. From the results of the replication, the noise did not function as a contingent reinforcer as Flanagan, Goldiamond, and Azrin had concluded. Had they reckoned with the distraction principle, or had they employed a control condition, there would be one bit less chaff in the harvest of research on stuttering.

Try as he may, no experimenter is immune from the pitfalls of research in stuttering, and it is always possible that some of our own cherished findings will be toppled by subsequent work. So it be! This is the way any field progresses. Were it not for the relentless march of research, we would still be changing handedness. I would be typing with one hand to protect my cerebral dominance, and this book would have taken twice as long.

A SUMMARY OF METHODOLOGICAL RECOMMENDATIONS

1. Obtain a Clinic-free Sample, If Possible

If this is not possible, obtain sample from different clinics, preferably including clinics with different orientations. Carry out a study that includes, where possible, those who did not go for help in a clinic. We might obtain samples from public schools, from industry, from entering-college populations, etc. A speech survey by the author of all incoming students at the UCLA Health Service in February, 1950, indicated that recovered stutterers may outnumber active stutterers, as later study confirmed.

2. Gather a Control Group in the Same Fashion as the Experimental Group

3. Control for Experimenter Bias

There must be a check on the experimenter's judgment such that his knowledge of the intent of the study does not affect the results. Rosenthal (1963) has shown that the experimenter pervasively shapes the results.

4. Choose the Sample from a Larger Pool or Population of Stutterers

This can be done by using names of stutterers from different clinics and a table of random numbers, so that only certain ones are selected. Such a procedure would be more desirable than using all the stutterers from one or two clinics. In practice this recommendation is often difficult.

5. Control the Inflation of Probabilities or Take Them into Account

Where possible, studies should be planned so that a few exact *prior* hypotheses may be tested. In a comparison of physiological measures on stutterers and nonstutterers, for example, or on personality measures, critical hypotheses must be stated in advance of gathering the sample and observing its characteristics. Moreover, if a large number of hypotheses are stated, the resultant inflation of probabilities must be reckoned with in the interpretation of the findings.

6. Make Explicit the Important Assumptions Underlying a Study

Where possible, simple companion experiments on at least a pilot basis should be carried out to demonstrate the tenability of these assumptions. Where this is not feasible, some justification should be presented based on logical or clinical grounds, or based on research studies already in the literature. Frequently a study rests upon an assumption more difficult to accept on *a priori* grounds than the main hypothesis under investigation. Thus we find some experimenters assuming something far-fetched in order to carry out an experimental procedure to demonstrate something fairly obvious.

7. Replicate More Studies

Not enough studies are repeated—a point that has been developed above.

8. Choose Samples Neither Too Large Nor Too Small

Consider both Type I and Type II errors in selecting the sample size. Type I involves reporting a difference where none exists; Type II involves missing a difference that does exist. The samples should not be too large, for if one has to build up a tremendous sample to obtain statistical significance, the effect discovered may be so small as to be of little importance. Nor should the sample be too small, for then one is likely to commit a Type II error; that is, there may be a real difference that is not revealed because small samples require results of greater absolute magnitude in order to achieve significance.

9. Conduct More Survey and Exploratory Studies

Too often the process of verification has been stressed at the expense of the process of discovery. Science marches forward from these twin processes. For example, in stuttering we probably have far too many studies trying to show physiological differences (see Chapter 5) and too few cross-cultural studies (see Chapter 4). Recent work by Goldman (1967) on cultural factors influencing the sex ratio is especially promising.

10. Rigor Must Not Become Rigor Mortis

Researchers should not become so inhibited by the foregoing that they cease carrying out the studies. We must be careful that attention to all these dangers does not lead to a creeping paralysis. There is real danger (and the author is quite conscious of this in citing all the need for rigor and statistical control) of confining all studies to trivia in order to demonstrate rigor. We must have scientific and clinical meaningfulness as well as operational meaning and rigor. We will not advance even at our present rate if we fall into the trap that has ensnared certain fields of psychology, i.e., confining ourselves to trivia in order to assure ourselves that we are rigorous and scientific. Sometimes we should be willing, in an exploratory study, to test clinically rich hypotheses even when some difficult assumptions are involved. Better occasional inelegance than utter sterility. We should deal with problems in the most rigorous manner available but should not neglect important problem areas when perfect rigor is not possible. When our methodological restrictions become too severe, rigor becomes *rigor mortis.*

CATEGORIES FOR FUTURE STUDY

Possibly we should approach research in stuttering not so completely in terms of ideas—general, theoretical or clinical hypotheses to be tested about the stutterer—but rather in terms of the study of categories of individual stutterers. Here we shall list some of the categories that should be especially fruitful in providing research leads that could ultimately develop questions for experimental answer.

There is no suggestion that all of the following are separate, homogeneous subtypes of stutterers. Rather, these are categories of individual stutterers, whose case histories or patterns of onset, development, and response to treatment distinguish them from one another in important respects. Not all the categories are mutually exclusive, and some stutterers fall into more than one category. Nonetheless, more intensive study of stutterers within these groupings, probably by systematic cross-comparisons, holds promise of telling us something new about the disorder.

1. Disfluent Normals

Children who go through the stage of syllable repetition and then outgrow it without even being labeled as primary stutterers.

2. Fluent Normals

Children who seem to go through the entire course of speech development and personality development without ever showing marked hesitancy in their speech.

3. Recovered Primary Stutterers

Children who become stutterers and become labeled and treated as stutterers for a discernible period. Somehow, then, the label does not stick, and the stuttering disappears before the age of 6 or 7.

4. "Family Onset" Cases

Children who follow the more typical pattern of the onset of stuttering at the age of 3 within the family situation.

5. "School Onset" Cases

Children who do not begin to stutter until they begin to go to school; that is, their stuttering begins not in the home where it is easy for speech pathologists to assign guilt to the parents, but in the school, probably in response to some early school situation. From our studies of onset and recovery, a few cases begin this way.

6. "Late Onset" Cases

Children who begin to stutter at the age of 8 or 10 or 12. Van Riper has hypothesized some differences between these stutterers and other stutterers. In this connection, it is important that careful case histories be taken, for it is possible for a child to do considerable primary stuttering for years and then have some dramatic event or shock aggravate the stutter-

343

ing enough so that the onset of stuttering is assigned to the dramatic event.

7. Pubescent Recoveries

Those whose stuttering disappears at the onset of adolescence or at puberty. Because of the reactivation of Oedipal conflicts as the individual passes psychosexual stages at this age, or possibly because of physiological and/or role change, this is an interesting phenomenon. In our studies of spontaneous recovery from stuttering, the years 11–14 were significant times of improvement.

8. Reactivated Stutterers (Relapsed Recoveries)

Individuals, usually men in service, who stuttered early in life, whose stuttering disappeared and then reappeared during stress in adult life.

9. "Adult Onset" Cases

Those who really began to stutter in later life. In the writer's experience, a true onset of stuttering for the first time in adult life is rare. Those that do occur seem to involve processes of severe decompensation and personality breakdown. In one case a captain who had been a company commander in Italy would break into tears at frequent intervals and sob that he, who used to be a company commander, would now not even make a good private. Such cases, incidentally, do not seem to fit very well the concept of diagnosogenesis as an etiological factor in stuttering. Discernible personality differences that developed very quickly in this case did not seem to hinge upon labeling behavior.

10. Plodding or Constant Stutterers

Stutterers who continue to stutter very consistently throughout all speech situations and who have stuttered almost from the onset of speaking.

11. Cyclical Stutterers

Many stutterers show marked wavelike variations in stuttering frequency, so that they may speak quite fluently for a period of an hour, a day, or a week, and be severely blocked during the next hour, day, or week. This is of course a very common breed of stutterer; therefore all the more worthy of more intensive investigation. Quarrington (1956) has reported data showing that cyclical variation is a major feature of the disorder.

12. Inner Stutterers, or Interiorized Stutterers

Every clinic encounters people who feel themselves to be stutterers, who show fear and anticipation of blocking, but who show very little in the way of overt speech differences. Many of these persons are actually more fluent than some of the officially normal examining clinicians, yet they suffer agonies in anticipation of something that never quite seems to happen to them. We are reminded of Wyneken's old characterization of the stutterer as a *sprachzweifler*—a doubter of speech. Certainly these individuals are displaying obsessive and phobic characteristics with respect to the act of speaking. On theoretical grounds, those showing such symptoms should be expected to show many of the personality characteristics of the obsessive compulsive individual, i.e., psychasthenic characteristics. Such cases would fit very well into psychoanalytic conceptions of the personality of the stutterer, and we wonder whether some of the psychoanalytic theories on stuttering were not derived from study of a few such individuals. Therapeutically, inner stutterers are particularly interesting in that they often derive great benefit from group therapy contact with other, more typical stutterers. Actually, the change in their personality and feelings often far exceeds any changes in overt speech characteristics, for to begin with there may have been little room for overt speech improvement. That inner stutterers—or perhaps we should say phobic normal speakers—can profit from group speech therapy may illustrate the basic psychotherapeutic nature of speech therapy groups. Further discussion of interiorization may be found in Freund (1966) and Douglas and Quarrington (1952).

13. Highly Disfluent Normal Speakers

These are the opposite of the inner stutterers. They are individuals who regard themselves as normal speakers, and have always been regarded as normal speakers, yet who have an unusually high proportion of disfluency and stuttering characteristics in their speech. Many in this category seem to stumble along so comfortably that they are able to use speech as part of their vocation and never seem to exhibit any fear or discomfort with their relatively nonfluent speech.

14. Highly Fluent Speakers

The personality as well as the speech characteristics of successful speakers should throw indirect light on the problem of the stutterer. Ferullo (1963) found that better speakers revealed a significantly higher degree of self-acceptance and personality integration than poorer speakers.

It might be interesting to compare the successful speaker's use of silence, for example, with the stutterer's comparative intolerance for periods of silence in his own speech.

15. Recovered Stutterers

Those who stuttered early in life and recovered, with or without therapy, without ultimate relapse. Four out of five who become stutterers recover spontaneously, though for those who were ever severe, it is only one out of two.

16. Psychotic Stutterers

Since stuttering is presumably an anxiety condition, the co-existence of stuttering and psychosis is puzzling and worthy of further investigation.

17. Psychopathic Stutterers

Guilt has been specified as an important source of anxiety in the stutterer. If any significant number of psychopathic stutterers can be found, it might be revealing to explore their mechanisms for handling guilt. The MMPI patterns of stutterers might turn up enough individuals with high Psychopathic Deviation scores to provide an intriguing sample for study of the handling of pressures toward conformity.

18. Persons with Stuttering as an Incidental Problem

This category includes all those in whom some symptom other than stuttering is the main presenting complaint. What can we learn of stuttering when it is a relatively minor part of the picture?

19. Stutterers Who Never Seek Treatment

Our scientific understanding of stuttering would be broadened by study of this largely unknown group, which probably differs in important ways from the group that seeks treatment and thus provides samples for research. Possibly these stutterers do not differ from treatment-seeking stutterers in personality or in any systematic way whatsoever, except that they have been subjected to so many abortive efforts that they have given up hope of ever finding relief. Possibly these are individuals whose avoidance drive is so strong that they cannot face the problem even to the extent of acknowledging the need for therapy.

FINAL COMMENT AND SUMMARY

Because our present knowledge of stuttering is so much like the top of the iceberg, with the major part remaining to be explored, the foregoing suggestions in terms of possible categories of stutterers represent primarily an example of one avenue of further research. The whole of this book is devoted to indicating other needed approaches, conceived from the vantage point of other disciplines and carried out at different levels of analysis.

In this chapter we have examined the status of our research knowledge on stuttering, summarized major points of our present knowledge and agreement, considered questions of methodology especially pertinent to research on the problem of stuttering, considered reasons for poor productivity among research workers on the problem of stuttering, pointed up a number of methodological hazards that have plagued previous followers of the trail, suggested an approach to studying categories or subgroups of individual stutterers, and attempted to accelerate movement toward a science of communication disorders. While it is not doubted that portions of the specific content of a chapter such as this will be rendered useless as our science advances, it is hoped that the emphasis on method, at least, will have more lasting impact. Only by improving our method shall we be enabled to explore the remainder of our iceberg, and to cause it ultimately to melt away.

References

References that are listed here only by author and year of publication appear in complete form in the Bibliography.

American Speech and Hearing Association, White House Conference Report. (1957) Speech disorders and speech correction. *Journal of Speech and Hearing Disorders, 17,* 129–137.

Andrews, G., and Harris, M.   (1964)

Aron, M. L.   (1960)

Aron, M. L.   (1962)

Auer, J. J.   (1958) *Introduction to research in speech.* New York: Harper & Row.

Bandura, A.   (1969) *Principles of behavior modification.* New York: McGraw-Hill.

Beech, H. R., and Fransella, F.   (1968)

Berlin, A. J.   (1954)

Biggs, B. E., and Sheehan, J. G. (1969)

Bloodstein, O. N. (1950)

Bloodstein, O. N. (1958)

Brookshire, R. and Martin, R. (1967) The differential effects of three verbal punishers on the disfluencies of normal speakers. *Journal of Speech and Hearing Research, 10,* 496–505.

Brutten, E. J., and Shoemaker, D. J. (1967)

Cronbach, L. J. (1949) Statistical methods applied to Rorschach scores: A review. *Psychological Bulletin, 46,* 393–429.

Dickson, S. (1968) Spontaneous remission and retention of incipient stuttering symptoms. Paper read before annual meeting of American Speech and Hearing Association, Denver.

Douglas, E., and Quarrington, B. (1952)

Dunlap, K. (1932) *Habits, their making and unmaking.* New York: Liveright.

Ferullo, R. J. (1963) The self-concept in communication. *Journal of Communication, 13,* 77–86.

Frederick, C. J., III. (1955) An investigation of learning theory and reinforcement as related to stuttering behavior. Ph.D. thesis, University of California, Los Angeles.

Freund, H. (1966)

Goldman, R. (1967)

Goodstein, L. D. (1958) Functional speech disorders and personality: A survey of the research. *Journal of Speech and Hearing Research, 1,* 359–376.

Gray, B. B., and England, G. (1969)

Gregory, H. H. (1968)

Hilgard, E., and Marquis, D. G. (1940) *Conditioning and learning.* New York: Appleton.

Johnson, W., et al. (1959)

Johnson, W., Darley, F., and Spriestersbach, D. C. (1962) *Diagnostic methods in speech pathology.* New York: Harper & Row.

Johnson, W., et al. (1967) *Speech handicapped school children.* 3rd edition. New York: Harper & Row.

Lemert, E. M. (1951) *Social pathology.* New York: McGraw-Hill, chap. 6.

Luper, H. L. (1968)

Madison, L. R., and Norman, R. D. (1952)

Martyn, M. M., and Sheehan, J. G. (1968)

Norton, D. W. (1952) An empirical investigation of the

effects of non-normality and heterogeneity upon the F-test of analysis of variance. Ph.D. thesis, University of Iowa. Summarized in E. F. Lindquist, *Design and analysis of experiments in psychology and education*. Cambridge, Mass.: Riverside Press, pp. 78–90.

Quarrington, B. (1956)

Rosenthal, R. (1963) On the social psychology of the psychological experiment: The experimenter's hypothesis as unintended determinant of experimental results. *American Scientist, 51*, 268–283.

Rosenthal, R. (1966) *Experimenter Effects in Behavioral Research*, New York: Appleton.

St. Onge, K. R. (1963) The stuttering syndrome. *Journal of Speech and Hearing Research, 6*, 195–197.

Sapir, E. (1915) Abnormal types of speech in Nootka. Ottawa: Government Printing Bureau.

Schuell, H. (1946) Sex differences in relation to stuttering. *Journal of Speech Disorders, 11*, 277–298.

Shearer, W. M., and Williams, J. D. (1965)

Sheehan, J. G. (1946) A study of the phenomena of stuttering. M.A. thesis, University of Michigan, Ann Arbor.

Sheehan, J. G. (1951)

Sheehan, J. G. (1953)

Sheehan, J. G. (1958a)

Sheehan, J. G. (1958b)

Sheehan, J. G. (1960) Cultural factors in stuttering: Stuttering in native Africans. Paper read before annual meeting of American Speech and Hearing Association, Los Angeles.

Sheehan, J. G. (1968)

Sheehan, J. G., Cortese, P. A., and Hadley, R. G. (1962)

Sheehan, J. G., and Martyn, M. M. (1966)

Sheehan, J. G., and Martyn, M. M. (1967)

Sheehan, J. G., and Martyn, M. M. (1970) Stuttering and its disappearance. *Journal of Speech and Hearing Research, 13*, No. 2. Reprinted in E. P. Trapp, and P. Himelstein, Eds., *Readings on the exceptional child: Research and theory* (Revised). New York: Appleton, 1970.

Skinner, B. F. (1953) *Science and human behavior*. New York: Macmillan.

Skinner, B. F. (1957a) The experimental analysis of behavior. *American Scientist, 45*, 343–371.

Skinner, B. F. (1957b) *Verbal behavior*. New York: Appleton.

Stewart, J. L. (1960) Studies of North American Indians

of the Plains, Great Basin, and Southwest. Paper read before annual meeting of American Speech and Hearing Association, Los Angeles.

Stunden, A. A. (1966) Computer simulation of therapy: The client-therapist match. *Journal of the American Speech and Hearing Association, 8,* 100–104.

Tate, M. W., and Clelland, R. C. (1957) *Nonparametric and shortcut statistics.* Danville, Ill.: Interstate.

Van Riper, C. (1963)

Weiss, D. A. (1950)

Williams, D. E. (1968)

Wingate, M. E. (1964)

Wingate, M. E. (1965) Panel comment at American Speech and Hearing Association, Chicago.

Wyllie, J. (1894) *The disorders of speech.* Edinburgh: Oliver and Boyd.

BIBLIOGRAPHY, 1950-1970

No scholarly task is more onerous than the compilation of a fairly extensive bibliography. It seems unending, and it is never entirely complete or completed. Errors have a fiendish capacity for inserting themselves at every stage of publication. Nevertheless, to the serious student of the complex disorder of stuttering, which cuts across the interests of many disciplines, a comprehensive bibliography is a tool of the utmost necessity. Having appreciated and relied upon the massive bibliography prepared by Dr. Charles Elliott for the years prior to 1950 (see the item under this name in the present compilation), I have felt it necessary to do what I could to bring the references up to date. I make no claims for all-inclusiveness (the Russian references are especially limited). Nevertheless, it is my hope that my own work might speed the efforts of others to understand stuttering.

Charles Van Riper

Abbott, T. B.   (1957)   A study of observable mother-child relationships in stuttering and non-stuttering groups. *Dissertation Abstracts, 17,* 148–149.

Adamczyk, B.   (1959)   Use of instruments for the production of artificial feedback in the treatment of stuttering *Folia Phoniatrica, 11,* 216–218. (German)

Adamczyk, B. (1963a) Correction of speech in stutterers by means of a telephone with the use of an artificial echo. I. *Otolaryngologia Polska, 17,* 479–481. (Polish)

Adamczyk, B. (1963b) Correction of speech in stutterers by means of a telephone with the use of an artificial echo. II. *Otolaryngologia Polska, 17,* 482–484. (Polish)

Adams, M. R. (1967) An exploratory investigation of the effect of an auditory extinction procedure on the consistency of stuttering. *Dissertation Abstracts, 28*(6–B), 2654.

Adams, M. R., and Dietze, D. A. (1965) A comparison of the reaction of stutterers and non-stutterers to items on a word association test. *Journal of Speech and Hearing Research, 8,* 195–202.

Adler, S. (1961) An integration of some research studies on stammering. *Rehabilitation Literature, 22,* 34–41.

Adler, S. (1966) *A clinician's guide to stuttering.* Springfield, Ill.: Charles C Thomas.

Agner, I. (1964) 1000 Bears—And we have no revolver: Course of play therapy with a 5-year-old boy. *Praxis der Kinderpsychologie und Kinderpsychiatrie* (Supplement), *6,* 28–36. (German)

Ainsworth, S. (1957) Integrating theories of stuttering. In L. E. Travis, *Handbook of speech pathology.* New York: Appleton.

Ainsworth, S. (1963) Speech handicapped; stuttering. *Review of Educational Research, 33,* 24–26.

Amirov, R. Z. (1960) Trigeminal 'naia trikhkompone naia metodika i zucheniia vysshei nervnoi deiatel'nosti cheloveka. Trigeminal, tricomponent method of studying higher nervous activity in man. *Zhurnal Vysshei Nervnoi deiatel 'nosti, 10,* pp. 468–472.

Anderson, Elwood G. (1968) A comparison of emotional stability in stutterers and nonstutterers. *Dissertation Abstracts, 28*(8–B), 3511.

Andrews, G. (1967) Stuttering: Theoretical and therapeutic considerations. II. Syllable timed speech, group psychotherapy and recovery from stuttering. *Australian Psychologist, 2*(1), 167 (abstract).

Andrews, G., and Harris, M. (1964) *The syndrome of stuttering.* London: Spastics Society Medical Education and Information Unit.

Andrews, J. G. (1965) The nature of stuttering. *Journal of the Australian College of Speech Therapists, 15,* 6–15.

Arend, R., Handzel, L., and Weiss, B. (1962) Dysphatic stuttering. *Folia Phoniatrica, 14,* 55–66.

Arnfred, A. H. (July 12, 1956) Word blindness and stuttering as developmental disorders. *Ugeskrift for Laeger,* p. 118. (Danish)

Arnott, D. W. A. (1958) Stammering. *Bulletin, Post Graduate Communications in Medicine* (University of Sydney, Australia), pp. 339–345.

Aron, M. L. (1960) Some general aspects concerning stuttering which indicate fields of research. *Journal of the South African Logopedic Society, 6,* 3–7.

Aron, M. L. (1962) Nature and incidence of stuttering among a Bantu group of school-going children. *Journal of Speech and Hearing Disorders, 27,* 116–128.

Aron, M. L. (1965) The effects of the combination of trifluoperazine and amylobarbitone on the adult stutterer. *Medical Proceedings* (South Africa), *11,* 227–233.

Aron, M. L. (1967) The relationships between measurements of stuttering behaviour. *Journal of the South African Logopedic Society, 14*(1), 15–34.

Azrin, N., Jones, R. J., and Flye, B. (1968) A synchronization effect and its application to stuttering by a portable apparatus. *Journal of Applied Behavioral Analysis, 1,* 283–295.

Bakwin, R., and Bakwin, H. (1952) Cluttering. *Journal of Pediatrics, 40,* 393–396.

Baldwin, M. (1954) Notes on play sessions with two stammering boys. *Speech* (London), *18,* 17–23.

Balkanyi, C. (1961) Psycho-analysis of a stammering girl. *International Journal of Psycho-Analysis, 42,* 97–109.

Balkanyi, C. (1968) La fonction verbale: point de vue psychanalytique, *Reeduc. orthophon., 34,* 71–86.

Bar, A. (1967) Effects of listening instructions on attention to manner and content of stutterers' speech. *Journal of Speech and Hearing Disorders, 10,* 87–92.

Barbara, D. A. (1954) *Stuttering: A psychodynamic approach to its understanding and treatment.* New York: Julian Press.

Barbara, D. A. (1956a) The classroom teacher's role in stuttering. *Speech Teacher, 5,* 137–139.

Barbara, D. A. (1956b) Understanding stuttering. *New York State Journal of Medicine, 45,* 1798–1802.

Barbara, D. A. (1957) Some aspects of stuttering in light of Adlerian psychology. *Journal of Individual Psychology, 13,* 188–193.

Barbara, D. A. (1962) Psychotherapy of the adult stutterer. In D. A. Barbara, ed., *The psychotherapy of stuttering.* Springfield, Ill.: Charles C Thomas.

Barbara, D. A. (1965) An experiment into the team approach to group therapy with stutterers. In D. A. Barbara, ed., *New directions in stuttering: Theory and practice.* Springfield, Ill.: Charles C Thomas.

Barbara, D. A., Goldard, N. and Oram, C. (1961) Group psycho-analysis with adult stutterers. *American Journal of Psychoanalysis, 21,* 40–57.

Barbara, D. A., ed. (1962) *The psychotherapy of stuttering,* Springfield, Ill.: Charles C Thomas.

Barbara, D. A., ed. (1965a) *New directions in stuttering: Theory and practice.* Springfield, Ill.: Charles C Thomas.

Barbara, D. A., ed. (1965b) *Questions and answers on stuttering.* Springfield, Ill.: Charles C Thomas.

Barnes, M. L. (1952) A study of attitudes of parents and teachers toward children who stutter. *Speech Monographs, 19,* 189.

Bastard, P. C. (1963) Vocational guidance of persons with normal intelligence but having a speech defect. *Revue de Neuropsychiatrie Infantile et d'Hygiene Mentale de l'Enfance, 11,* 245–250. (French)

Bäumler, F. (1957) Multidimensional treatment of stuttering children and adolescents in speech therapy groups. *Zeitschrift für Psychotherapie und Medizinische Psychologie, 7,* 99–104.

Baurand, G., and Striglioni, L. (1968) Importance du facteur parental dans le symptome begaiement. *Journal Francais ORL, 17,* 209–216.

Bayly, R. B. (1965) Comments from a stutterer. *Today's Speech, 13,* 2–3.

Bearss, M. L. (1952) An investigation of the effect of penalty on the expectance of frequency of stuttering. *Speech Monographs, 19,* 189–190.

Bed rest best way to unwind stammering child. (December, 1959) *Science News-Letter,* pp. 88–89.

Beebe, H. (1957) Sentence mindedness. *Folia Phoniatrica, 9,* 44–48.

Beebe, H., and Froeschels, E. (1960) Symptomatology in stuttering: An aid to the case history. *Aktuelle Probleme der Phoniatric und Logopaedie; Supplementa ad Folia Phoniatrica, 1,* 179–183.

Beech, H. R., and Fransella, F. (1968) *Research and experiment in stuttering.* London: Pergamon Press.

Beech, H. R., and Fransella, F. (1969) Explanation of the "Rhythm Effect" in stuttering. In B. Gray and G. England, eds., *Stuttering and the conditioning therapies.* Monterey, Calif.: Monterey Institute for Speech and Hearing.

Beech, Reginald. (1967) Stuttering and stammering. *Psychology Today, 1,* 48–51, 61.

Belleti, M. F., and Facchine, G. M. (1965) Medical-psycho-educational observations and a schematic of the principal aspects of stuttering in school girls. *Bellettino Societa Italiana di Fonetica Sperimentale, Fonetica Biologica, Foniatria Audiologia. 14,* 14–28.

Bellussi, G., and Granone, F. (1949) Narcotherapy in stuttering. *Rivista Oto-Neuro-Oftalmolgica, 24,* 497–506.

Ben-Israel, L. (1957) Derekh hadasha beripuy hagimgum. (A new way to heal stuttering). *Ofakim, 11,* 155–160.

Berges, J. (1964) Indications of relaxation in the child. *Revue de Neuropsychiatrie Infantile et d'Hygiene Mentale de l'Enfrance, 12,* 483–487. (French)

Berlin, A. J. (1954) An exploratory attempt to isolate types of stuttering. *Dissertation Abstracts, 14,* 2433–2434. Abstract of doctoral dissertation, Northwestern University, 1954.

Berlin, C. I. (1960) Parents' diagnoses of stuttering. *Journal of Speech and Hearing Research, 3,* 372–379.

Berlin, S., and Berlin, C. (1964) Acceptability of stuttering control patterns. *Journal of Speech and Hearing Disorders, 29,* 436–441.

Berlinsky, S. L. (1954) A comparison of stutterers and non-stutterers in four conditions of experimentally induced anxiety. *Dissertation Abstracts, 14,* 719. Abstract of doctoral dissertation, University of Michigan, 1954.

Bernhardt, R. B. (1954) Personality conflict and the act of stuttering. *Dissertation Abstracts, 14,* 709. Abstract of doctoral dissertation, University of Michigan, 1954.

Berry, M. F. (1965) Historical vignettes of leaders in speech and hearing. III. Stuttering. *Asha, 7,* 78–79.

Berwick, N. H. (1955) Stuttering in response to photographs

of certain selected listeners. In W. Johnson and R. Leutenneger, eds., *Stuttering in children and adults.* Minneapolis: University of Minnesota Press.

Bibik, V. A. (1966) The use of tranquilizers in the treatment of stuttering in children. *Zhurnal Nevropatologii i Psikhiatrii, 66,* 1089–1090.

Biesalski, I. (1964) Experiences with a youth hostel for speech therapy. *Zeitschrift fur Laryngologie, Rhinologie, Otologie und Ihre Grenzgebietl, 43,* 254–257.

Biggs, B. E., and Sheehan, J. G. (1969) Punishment or distraction? Operant stuttering revisited. *Journal of Abnormal Psychology, 74,* 256–262.

Bignardi, F., and Spettoli, L. (1955) Stuttering and contrasted left-handedness: Clinical study. *Giornale de Psichiatria e di Neuropatologie, 83,* 357–361. (Italian)

Blankenship, J. (1964) Stuttering in normal speech. *Journal of Speech and Hearing Research, 7,* 95–96.

Blanton, S. (1965) Stuttering. In D. A. Barbara, ed., *New directions in stuttering: Theory and practice.* Springfield, Ill.: Charles C Thomas.

Bloch, J. (1962) Case history of an 18 year old stutterer. *Journal of the South African Logopedic Society, 9,* 24–27.

Bloch, P. (1958) The problem of stuttering. Rio de Janeiro: Colecao Fala. (Portuguese)

Bloodstein, O. N. (1950a) Hypothetic conditions under which stuttering is reduced or absent. *Journal of Speech and Hearing Disorders, 15,* 142–153.

Bloodstein, O. N. (1950b) Rating scale study of conditions under which stuttering is reduced or absent. *Journal of Speech and Hearing Disorders, 15,* 29–36.

Bloodstein, O. N. (1958) Stuttering as an anticipatory struggle reaction. In J. Eisenson, ed., *Stuttering: A symposium,* New York: Harper & Row.

Bloodstein, O. N. (1959) *A handbook on stuttering for professional workers.* Chicago: National Society for Crippled Children and Adults.

Bloodstein, O. N. (1960a) Development of stuttering. I., *Journal of Speech and Hearing Disorders, 25,* 219–237.

Bloodstein, O. N. (1960b) Development of stuttering. II. *Journal of Speech and Hearing Disorders, 25,* 366–376.

Bloodstein, O. N. (1961a) Development of stuttering. III. *Journal of Speech and Hearing Disorders, 26,* 67–82.

Bloodstein, O. N. ((1961b) Stuttering in families of adopted stutterers. *Journal of Speech and Hearing Disorders, 26,* 395–396.

Bloodstein, O. N. (1969) *A handbook on stuttering.* Chicago: National Easter Seal Society.

Bloodstein, O. N., Alper, J., and Zisk, P. (1965) Stuttering as an outgrowth of normal disfluency. In D. A. Barbara, ed., *New directions in stuttering: Theory and practice.* Springfield, Ill.: Charles C Thomas.

Bloodstein, O. N., and Bloodstein, A. (1955) Interpretations of facial reactions to stuttering. *Journal of speech and hearing disorders, 20,* 148–55.

Bloodstein, O. N., and Gantwerk, B. F. (1967) Grammatical function in relation to stuttering in young children. *Journal of Speech and Hearing Research, 10,* 786–789.

Bloodstein, O. N., Jaeger, W., and Tureen, J. (1952) Diagnosis of stuttering by parents of stutterers and nonstutterers. *Journal of Speech and Hearing Disorders, 17,* 308–315.

Bloodstein, O. N., and Schreiber, L. R. (1957) Obsessive-compulsive reactions in stutterers. *Journal of Speech and Hearing Disorders, 22,* 33–39.

Bloodstein, O. N., and Smith, S. M. (1954) A study of diagnosis of stuttering with special references to the sex ratio. *Journal of Speech and Hearing Disorders, 19,* 459–466.

Bloom, J. (1958) Child training and stuttering. Ph.D. dissertation, University of Michigan, Ann Arbor.

Bluemel, C. S. (1957) *Riddle of stuttering.* Danville, Ill.: *Interstate.*

Bluemel, C. S. (1958) Stuttering: A psychiatric viewpoint. *Journal of Speech Disorders, 23,* 263–267.

Bluemel, C. S. (1959) If a child stammers. *Mental Hygiene, 43,* 390–393.

Bluemel, C. S. (1960) Concepts of stammering: A century in review. *Journal of Speech and Hearing Disorders. 25,* 24–32.

Bluemel, C. S. (1962) Organization of speech as basic therapy. In D. A. Barbara, ed., *The psychotherapy of stuttering.* Springfield, Ill.: Charles C Thomas.

Boehmler, R. M. (1958) Listener responses to non-fluencies. *Journal of Speech and Hearing Research, 1,* 132–141.

Boland, J. L., (1951) Type of birth as related to stuttering. *Journal of Speech and Hearing Disorders, 16,* 40–43.

Boland, J. L. (1952) A comparison of stutterers and non-stutterers on several measures of anxiety. *Speech Monographs, 20,* 144. Abstract of doctoral dissertation, University of Michigan, 1952.

Bolin, B. J. (1953) Left-handedness and stuttering as a sign diagnostic for epileptics. *Journal of Mental Science, 99,* 483–488.

Borel-Maisonny, S. (1966) Delayed speech with disposition toward stuttering. *Pedo-psychiatrie, 1,* 23–29. (French)

Borel-Maisonny, S. (1966) Retard de parole evoluant vers un begaiement: Etude du quelques cas typiques. *Annales Medico-Psychologiques, 2*(4), 531.

Bormann, E. G. (1969) Ephphatha, or, some advice to stammerers. *Journal of Speech and Hearing Research, 12,* 453–461.

Brady, J. P. (1968) A behavioral approach to the treatment of stuttering. *American Journal of Psychiatry, 125,* 843–848.

Brady, J. P. (1969) Studies on the metronome effect on stuttering. *Behaviour Research and Therapy, 7,* 197–204.

Brankel, O. (1958) Sinn und Grenzen d. autogenen Trainings im Rahmen der Stotterbehandlung. *Folia Phoniatrica, 10,* 112–119.

Brankel, O. (1960) The pathophysiology of stuttering in the light of the doctrine of internal image. *Aerztliche Forschung, 15*(1), 341–347. (German)

Brankel, O. (1961) Pneumotachographic studies in stutterers. *Folia Phoniatrica, 13,* 136–143. (German)

Brankel, O. (1963) Die Bedeutung der synchronen Erfassung von skustischen, pneumotachographischen, myographischen, und elektromyographischen Symptomenbildern Beim Stottern. *Folia Phoniatrica, 15,* 177–182.

Brodnitz, F. S. (1951) Stuttering in different types of identical twins. *Journal of Speech and Hearing Disorders, 16,* 334–336.

Brody, M. V., and Harrison, S. I. (1954) Group psychotherapy with male stutterers. *International Journal of Group Psychotherapy, 4,* 154–162.

Brody, M. W., and Harrison, S. I. (1966) Stutterers. In S. R. Slavson, ed., *The fields of group psychotherapy.* New York: Wiley.

Brook, F. (1957) *Stammering and its treatment.* London: Pitman.

Brookshire, R. H. (1969) Effects of random and response contingent noise upon disfluencies of normal speakers, *Journal of Speech and Hearing Research, 12,* 126–134.

Brookshire, R. H., and Eveslage, R. A. (1969) Verbal punishment of disfluency following augmentation of disfluency by random delivery of aversive stimuli. *Journal of Speech and Hearing, 12,* 383–388.

Browning, R. M. (1967) Behavior therapy for stuttering in a schizophrenic child. *Behaviour Research and Therapy, 5,* 27–35.

Bruckner, P. (1956) Beiträge zur Pathocharakterologie Stotternder jugendlicher. Contributions to the patho-characterology of young stutterers.) *Praxis der Kinderpsychologie und Kinderpsychiatrie, 5,* 202–6.

Bruno, G., Camarda, V. and Curi, L. (1965) Contribution to the study of organic causal factors in the pathogenesis of stuttering. *Bolletino delle Malattie dell' Orecchio, della Gola, del Naso, 83,* 753–758. (Italian)

Brutten, E. J. (1957) A colorimetric anxiety measure of stuttering and expectancy adaptation. *Dissertation Abstracts, 17,* 2707–2708.

Brutten, E. J. (1963) Palmar sweat investigation of disfluency and expectancy adaptation. *Journal of Speech and Hearing Research, 6,* 40–48.

Brutten, E. J. (1969) Stuttering: reflections on a two-factor approach to behavior modification. In B. Gray and G. England, eds., *Stuttering and the conditioning therapies.* Monterey, Calif.: Monterey Institute for Speech and Hearing.

Brutten, E. J., and Gray, B. B. (1961) Effects of word cue removal on adaptation and adjacency: A clinical paradigm. *Journal of Speech and Hearing Disorders, 26,* 385–389.

Brutten, E. J., and Shoemaker, D. J. (1967) *The modification of stuttering.* Englewood Cliffs, N. J.: Prentice-Hall.

Brutten, E. J., and Shoemaker, D. J. (1969) Stuttering: the disintegration of speech due to conditioned negative emotion. In B. Gray and G. England, eds., *Stuttering and the Conditioning Therapies.* Monterey, Calif.: Monterey Institute for Speech and Hearing.

Bryngelson, B. (1952) Suggestions in the theory and treatment of dysphemia and its symptom, stuttering. *The Speech Teacher, 1,* 131–136.

Bryngelson, B. (1955) A study of the speech difficulties of thirteen stutterers. In W. Johnson and R. Leutenegger, eds., *Stuttering in children and adults.* Minneapolis: University of Minnesota Press.

Bryngelson, B. (1958) Inside the skin. *Journal of Speech Disorders, 23,* 229–236.

Bryngelson, B. (1964) *Personality development through speech.* Minneapolis, Minn.: Denison.

Bryngelson, B. (1966) *Clinical group therapy for problem people: A practical treatise for stutterers and normal speakers.* Minneapolis, Minn.: Denison.

Bryngelson, B., Chapman, M. E., and Hansen, O. K. (1966) *Know yourself guide for those who stutter.* 4th ed. Minneapolis, Minn.: Burgess Publishing.

Bundeson, H. N. (January 1950) The child who stutters. *Ladies Home Journal,* pp. 24–25.

Bünzli-Zehnder, M. (1952) Cure of stuttering by psychotherapy. *Schweizer Archic für Neurologie und Psychiatrie,* 70, 399–406. (German)

Burke, B. D. (1969) Reduced auditory feedback and stuttering. *Behaviour Research and Therapy,* 7, 309–316.

Burke, B. D., and Yates, A. J. (1967) Stuttering: Theoretical and therapeutic considerations. I. Some implications of recent research findings to the theory of stuttering. *Australian Psychologist,* 2(1), 167 (abstract).

Burr, H. G., and Mullendore, J. M. (1960) Recent investigations on tranquilizers and stuttering. *Journal of Speech and Hearing Disorders,* 25, 33–37.

Burtscher, H. T., Jr. (1952) The operation of frustration in the transition to and the development of secondary stuttering. *Speech Monographs,* 19, 191.

Busse, E. W., and Clark, R. M. (1957) The use of the encephalogram in diagnosing speech disorders. *Folia Phoniatrica,* 9, 182–187.

Butler, B. R., Jr. (1965) The stuttering problem considered from an automatic control point of view. *Clearinghouse for Federal Scientific and Technical Information,* U. S. Department of Commerce, Springfield, Va. AD-622–685.

Cali, G., Pisani, F. and Tagliareni, F. (1965) Stuttering and electroencephalographic curves. *Clinica Otorinolaringoiatrica,* 17, 316–328. (Italian)

Carp, F. M. (1962) Psychosexual development of stutterers. *Journal of Projective Techniques and Personality Assessment,* 26, 388–391.

Carr, B. M. (1969) Speculation of vocal adaption of stutterers and nonstutterers. *Journal of Speech and Hearing Research,* 12, 665–666.

Chaney, C. F. (1969) Loci of disfluencies in the speech of

nonstutterers. *Journal of Speech and Hearing Research,* *12,* 667–668.

Chapin, A. B., and Kessler, H. E. (1950) Dental caries in individuals who stutter. *Dental Items of Interest, 72,* 162–167.

Chapman, M. (1959) *Self inventory: Group therapy for those who stutter.* Minneapolis, Minn.: Burgess Publishing.

Chase, R. A. (1958) Effect of delayed auditory feedback on the repetition of speech sounds. *Journal of Speech and Hearing Disorders, 23,* 583–590.

Cherepanov, I. M. (1967) Vliyanie fotostimulyatsii na bioelektricheskuyu aktivnost' golovnogo mozga i tonus myshts rechevogo apparate u bol'nykh logonevrozami. (Influence of photostimulation on bioelectrical activity of the brain and tonus of muscles of the speech apparatus in logoneurotics). *Zhurnal Nevropatologii i Psikhiatrii, 67,* 1477–1481. (Russian)

Cherry, C., and Sayers, B. M. (1956) Experiments upon the total inhibition of stammering by external control, and some clinical results. *Journal of Psychosomatic Research, 1,* 233–246.

Cherry, C., Sayers, B., and Marland, P. (1956) Some experiments on the total suppression of stammering; and a report on some clinical trials. *Bulletin of the British Psychological Society, 30,* 43–44. Abstract.

Cheveleva, N. A. (1961) O zaniatiiakh po ispravleniiu zaikaniia v proteesse ruchnogo truda. (Correction of stuttering by means of manual work.) *Doklady Akademia Petagogicheskikh Nauk RSFSR* (Institute of Defectology RSFSR Academy of Pedagogical Sciences), no. 6, 117–120.

Cheveleva, N. A. (1967) O metodakh preodoleniya zaikaniya, *Spetsial'naya Shkola, 3,* 9–15.

Cheveleva, N. A. (1968) Primenenie metoda ustraneniya zaikaniya u detei v protsesse ruchnoi i uchebnoi deyatel' nosti. (Application of the method for eliminating stuttering in young children in the process of manual and educational activity.) *Spetsial'naya Shkola, 4,* 80–84. (Russian)

Chevrie-Muller, C. (1964) Study of laryngeal functions in stutterers by the glottographic method (apropos of 28 cases). *Revue de Laryngologie, Otologie, Rhinologie, 85,* 763–774. (French)

Chotlos, J. W. (1955) Covariation in frequency of types of stuttering reactions. In W. Johnson and R. Leutenneger, eds., *Stuttering in children and adults.* Minneapolis: University of Minnesota Press.

Christensen, A. (1952) A quantitative study of personality dynamics in stuttering and nonstuttering siblings. *Speech Monographs, 19,* 144–45.

Chworowsky, C. R. (1952) A comparative study of the diadochokinetic rates of stutterers and non-stutterers in speech related and non-speech related movements. *Speech Monographs, 19,* 192.

Ciabrini, J., Hekimoglou, A., and Terrier, S. (1968) Approches du begaiement. *Reeduc. orthophon., 34,* 92–108.

Clark, R. M., and Fitzpatrick, J. A. (1962) The use of self-concept as an adjunct to diagnosis and psychotherapy. In D. A. Barbara, ed., *The psychotherapy of stuttering.* Springfield, Ill.: Charles C Thomas.

Clark, R. M., and Murray, F. P. (1965) Alterations in self-concept: A barometer of progress in individuals undergoing therapy for stuttering. In D. A. Barbara, ed., *New directions in stuttering: Theory and practice.* Springfield, Ill.: Charles C Thomas.

Clark, R. M., and Snyder, M. (1955) Group therapy for parents of preadolescent stutterers. *Group psychotherapy, 8,* 226–231.

Clawson, T. A., Jr. (1964) Hypnosis in medical practice. *Amercan Journal of Clinical Hypnosis, 6,* 232–236.

Coelho, C. A. (1961) Report from India. *Journal of Speech and Hearing Disorders, 26,* 90–94.

Cohen, E. (1953) A comparison of oral and spontaneous speech of stutterers with special reference to adaptation and consistency effects. *Speech Monographs, 20,* 144. Abstract of doctoral dissertation, State University of Iowa, 1952.

Connett, M. H. (1955) Experimentally induced changes in the relative frequency of stuttering on a specified sound. In W. Johnson and R. Leutenegger, eds., *Stuttering in children and adults.* Minneapolis: University of Minnesota Press.

Conway, J. K., *et al.* (1963) Positional effects in the stuttering of contextually organized verbal material. *Journal of Abnormal and Social Psychology, 67,* 299–303.

Cooper, E. B. (1965a) An inquiry into the use of interpersonal communication as a source for therapy with stutterers. In D. A. Barbara, ed., *New directions in stuttering: Theory and practice.* Springfield, Ill.: Charles C Thomas.

Cooper, E. B. (1965b) Structuring therapy for therapist and stuttering child. *Journal of Speech and Hearing Disorders, 30,* 75–79.

Cooper, E. B. (1966) Client-clinician relationships and concomitant factors in stuttering therapy. *Journal of Speech and Hearing Research, 9,* 194–207.

Cooper, E. B. (1968) A therapy process for the adult stutterer. *Journal of Speech and Hearing Disorders, 33*(3), 246–260.

Correll, R. E. (1956) Frequency analyses of EEG's of stutterers and normal speakers during photic stimulation. *Proceedings of the Iowa Academy of Science. 63,* 586–590.

Counihan, D. (1964) Stuttering: Etiology and prevention. *Clinical Pediatrics, 3,* 229–232.

Crayhay, S. (1967) Les facteurs psychologiques dans le begaiement. (Psychological factors in stuttering.) *Acta Neurologica Psychiatrica Beligica, 67*(11), 946–958. (French)

Cullinan, W. L., and Prather E. M. (1968) Reliability of "live" ratings of the speech of stutterers. *Perceptual and Motor Skills, 27,* 403–409.

Cullinan, W. L., Prather, E. M., and Williams, D. E. (1963) Comparison of procedures for scaling severity of stuttering. *Journal of Speech and Hearing Research, 6,* 187–194.

Cure for stammering? (November 21, 1955) *Newsweek,* p. 46.

Curlee, R. F. (1967) An experimental study of the effect of punishment of the expectancy to stutter on the frequency of subsequent expectancies and stuttering. *Dissertation Abstracts, 23*(5-B), 2173.

Curlee, R. F., and Perkins, W. H. (1968) The effect of punishment of expectancy to stutter on the frequencies of subsequent expectancies and stuttering. *Journal of Speech and Hearing Research, 11*(4), 787–795.

Curlee, R. F., and Perkins, W. H. (1969) Conversational rate control therapy for stuttering. *Journal of Speech and Hearing Disorders, 34,* 245–250.

Curry, F. K., and Gregory, H. H. (1969) The performance of stutterers on dichotic listening tasks thought to reflect cerebral dominance. *Journal of Speech and Hearing Research, 12,* 73–82.

Curtis, W. S. (1960) The effects of side-tone filtering on certain speech characteristics of stutterers. Ph.D. dissertation, Purdue University, Lafayette, Ind.

Czarnecka-Palinska, W., et. al. (1963) Experimental therapeutic colonies for stuttering children. *Otolaryngologia Polska, 17,* 485–486. (Polish)

Daly, D. A. and Cooper, E. B. (1967) Rate of stuttering adaptation under two electro-shock conditions. *Behaviour Research and Therapy, 5,* 49–54.

Daskalov, D. C. (1962) On the problem of the basic principles and methods of prevention and treatment of stammering. *Zhurnal Nevropatologii i Psikhiatrii imeni S. S. Korsakova, 62,* 1047–1052. (Russian)

Decrois, G., VanRapenbusch, R., and Depoorter, R. (1953) Neurovegitative dystonias in stutterers. *Revue de Laryngologie, Otologie, Rhinologie Supplement, 74,* 174–178. (French)

DeFranco, F., and Ragonese, G. (1960) Studies on stuttering. Cerebral bioelectric activity and somato-agnosia. *Giornale di Psichiatria e di Neuropatologia, 88,* 1031–1048.

DeFranco, F., and Sacco, F. (1960) Studies on stuttering. The psychomotoricity of stutterers. *Giornale di Psichiatria e di Neuropatologia, 88,* 1049–1065. (Italian)

DeFranco, F., and Sacco, F. (1961a) Studies on balbuties. Perceptive organization and spatial intelligence of stammering patients. *Rassegna di Studi Psichiatrici, 50,* 1–16. (Italian)

DeFranco, F., and Sacco, F. (1961b) Studies on balbuties. Abstract thinking of the stammering patient. *Rassegna di Studi Psichiatrici, 50,* 17–36. (Italian)

DeHirsch, K., and Langford, W. S. (1950) Clinical note on stuttering and cluttering in young children. *Pediatrics, 5,* 934–940.

Delacato, C. H. (1963) *The diagnosis and treatment of speech and reading problems.* Springfield, Ill.: Charles C Thomas.

Densem, A. E. (1955) The treatment of stammering. *New Zealand Speech Therapists Journal, 10,* 3–10.

DePlatero, D. M. (1967) La prueba del dibujo de la figura humana en el nino tartamudo, *Revista de Psiquiatria y Psicologia Medica, 8,* 27–34.

Depoorter, M. (1957) Guerison d'un begaiement particulier.

Journal Francais d'Oto-rhino-laryngologie, 6, 397–415.

Des, R. (1952) Electroencephalographic study of stutterers during sleep. *Speech Monographs, 19,* 192–193.

De Santis, M. (1958) Endocrine research into cases of stammering. *Valsalva, 35,* 328–333.

DeSouza Bittancourt, R. (1954) O desenvolmimen to da linguagem e seus desturbios. Consideracoes sobre a gagueira. (The development of speech and its disturbances. Considerations about stammering.) *Boletim do Instituto de Psicologie, Rio de Janeiro,* 4(7–8), 16–21.

Diatkine, R. (1951) Stuttering. *Evolution Psychiatrique,* no. 4, 525–544.

Diatkine, R. (February 1961) Stammering, its origins and treatment. *Semaine Thérapeutique, 37,* 142–43. (French)

DiCarlo, L. M., Katz, J., and Batkin, S. (1959) An exploratory investigation of the effect of meprobamate on stuttering behavior. *Journal of Nervous and Mental Diseases, 128,* 558–561.

Diehl, C. F. (1958) *A compendium of research and theory on stuttering.* Springfield, Ill.: Charles C Thomas.

Diehl, C. F. (1962) Patient-therapist relationship. In D. A. Barbara, ed., *The psychotherapy of stuttering.* Springfield, Ill.: Charles C Thomas.

Dixon, C. C. (1955) Stuttering adaptation in relation to assumed level of anxiety. In W. Johnson and R. Leutenegger, eds., *Stuttering in children and adults.* Minneapolis: University of Minnesota Press.

Dixon, C. C. (1957) The effect of interjected non-propositional verbalization during oral reading on stuttering frequency. *Journal of Educational Research, 51* 153–155.

Donohue, I. R. (1955) Stuttering adaptation during three hours of continuous oral reading. In W. Johnson and R. Leutenegger, eds., *Stuttering in children and adults.* Minneapolis: University of Minnesota Press.

Dosuzkov, B. (1960) On the relationship between stuttering and other neuroses. *Ceskoslovenska Psychiatric, 56,* 395–402. (Czech)

Dosuzkov, T. (1962) The anal and urethral control in children who suffer from idiopathic stuttering. *Abstracts of the Twelfth Congress of the International Association of Logopaedics and Phoniatrics.*

Douglas, E. (1954) Development of stuttering and its diagnosis. *Canadian Medical Association Journal, 71,* 366–371.

Douglass, E. (1951) Symptomatology and development of stuttering. *Canadian Medical Association Journal, 64,* 397–400.

Douglass, E., and Quarrington, B. (1952) Differentiation of interiorized and exteriorized secondary stuttering. *Journal of Speech and Hearing Disorders, 17,* 377–385.

Douglass, R. L. (1952) An experimental electroencephalographic study of stimulus reaction in stutterers. *Speech Monographs, 19,* 146.

Downton, W. (1955) The effect of instructions concerning mode of stuttering on the breathing of stutterers. In W. Johnson and R. Leutenegger, eds., *Stuttering in Children and Adults.* Minneapolis: University of Minnesota Press.

Eastman, D. F. (1960) An exploratory investigation of the psychoanalytic theory of stuttering by means of the Blacky pictures test. Ph.D. dissertation, University of Nebraska, Lincoln.

Egland, G. O. (1955) Repetitions and prolongations in the speech of stuttering and non-stuttering children. In W. Johnson and R. Leutenegger, eds., *Stuttering in children and adults.* Minneapolis: University of Minnesota Press.

Eisenson, J. (1958) A perseverative theory of stuttering. In J. Eisenson, ed., *Stuttering: A symposium.* New York: Harper & Row.

Eisenson, J. (1966) Observations of the incidence of stuttering in a special culture. *Asha, 8,* 391–394.

El-Kholy, W. (1950–1951) Stuttering and stammering. *Egyptian Journal of Psychology, 3,* 31–40.

Elliott, C. S. (1951) *Bibliography of stuttering: Tentative edition.* Evanston, Ill.: Book Box.

Emerick, L. L. (1960a) Extensional definition and attitude toward stuttering. *Journal of Speech and Hearing Research, 3,* 181–186.

Emerick, L. L. (1960b) Social distance scale for stutterers. *Journal of Speech and Hearing Disorders, 25,* 408–409.

Emerick, L. L. (1963) Clinical observation on the "final" stuttering. *Journal of Speech and Hearing Disorders, 28,* 194–195.

Emerick, L. L. (1966a) Bibliotherapy for stutterers: Four case histories. *Quarterly Journal of Speech, 52,* 74–79.

Emerick, L. L. (1966b) Social distance and stuttering. *Southern Speech Journal, 31*, 219–222.

Emerick, L. L. (1967) An evaluation of three psychological variables in tonic and clonic stutterers and in non-stutterers. *Dissertation Abstracts, 28*(1-A), 317.

Emonds, P. L. F. (1953–1954) Het stotteren. (Stuttering.) *Gawein, 2*, 1–17, 43–47.

Fahmy, M. (1950) The theory of habit control and negative practice as a curative method in the treatment of stammering. *Speech* (London), *14*, 24–30.

Fahmy, M. (1951) Stuttering. *Egyptian Journal of Psychology, 3*, 399–404.

Falck, F. J. (1964) Stuttering and hypnosis. *International Journal of Clinical and Experimental Hypnosis, 12*, 67–74.

Fawcus, R., and Fawcus, M. A. (1962) Some observations on group work with adult stammerers. *Journal of South African Logopedic Society, 9*, 16–23.

Fernau-Horn, H. (1952) Circle of inhibition and expiration in pathogenesis and therapy of stuttering. *Medizinische Monatsschrift, 6*, 323–327. (German)

Fiedler, F. E., and Wepman, J. M. (1951) An exploratory investigation of the self-concept of stutterers. *Journal of Speech and Hearing Disorders, 16*, 110–114.

Fierman, E. Y. (1955) The role of cues in stuttering adaptation. In W. Johnson and R. Leutenegger, eds., *Stuttering in children and adults*. Minneapolis: University of Minnesota Press.

Finkelstein, P., and Weisberger, S. E. (1954) The motor proficiency of stutterers. *Journal of Speech and Hearing Disorders. 19*, 52–57.

Fish, C. H., and Bowling, E. (1965) The effect of treatment with d-amphetamine and a tranquilizing agent, trifluoperazine. A preliminary report on an uncontrolled study. *California Medicine, 103*, 337–339.

Fisher, Martin N. (1968) The anal-obsessive character structure of the stutterer and its effects upon meaning. *Dissertation Abstracts, 28*(11-B), 4745–4746.

Fitzsimons, R. (1962) *A new boy on Hillside Street.* New York: Springer Publishing.

Flanagan, B. (1959) Instatement of stuttering in normally fluent individuals through operant procedures. *Science, 130*, 979–981.

Flanagan, B., Goldiamond, I., and Azrin, N. (1958) Operant stuttering: The control of stuttering behavior through response-contingent consequences. *Journal of Experimental Analysis of Behavior, 1,* 173–177.

Fleming, M. (1957) Relationship between stammering and aphasia. *Journal of South African Logopedic Society, 4,* 3–6.

Flosdorf, P. (1960) Uber das Stottern. (On stuttering.) *Jahrbuch für Psychologie, Psychotherapie und Medizinesche Anthropologie, 7,* 126–174.

Forte, M., and Fried, B. (1962) Theories of stuttering. *Megamot, 12,* 158–167.

Fowler, R. D. (1962) The role of the psychologist in the treatment of stuttering. In D. A. Barbara, ed., *The psychotherapy of stuttering.* Springfield, Ill.: Charles C Thomas.

Fox, D. R. (1966) Electroencephalographic analysis during stuttering and non-stuttering. *Journal of Speech and Hearing Research, 9,* 448–497.

Fransella, F. (1965) An experimental evaluation of the speech correction semantic differential. *Speech Monograph, 32,* 448–451.

Fransella, F. (1967) Rhythm as a distractor in the modification of stuttering. *Behavior Research and Therapy, 5*(3), 253–255.

Fransella, F. (1969) The stutterer as subject or object. In B. Gray and G. England, eds., *Stuttering and the conditioning therapies.* Monterey, Calif.: Monterey Institute for Speech and Hearing.

Fransella, F., and Beech, H. R. (1965) An experimental analysis of the effect of rhythm on the speech of stutterers. *Behaviour Research and Therapy, 3,* 195–201.

Frasier, J. (1955) An exploration of stutterers' theories of their own stuttering. In W. Johnson and R. Leutenegger, eds., *Stuttering in children and adults.* Minneapolis: University of Minnesota Press.

Freed, G. H. (December 31, 1957) Anti-stammering device. U. S. Patent Office, No. 2, 818, 065.

Freud, E. D. (1957) What causes stuttering? *Acta Psychiatrica et Neurologica Scandinavica, 33,* 137–150.

Freund, H. (1952) Studies in the relationship between stuttering and cluttering. *Folia Phoniatrica, 4,* 146–158.

Freund, H. (1953) Psychopathological aspects of stuttering. *American Journal of Psychotherapy, 7,* 689–705.

Freund, H. (1955) Psychosis and stuttering. Journal of Nervous and Mental Diseases, 122, 161–172.

Freund, H. (1960) Reflexions on subconscious phenomena in stuttering. *Aktuelle Probleme der Phoniatrie und Logopaedie; Supplementa ad Folia Phoniatrica, 1,* 184–189.

Freund, H. (1966) *Psychopathology and the problems of stuttering.* Springfield, Ill.: Charles C Thomas.

Frick, J. V. (1952) An exploratory study of the effect of punishment (electric shock) upon stuttering behavior. *Speech Monographs, 19,* 146–147.

Frick, J. V. (1955) Spontaneous recovery of the stuttering response as a function of the degree of adaptation. In W. Johnson and R. Leutenegger, eds., *Stuttering in children and adults.* Minneapolis: University of Minnesota Press.

Friedman, G. M. (1955) A test of attitude toward stuttering. In W. Johnson and R. Leutenegger, eds., *Stuttering in children and adults.* Minneapolis: University of Minnesota Press.

Fritzell, B. (1963) On stuttering and studies on stuttering in Marburg (Anton Schilling). *Svenska Lakartidningen, 60,* 3396–3405. (Swedish)

Froeschels, E. (1950) A technique for stutterers—"Ventriloquism." *Journal of Speech and Hearing Disorders, 15,* 336–337.

Froeschels, E. (1951) Stuttering and psychotherapy. *Folia Phoniatrica, 3,* 1–9.

Froeschels, E. (1952a) Chewing method as therapy. *American Medical Association Archives in Otolaryngology, 56,* 427–434.

Froeschels, E. (1952b) The significance of symptomatology for the understanding of the essence of stuttering. *Folia Phoniatrica, 4,* 217–230.

Froeschels, E. (1953) Basic thinking disorders in stutterers. *Monatsschrift für Psychiatrie und Neurologie, 125,* 135–139. (German)

Froeschels, E. (1954) Imitation stuttering. *Folia Phoniatrica, 6,* 178–185.

Froeschels, E. (1955a) Contributions to the relationship between stuttering and cluttering. *Logopaedie en Phoniatrie, 4,* 1–6.

Froeschels, E. (1955b) Core of stuttering. *Acta-Oto-Laryngologica, 45,* 115–119.

Froeschels, E. (1957) A sign of stuttering not described before. *Logopaedie en Phoniatrie, 10,* 1–6.

Froeschels, E. (1961) New viewpoints on stuttering. *Folia Phoniatrica, 13,* 187–201.

Froeschels, E. (1964) Speech structure and stuttering. *The Voice, 8,* 20–21.

Froeschels, E., and Rieber, R. W. (1963) The problem of auditory and visual imperceptivity in stutterers. *Folia Phoniatrica, 15,* 13–20.

Früh, K. F. (1965) *Cybernetics of voice production and stuttering.* Stuttgart: Eugen Rentsch Verlag. (German)

Garde, E. J. (1957) Physio-pathologie et therapeutique des begaiements. *Semaine des Hospitaux de Paris, 33,* 1406–1407.

Gaitonde, M. R. (1954) Stammering: Treatment of twenty-seven cases. *Indian Journal of Medical Sciences, 8,* 831–835.

Gedda, L., Branconi, L., and Bruno, G. (1960) Su alcuni casi di balbuzis in coppie gemellari mono-e dizigotiche. Some cases of stammering in monozygotic and dizygotic twin pairs. *Acta Geneticae Medical et Gemellologiae, 9,* 407–426.

Geisler, E. (1955) Etiology and therapy of stuttering during childhood. *Archiv für Kinderheilkunde, 152,* 11–30. (German)

Geller, A. (1962) The need for a total evaluation of the patient: A case history of stuttering and epilepsy. *Chicago Medical School Quarterly, 22,* 106–113.

Gherarducci, D., and Jaria, A. (1956) Personality of stuttering children studied by means of mental tests. *Rivista di Patologia Nervosa e Mentale. 77,* 521–523. (Italian)

Gildston, P. (1967) Stutterers' self-acceptance and perceived parental acceptance. *Journal of Abnormal Psychology, 72,* 59–64.

Gilmore, M. L. (October 1961) Stop your stuttering. *PTA Magazine,* pp. 7–8.

Girone, D., and Bruno, G. (1957) Some characteristics of the glycemic curve in stutterers, *Folia Phoniatrica, 9,* 87–89.

Glasner, P. J. (1962) A holistic approach to the problem of stuttering in the young child. In D. A. Barbara, ed., *Psychological and psychiatric aspects of speech and hearing.* Springfield, Ill.: Charles C Thomas.

Glasner, P. J., and Dahl, M. F. (1952) Stuttering—Prophylactic program for its control. *American Journal of Public Health, 42,* 1111–1115.

Glasner, P. J., and Rosenthal, D. (1957) Parental diagnosis of stuttering in young children. *Journal of Speech Disorders, 22,* 288–295.

Glasner, P. J., and Vermilyea, F. D. (1953) An investigation of the definition and use of the diagnosis, "primary stuttering." *Journal of Speech and Hearing Disorders, 18,* 161–167.

Glauber, H. M. (1953) The impact of a shift in the psychological constellation of the family on the treatment of a stuttering boy. *American Journal of Orthopsychiatry, 22,* 755–774.

Glauber, I. P. (1952) Dynamic therapy for the stutterer. In G. Bychowski and J. L. Despert, eds., *Specialized techniques in psychotherapy.* New York: Basic Books.

Glauber, I. P. (1953) The treatment of stuttering. *Social Casework, 24,* 162–167.

Glauber, I. P. (1954) The nature of stuttering. *Social Casework, 34,* 95–103.

Glauber, I. P. (1958a) Freud's contributions on stuttering: Their relation to some current insights. *Journal of the American Psychoanalytic Association, 6,* 326–347.

Glauber, I. P. (1958b) The psychoanalysis of stuttering, in J. Eisenson, ed., *Stuttering: A symposium,* New York: Harper & Row.

Glauber, I. P. (1959) Notes on the early stages in the development of stuttering. *Journal of Hillside Hospital, 8,* 54–64.

Glauber, I. P. (1968) Dysautomatization: A disorder of preconscious ego functioning. *International Journal of Psycho-Analysis, 49*(1), 89–99.

Goda, S. (1961) Stuttering manifestations following spinal meningitis. *Journal of Speech and Hearing Disorders, 26,* 392–393.

Goldburgh, S. J., and Penney, J. F. (1966) Stuttering: An integrated view. *Diseases of the Nervous System, 27,* 42–46.

Goldiamond, I. (1960a) Blocked speech communication and delayed feedback: An experimental design. Technical Report No. 1, Progress Report. Operational Applications Laboratory, Air Force Cambridge Research Center, Bedford, Mass.

Goldiamond, I. (1960b) The temporal development of fluent and blocked speech communication. Final Report and Technical Report, Numbers 2, 3, 4. Operational Applications Laboratory, Air Force Cambridge Research Center, Bedford, Mass.

Goldiamond, I. (1964) Stuttering and fluency as manipulable operant response classes. In L. Krasner and L. P. Ullmann, eds., *Research in behavior modification: New developments and their clinical applications.* New York: Holt, Rinehart and Winston.

✓ Goldman, P. M. (January 10, 1965) Children's problems that go away. *New York Times Magazine,* p. 58.

Goldman, R. (1967) Cultural influences on the sex ratio in the incidence of stuttering. *American Anthropologist, 69,* 78–81.

Goldman, R., and Shames, G. H. (1964a) A study of goal setting behavior of parents of stutterers and nonstutterers. *Journal of Speech and Hearing Disorders, 29,* 192–194.

Goldman, R., and Shames, G. H. (1964b) Comparisons of the goals that parents of stutterers and parents of nonstutterers set for their children. *Journal of Speech and Hearing Disorders, 29,* 381–389.

Golub, A. J. (1952) The influence of constant and varying word stimuli on stuttering adaptation. *Speech Monographs, 19,* 193.

Golub, A. J. (1953) The heart rates of stutterers and nonstutterers in relation to frequency of stuttering during a series of oral readings. *Speech Monographs, 20,* 146. Abstract of doctoral dissertation, State University of Iowa, 1952.

✓ Gondaira, T. (1960) A case study of a boy with stuttering and physical malformation. *Japanese Journal of Child Psychology, 1,* 340–350.

Goodstein, L. D. (1956) MMPI profiles of stutterers' parents: A follow-up study. *Journal of Speech Disorders, 21,* 430–435.

Goodstein, L. D., and Dahlstrom, W. G. (1956) MMPI difference between parents of stuttering and nonstuttering children. *Journal of Consulting Psychology, 20,* 365–370.

Goss A. E. (1952) Stuttering behavior and anxiety as function of duration of stimulus words. *Journal of Abnormal and Social Psychology, 47,* 38–50.

Goss, A. E. (1956) Stuttering behavior and anxiety as a function of experimental training. *Journal of Speech Disorders, 21,* 343–351.

Gottlober, A. B. (1953) *Understanding stuttering.* New York: Grune & Stratton.

Gottsleben, R. H. (1955) The incidence of stuttering in a group of mongoloids. *Training School Bulletin, 51,* 209–218.

Gould, E. (1966) Some reactions of stutterers to imposed silence. *Dissertation Abstracts, 26,* 5547–5548.

Gould, E., and Sheehan, J. G. (1967) Effect of silence on stuttering. *Journal of Abnormal Psychology, 72,* 441–445.

Graf, O. I. (1955) Incidence of stuttering among twins. In W. Johnson and R. Leutenegger, *Stuttering in children and adults.* Minneapolis: University of Minnesota Press.

Gray, B. B. (1965a) Theoretical approximations of stuttering adaptation. *Behaviour Research and Therapy, 3,* 171–185.

Gray B. B. (1965b) Theoretical approximations of stuttering adaptation: Statement of predictive accuracy. *Behavior Research and Therapy, 3,* 221–227.

Gray, B. B., and Brutten, E. J. (1965) The relationship between anxiety, fatigue, and spontaneous recovery in stuttering. *Behavior Research and Therapy, 2,* 251–259.

Gray, B. B., and Karmen, J. L. (1967) The relationship between non-verbal anxiety and stuttering adaptation. *Journal of Communication Disorders, 1,* 141–151.

Gray, B., and England, G. (1969) Stuttering: The measurement of anxiety during reciprocal inhibition. In B. Gray and G. England, eds., *Stuttering and the conditioning therapies.* Monterey, Calif.: Monterey Institute for Speech and Hearing.

Gray, B., and England, G., eds. (1969) *Stuttering and the conditioning therapies.* Monterey, Calif.: Monterey Institute for Speech and Hearing.

Gray, K. C. (1968) Anticipation and stuttering: A pupillographic study. *Dissertation Abstracts, 29,* 406–407.

Gregory, H. H. (1964a) Speech clinic helps the adult stutterer. *Rehabilitation Record, 5,* 9–12.

Gregory, H. H. (1964b) Stuttering and auditory central nervous system disorders. *Journal of Speech and Hearing Research, 7,* 335–341.

Gregory, H. H. (1968) Applications of learning theory concepts in the management of stuttering. In H. H. Gregory, ed., *Learning theory and stuttering therapy*. Evanston, Ill.: Northwestern University Press.

Gregory, H. H. (1969) *An assessment of the results of stuttering therapy*. This is a final report, research and demonstration project 1725-S, Social and Rehabilitation Service, U.S. Dept. of H. E. and W.

Griffith, F. A. (1969) Uses of the Sheehan Sentence Completion Test in speech therapy for stuttering. *Journal of Speech and Hearing Disorders, 34,* 342–349.

Grossman, D. J. (1952) A study of the parents of stuttering and non-stuttering children using the Minnesota multiphasic personality inventory and the Minnesota scale of parents' opinions. *Speech Monographs, 19,* 193–194.

Gruber, L. (1958) An experimental investigation of the effect of severity of stuttering upon listener judgments of the suitability of individuals for various types of employment. *Speech and Hearing Therapist* (Indiana), *17,* 9–11.

Gruber, L. (1965) Sensory feedback and stuttering. *Journal of Speech and Hearing Disorders, 30,* 373–380.

Guantieri, G. (1963) Contribution to the study of the etiopathogenesis and therapy in stuttering: Psychological investigation of a case. *Annali di Larengologia, Otologia, Renologia, Faringologia, 62,* 338–346. (Italian)

Gumpertz, P. (1961) Moderne Betrachungenz. Stotterproblem. *Die Sprachheilkunde, 61,* 1–7.

Gundermann, H., and Weuffen, M. (1965) Usefulness of stuttering courses. *Zeitschrift fur Laryngologie, Rhinologie, Otologie, und irhe Grenzgebiete, 44,* 517–521. (German)

Guns, P. (November 1955) Stammering and stuttering. *Revue de Laryngologie, Otologie, Rhinologie,* Supplement, *76,* 695–707. (French)

Gutzman, H. J. (1954) Experiments with treatment of speech disorders with glutamic acid. *Folia Phoniatrica, 6.*

Gutzman, H. J. (1962) On the possibility or necessity of medical treatment of stuttering. *Deutsches Medizinisches Journal, 13,* 467–469. (German)

Habermann, G. (December 9, 1963) On the treatment of stuttering with methylpentynol (Subcorticalum). Studies on school children with speech disorders. *Archiv fur Ohren-Nasen und Kehlkopfheilkunde Vereinigt mit Zeitschrift fur Hals-, Nasen und Ohrenheilkunde, 172,* 680–684. (German)

Hackett, John D. (1968) Schizophrenia: A different, but comparable model. *Diseases of the Nervous System,* Supplement, *29*(5), 133–143.

Hagspihl, K. (1954) Analytic psychotherapy with a young stutterer and exhibitionist. *Praxis der Kinderpsychologie under Kinderpsychiatrie, 3,* 37–45.

Hahn, E. F. (1956) Stuttering: Significant theories and therapies. 2nd ed. Stanford, Calif.: Stanford University Press.

Hale, L. L. (1951) Consideration of thiamin supplement in prevention of stuttering in preschool children. *Journal of Speech and Hearing Disorders, 16,* 327–33.

Ham, R. E. (1957) Certain effects on speech of alterations in the auditory feedback of speech defectives and normals. *Dissertation Abstracts, 17,* 1623–1624.

Hamre, C. E., and Wingate, M. E. (1967) Pyknolepsy and stuttering. *Quarterly Journal of Speech, 53,* 374–377.

Handzel, L., and Weiss, B. (1959) Modern therapy of stuttering. *Polski Tygodnik Lekarski, 14,* 1308–1312. (Polish)

Haney, H. R. (1951) Motives implied by the act of stuttering as revealed by prolonged experimental projection. *Speech Monographs, 18,* 129.

Hanicke, O., et al. (1964) Contributions to modern views on and treatment of stuttering. *Deutsche Gesundheitswesen, 19,* 545–549.

Haroldson, S. K., Martin, R. R., and Starr, C. D. (1968) Time-out as a punishment for stuttering. *Journal of Speech and Hearing Research, 11,* 560–566.

Harris, L. L. (1951) A clinical study of nine stuttering children in group psychotherapy. *Speech Monographs, 18,* 129–130.

Heese, G. (1960) *Sur Verhustung und Behandlung des Stotterns.* Berlin: Marbold.

Hejna, R. F. (1955) A study of the loci of stuttering in spontaneous speech. *Dissertation Abstracts, 15,* 1674–1675.

Hejna, R. F. (1960) Stuttering theory and research. *Journal of Speech and Hearing Disorders. 25,* 305–306.

Hejna, R. F. (1963) *Interviews with a stutterer.* Danville, Ill.: Interstate.

Heltman, H. (1956) Don't teach your child to stutter. *Today's Health, 34,* 34–35.

Hemery, H. F. (1953) Stammering; management. *British Journal of Physical Medicine Including its Application to Industry, 16,* 142–148.

Henyer, G., Teyssevre, G., Enet, S., and Tatsoglon, M. (1954) Un cas de begaiement. *Praxis der Kinderpsychologie und Kinderpsychiatrie, 3,* 1–6.

Hift, E., and Kos, M. (1961) Psychotherapy of stuttering children. *Aktuelle Probleme der Phoniatrie und Logopaedie; Supplementa ad Folia Phoniatrica, 2,* 86–114. (German)

Higdon, H. (1968) Michigan's remarkable summer speech camp. *Today's Health, 46,* 34–37, 45–75.

Hirschbergh, J. (1965) Stuttering. *Orvosi Hetilap, 106,* 780–784. (Hungarian)

Holliday, A. R. (1958) An empirical investigation of the personality characteristics and attitudes of the parents of children who stutter. *Dissertation Abstracts, 19,* 569–570.

Holtzman, P. D. (1960) An old and new direction in stuttering research. In D. A. Barbara, ed., *Psychological and psychiatric aspects of speech and hearing.* Springfield, Ill.: Charles C Thomas.

Homefield, H. D. (1959) Creative role-playing as therapy for stuttering children: With special reference to the use of masks. Doctoral dissertation, New York University, New York.

Hommerich, K. W., and Korzendorfer, M. (1966) Research on the use of librium in the treatment of stuttering. *H.N.O., Wegweiser für die Fachurztliche Praxis, 15,* 211–218. (German)

Horlick, R. S., and Miller, M. H. (1960) A comparative personality study of a group of stutterers and hard of hearing patients. *Journal of General Psychology, 63,* 259–266.

Horowitz, E. (1962) A follow-up study of former stutterers. *Speech Pathology and Therapy, 5,* 25–33.

How to talk to a stutterer. (1958) *Science Digest, 43,* 19.

Hubbard, D. J. (1967) Characteristics of speaking behavior related to judgments of stuttering severity in school-age children. *Dissertation Abstracts, 28*(1–B), 375–376.

Imaseki, Y. (1964) Psychogalvanic reflex (galvanic skin reflex) of stutterers. *Folia Phoniatrica, 16,* 29–38.

Ingram, R. (1967) Stuttering: Theoretical and therapeutic considerations. III. Family dynamics and the recovery from stuttering. *Australian Psychologist, 2*(1), 167 (abstract).

Irving, R. W., and Webb, M. W.   (1961)   Teaching esophageal speech to a pre-operative severe stutterer. *Annals of Otology, Rhinology and Laryngology, 70,* 1069–1079.

Iwert, H.   (1968)   Das storungsumfeld des storrerers. (The stutterer's field of disturbances.) *Praxis der Kinderpsychologie und Kinderpsychiatrie, 17,* 251–257. (German)

Jakobovitz, L. A.   (1966)   Utilization of semantic satiation in stuttering: A theoretical analysis. *Journal of Speech and Hearing Disorders, 31,* 105–114.

Jameson, A. M.   (1955)   Stammering in children—some factors in the prognosis. *Speech* (London), *19,* 60–67.

Jamison, D. J.   (1955)   Spontaneous recovery of the stuttering response as a function of the time following adaptation. In W. Johnson and R. Leutenegger, eds., *Stuttering in children and adults,* Minneapolis: University of Minnesota Press.

Jan-Tausch, J.   (October 1961)   How can the teacher help the stutterer? *Instructor,* p. 30.

Jensen, P. J.   (1966)   Stuttering and iatrogenesis. *EENT Mon., 45,* 86–87, 89.

Johnson, W.   (1946)   *People in quandaries: The semantics of personal adjustment.* New York: Harper & Row.

Johnson, W.   (1950)   Open letter to the parent of a stuttering child. *Crippled Child, 30,* 7–9, 28.

Johnson, W.   (1950)   Rehabilitation of a stutterer. *Illinois Medical Journal, 98,* 341–343.

Johnson, W.   (1955a)   The descriptive principle and the principle of static analysis. In W. Johnson and R. Leutenegger, eds., *Stuttering in children and adults.* Minneapolis: University of Minnesota Press.

Johnson, W.   (1955b)   A study of the onset and development of stuttering. In W. Johnson and R. Leutenegger, eds., *Stuttering in children and adults.* Minneapolis: University of Minnesota Press.

Johnson, W.   (February 13, 1955)   For the stutterer, a sympathetic ear. *New York Times Magazine,* p. 42.

Johnson, W.   (1956a)   Perceptual and evaluational factors in stuttering. *Folia Phoniatrica, 8,* 211–233.

Johnson, W.   (1956b)   Stuttering. In W. Johnson et al., eds., *Speech handicapped school children.* Revised ed. New York: Harper & Row.

Johnson, W.   (January 5, 1957)   I was a despairing stutterer. *Saturday Evening Post,* 26–27.

Johnson, W. (1959a) New look at stuttering. *Child Study,* *36,* 14–18.

Johnson, W. (1959b) *Toward understanding stuttering.* Chicago, Ill.: National Society for Crippled Children and Adults.

Johnson, W. (1961a) Are speech disorders "superficial" or "basic"? *Asha, 3,* 233–236.

Johnson, W. (1961b) Counseling parents about the problem called stuttering or stammering. *Speech Pathology and Therapy, 4,* 7–10.

Johnson, W. (1961c) Measurements of oral reading and speaking rate and disfluency of adult male and female stutterers and nonstutterers. *Journal of Speech and Hearing Disorders,* Monograph Supplement No. 7, 1–20.

Johnson, W. (1961d) *Stuttering and what you can do about it.* Minneapolis: University of Minnesota Press.

Johnson, W., Brown, F., Curtis, J., Edney, C., and Keaster, J. (1967) *Speech handicapped school children.* 3rd ed. New York: Harper & Row.

Johnson, W., and Knott, J. R. (1955) A systematic approach to the psychology of stuttering. In W. Johnson and R. Leutenegger, eds., *Stuttering in children and adults.* Minneapolis, Minn.: University Press.

Johnson, W., Young, M. A., Sahs, A. L., and Bedell, G. N. (1959) Effects of hyperventilation and tetany of the speech fluency of stutterers and non-stutterers. *Journal of Speech and Hearing Research, 2,* 203–215.

Johnson, W., et al. (1959) *The onset of stuttering: Research findings and implications.* Minneapolis: University of Minnesota Press.

Johnson, W., et al. (1961) Studies of speech disfluency and rate of stutterers and non-stutterers. *Journal of Speech and Hearing Disorders,* Monograph Supplement No. 7, 1–62.

Johnson, W., ed. (1955) *Stuttering in children and adults: Thirty years of research at the University of Iowa.* Minneapolis: University of Minnesota Press.

Jones, E. L. (1955) Explorations of experimental extinction and spontaneous recovery in stuttering. In W. Johnson and R. Leutenegger, eds., *Stuttering in children and adults.* Minneapolis: University of Minnesota Press.

Jones, H. G. (1969) Behavior Therapy and stuttering: The need for a multifarious approach to a multiplex problem. In B. Gray and G. England, eds., *Stuttering and the conditioning therapies.* Monterey, Calif.: Monterey Institute for Speech and Hearing.

Jorswieck, E., and Stephen, O. (1966) Differentiating observations on the intelligence of stuttering and stammering children. *Praxis der Kinderpsychologie und Kinderpsychiatrie, 15,* 183–184.

Jussen, H. (1964) The stuttering problem in the American professional literature. *Sprachheilarbeit,. 9,* 162–178. (German)

Kaempffert, W. (March 1956) Stammer corrected. *Science Digest,* back cover.

Kapos, E., and Standlee, L. S. (1958) Behavioral rigidity in adult stutterers. *Journal of Speech Research, 1,* 294–296.

Karlin, I. W. (1950) Stuttering: Problems today. *Journal of the American Medical Association, 143,* 732–736.

Karlin, I. W. (1956) Stuttering: Evaluation and treatment. *New York Journal of Medicine, 56,* 3719, 3724.

Karlin, I. W. (1959) Stuttering: Basically an organic disorder. *Logos, 2,* 61–63.

Kehrer, H. E., and Stegat, H. (1968) Uber die behandlung von Stotterern nach verhaltenstherapeutischer methode. (On the treatment of stutterers by means of a behaviortherapeutic method (negative practice.) *Praxis der Kinderpsychologie und Kinderpsychiatrie, 17,* 164–170. (German)

Keisman, I. B. (1958) Stuttering and anal fixation. Doctoral dissertation, New York University, New York.

Kelham, R., and McHale, A. (1966) The application of learning theory to the treatment of stammering. *British Journal of Disorders of Communication, 1,* 114–118.

Kent, L. R. (1961a) Carbon dioxide therapy as a medical treatment for stuttering. *Journal of Speech and Hearing Disorders, 26,* 268–271.

Kent, L. R. (1961b) Retraining for the adult who stutters. *Journal of Speech and Hearing Disorders, 26,* 141–144.

Kent, L. R. (1963) Use of tranquilizers in the treatment of stuttering; reserpine, chlorpromazine, meprobamate, atarax. *Journal of Speech and Hearing Disorders, 28,* 288–294.

Kent, L. R., and Williams, D. E. (1959) Use of meprobamate as an adjunct to stuttering therapy. *Journal of Speech and Hearing Disorders, 24,* 64–69.

379

Kew, C. E. (1966) The nature, etiology, and treatment of stuttering. *Pastoral Counselor, 4,* 28–36.

King, P. T. (1954) Perseverative factors in a stuttering and non-stuttering population. *Speech Monographs, 21,* 211–212. Abstract of a doctoral dissertation, Pennsylvania State University, 1953.

King, P. T. (1961) Perseveration in stutterers and non-stutterers. *Journal of Speech and Hearing Research, 4,* 346–357.

Kinstler, D. B. (1959) An experimental study of the role of covert and overt maternal rejection and acceptance in the etiology of stuttering. Doctoral dissertation, University of Southern California, Los Angeles.

Kinstler, D. B. (1961) Covert and overt maternal rejection in stuttering. *Journal of Speech and Hearing Disorders, 26,* 145–155.

Kline, D. F. (1958) An experimental study of the frequency of stuttering in relation to certain goal-activity drives in basic human behavior. Doctoral dissertation, University of Missouri, Columbia.

Klinger, H. N. (1959) The effects of stuttering on audience listening comprehension. Doctoral dissertation, New York University, New York.

Knabe, J. M., Nelson, L. A., and Williams, F. (1966) Some general characteristics of linguistic output: Stutterers versus non-stutterers. *Journal of Speech and Hearing Disorders, 31,* 178–182.

Knepflar, K. (1965) Voluntary normal disfluency: A speech therapy technique for stutterers. *Asha, 8,* 401.

Knott, J. R., and Correll, R. E. (1954) Photic driving in stutterers. *EEG and Clinical Neurophysiology, 6,* 158. Abstract.

Knott, J. R., Correll, R. E., and Shepherd, J. N. (1959) Frequency analysis of electroencephalograms of stutterers and non-stutterers. *Journal of Speech and Hearing Research, 2,* 74–80.

Knox, A. (1962) Classroom teacher and the stuttering child. *Phi Delta Kappan, 44,* 136–137.

Kondas, O. (1965) Principle of interference in dissenting correction of stammering and dyslexia. *Psychologica, 16,* 57–58. (Czech)

Kondas, O. (1967) The treatment of stammering in children by the shadow method. *Behaviour Research and Therapy, 5,* 325–329.

Krichhauff, G. (1952) Therapeutic possibilities of the initial interview with neurotic children: Case of a stutterer. *Praxis der Kinderpsychologie und Kinderpsychiatrie, 1,* 44–47.

Krupnova, Z. A. (1967) Preodolenie zaikaniya u doshkol'nikov v protesse ruchnoi deyatel'nosti. *Spetsial'naya Shkola, 3,* 16–18.

Kuliev, E. M. (1967) Izuchenie osobennostei proizvol'nogo vnimaniya zaikayushchikhsya detei. (Study of the features of voluntary attention in stuttering children.) *Spetsial'naya Shkola, 5,* 119–126. (Russian)

Kurshev, V. A. (1961) O vneshnem tormozhenii i rastormazhivanii vo vzaimodeistvii signal 'nykh sistem u zaikaiushchikhsia. External inhibition and disinhibition in the interaction of signaling systems of stutterers. *Zhurnal Vysshei Nervoni Deyatel 'nosti, 11,* 985–990.

Kurth, E. (1964) Mehrdimensionale Untersuchungen an stotterenden Kindern. Multidimensional examinations of stuttering children. *Probleme und Ergebnisse der Psychologie, 12,* 49–58.

Kutash, S. B. (1951) Differential diagnosis and therapeutic follow-up in a case of neurotic stuttering. *Case Reports of Clinical Psychology, 2*(3), 7–16.

Ladell, R. M. (1957) The problem of the stammerer, *Practitioner* (London), *178,* 342–343.

Ladell, R. M., and Brown V. A. (August 1958) Why do you s-s-stutter? *American Mercury,* pp. 106–109.

Laeder, R., and Francis, W. C. (1968) Stuttering workshops: Group therapy in a rural high school setting. *Journal of Speech and Hearing Disorders, 33,* 38–41.

LaFollette, A. C. (1956) Parental environment of stuttering children. *Journal of Speech and Hearing Disorders, 21,* 202–207.

Landolt, H., and Luchsinger, R. (June 18, 1954) Language disorder, stuttering and chronic organic psychosyndrome; electroencephalographic results and studies of pathology of speech. *Deutsche Medizinische Wochenschrift, 79,* 1012–1015. (German)

Langova, J., and Moravek, M. (March 9, 1962) Experimental study on stuttering and stammering. *Caspois Lekaru Cesych, 101,* 297–300. (Czech)

Langova, J., and Moravek, M. (1964) Some results of experimental examinations among stutterers and clutterers *Folia Phoniatrica, 16,* 290–296.

Lanyon, R. I. (1965) The relationship of adaptation and consistency to improvement in stuttering therapy. *Journal of Speech and Hearing Research, 8,* 263–270.

Lanyon, R. I. (1966) The MMPI and prognosis in stuttering therapy. *Journal of Speech and Hearing Disorders, 31,* 186–191.

Lanyon, R. I. (1967) The measurement of stuttering severity. *Journal of Speech and Hearing Research, 10,* 836–843.

Lanyon, R. I. (1968) Some characteristics of nonfluency in normal speakers and stutterers. *Journal of Abnormal Psychology, 63,* 550–555.

Lanyon, R. I. (1969) Behavior change in stuttering through systematic desensitization. *Journal of Speech and Hearing Disorders, 34,* 263–270.

Lanzkron, J. (1960) A sex-linked neurosis . . . stuttering. *Medical Times, 88,* 743–744.

Lapidus, F. I. (December 1963) Psychological influences on the personality of the stutterer. *Zdravookhranenie Belorussii, 9,* 57–60. (Russian)

Lawrence, C. J. (1961) How nurses can help the child who stutters. *Nursing Outlook, 9,* 285–287.

Lay, C. H., and Paivio, A. (1969) The effects of task difficulty and anxiety on hesitation in speech. *Canadian Journal of Behavioral Science, 1*(1), 25–37.

Lazarus, A. (1960) Objective psychotherapy in the treatment of dysphemia. *Journal of the South African Logopedic Society, 6,* 8–10.

Lazarus, A. (1969) Case history of a stutterer treated as an obsessive-compulsive disorder by Broad-Spectrum behavior therapy. In G. Gray and G. England, eds., *Stuttering and the conditioning therapies.* Monterey, Calif.: Monterey Institute for Speech and Hearing.

Leach, E. (1969) Stuttering: clinical application of response-contingent procedures. In B. Gray and G. England, eds., *Stuttering and the conditioning therapies.* Monterey, Calif.: Monterey Institute for Speech and Hearing.

Leanderson, R. and Levi, L. (1966) A new approach to the experimental study of stuttering and stress. *Acta Oto-Laryngologica, Supplement* No. 224, 311–316.

Leary, T. G. (1950) Tragedy of stammering and its relation to reeducation. *Medical Journal of Australia, 2,* 8–10.

Lebrun, Y. (1967) Schizophasie et begaiement. (Schizophrenia and stammering.) *Acta Neurologica et Psychiatrica Belgica, 67*, 939–945. (French)

Lederer, W. J. (December 1957) B-B-B-Best friend I ever had in the Navy. *Readers Digest*, pp. 193–194.

Lee, B. S. (1951) Artificial stutterer. *Journal of Speech and Hearing Disorders, 16*, 53–55.

Lehambre, J. (July 1964) "Paradoxical intention," a psychotherapeutic procedure. *Acta Neurologica et Psychiatrica Belgica, 64*, 725–735. (French)

Leith, W. R. (1954) An investigation of the adaptation phenomenon and certain concomitant voice alterations in stutterers and non-stutterers. *Dissertation Abstracts, 14*, 2156–2157. Abstract of doctoral dissertation, Purdue University.

Lelkens, G. (1967) Gedragstherapie van het stotteren. Therapy of stuttering by means of correction of behavior. *Tijdschrift voor Psychologie Gawein*, pp. 344–358.

Lemert, E. M. (1952) Stuttering among the North Pacific Coastal Indians. *Southwestern Journal of Anthropology, 8*, 429–441.

Lemert, E. M. (1953) Some Indians who stutter. *Journal of Speech and Hearing Disorders, 18*, 168–174.

Lemert, E. M. (1962) Stuttering and social structure in two Pacific societies. *Journal of Speech and Hearing Disorders, 27*, 3–10.

Lennon, E. J. (1962) *Le begaiement: Therapeutiques modernes*, Paris: G. Doin et Cie.

Lepson, D. S. (1959) Speech anxiety (drive) level, degree of response competition, and mode of response in a forced-choice variation of paired associates learning. Doctoral dissertation, University of Pittsburgh, Pittsburgh, Pa.

Lerea, L. (1954) An exploratory study of the effects of experimentally induced success and failure upon the oral reading performance and the levels of aspiration of stutterers. *Dissertation Abstracts, 14*, 2401. Abstract of doctoral dissertation, University of Pittsburgh, 1954.

Lerman, J. W., Powers, G. R., and Rigrodsky, S. (1965) Stuttering patterns observed in a sample of mentally retarded individuals. *Training School Bulletin, 62*, 27–32.

Lerman, J. W., and Shames, G. H. (1965) The effect of situational difficulty on stuttering. *Journal of Speech and Hearing Research, 8*, 271–280.

Leutenegger, R. R. (1957) Adaptation and recovery in the

oral reading of stutterers. *Journal of Speech Disorders,* 22, 276–287.

Levina, R. Y. (1968) Study and treatment of stammering among children. *Journal of Learning Disabilities, 1,* 24–30.

Lewis, D., and Sherman, D. (1951) Measuring severity of stuttering. *Journal of Speech and Hearing Disorders, 16,* 320–326.

Lichtenstein, F. (1962) Guidance work with stutterers. *High Points, 44,* 44–50.

Like to stammer? (January 5, 1953) *Newsweek,* p. 59.

Loosli-Usteri, M. (1951) Stuttering cured by projective play method; case. *Encephale, 40,* 498–543. (French)

Lotzmann, G. von (1961) Zur annendung varuerter versogerungszeiten bei balbuties. *Folia Phoniatrica, 13,* 276–312. (French)

Love, L. A. (1968) Identification of brief pauses in the fluent speech of stutterers and non-stutterers. *Dissertation Abstracts, 29,* 1870.

Love, W. R. (1955) The effect of pentobarbital sodium (nembutal) and amphetamine sulfate (Benzedrine) on the severity of stuttering. In W. Johnson and R. Leutenegger, eds., *Stuttering in children and adults.* Minneapolis: University of Minnesota Press.

Lovett, D. W. (1956) Stress and psychopathology in stutterers and nonstutterers to isolated word stimuli. *Dissertation Abstracts, 28*(6-B), 2657.

Lovett, D. W. (1965) Stress and psychopathology in stutterers. *Canadian Journal of Psychology, 10,* 31–37.

Lovett, D. W., and Coleman, L. I. M. (1955) The psychophysics of communication. III. Discriminatory awareness in stutterers and its measurement by the critical Flicker fusion threshold. *A.M.A. Archives of Neurology and Psychiatry, 84,* 650–652.

Lowinger, L. (1952) The psychodynamics of stuttering: An evaluation of the factors of aggression and guilt feelings in a group of institutionalized children. *Dissertation Abstracts. 12,* 725.

Lubinsky, F. T. (1957) Negative practice in dysphemia therapy: A case history. *Journal of the South African Logopedic Society, 4,* 15–16.

Luchsinger, R. (1955) Ueber das eltern das sogenannte "stottern mit polterkimponente" und deren bezeihungen su aphasien. *Folia Phoniatrica, 7,* 12.

Luchsinger, R., and Arnold, G. *Voice-Speech-Language.* Belmont, Calif.: Wadsworth.

Luchsinger, R., and Dubois, C. (1963) Ein vergleich der sprachmelodie: Und lautstarkekurve bei normalen, gehirnkranken und stotterern. *Folia Phoniatrica, 15,* 21.

Luchsinger, R., and Landolt, H. (1951) Electroencephalographische untersuchungen bei stotterern mit und ohne polterkomponente, *Folia Phoniatrica, 3,* 135–151.

Luper, H. L. (1956) Consistency of stuttering in relation to the goal gradient hypothesis. *Journal of Speech Disorders, 21,* 336–342.

Luper, H. L. (1968) An appraisal of learning theory concepts in understanding and treating stuttering in children. In H. H. Gregory, ed., *Learning theory and stuttering therapy.* Evanston, Ill.: Northwestern University Press.

Luper, H. L., and Mulder, R. L. (1964) *Stuttering therapy for children.* Englewood Cliffs, N. J.: Prentice-Hall.

Lynch, E. M. (1955) Bibliotherapy for stutterers. In W. Johnson and R. Leutenegger, eds., *Stuttering in children and adults,* Minneapolis: University of Minnesota Press.

McAllister, A. H. (1958) The problem of stammering. *Speech Pathology and Therapy* (London), *1,* 3–8.

McCord, H. (1955) Hypnotherapy and stuttering. *Journal of Clinical and Experimental Hypnosis, 3,* 210–214.

McCrosky, R. L. (1956) The effect of speech on metabolism: A comparison between stutterers and non-stutterers. *Dissertation Abstracts, 16,* 1532.

McCulloch, J. W., et al. (1964) Some factors affecting the prevalence of stammering. *British Journal of Preventive and Social Medicine, 18,* 146–151.

McDearmon, J. (1966) C. S. Bleumel and the learning theory approach to stuttering. *Western Speech, 30,* 106–111.

McDearmon, J. R. (1968) Primary stuttering at the onset of stuttering: A reexamination of data. *Journal of Speech and Hearing Research, 11,* 631–637.

McDonald, E., and Frick, J. (1954) Store clerks reaction to stuttering. *Journal of Speech and Hearing Disorders, 19,* 306–311.

McHale, A. (1967) An investigation of personality attributes of stammering, enuretic and school-phobic children. *British Journal of Educational Psychology, 37,* 400–403.

Madison, L. (1956) An heuristic classification of stuttering. *Perceptual and Motor Skills, 6,* 21–24.

Madison, L., and Norman, R. D. (1952) A comparison of the performance of stutterers and non-stutterers on the Rosenzweig picture-frustration test. *Journal of Clinical Psychology, 8,* 179–183.

Mahaffey, J. Q. (August 1956) How Will Rogers changed my life. *Readers Digest,* p. 143.

Mahrer, A. R., and Young, H. H. (1962) The onset of stuttering. *Journal of General Psychology, 67,* 241–250.

Malkin, R. (July 1957) Nobody needs to stutter. *Parents Magazine,* pp. 48–49.

Malmivaara, K., and Kolho, P. (1962) The personality of stuttering children at the age of 5–7 years in the light of the Sceno and Rorschach tests. *Annales Paediatriae Fenniae, 7,* 17–23.

Mann, M. B. (1955) Nonfluencies in the oral reading of stutterers and non-stutterers. In W. Johnson and R. Leutenegger, eds., *Stuttering in children and adults,* Minneapolis: University of Minnesota Press.

Maraist, J. A., and Hutton, C. (1957) Effects of auditory masking upon the speech of stutterers. *Journal of Speech Disorders, 22,* 385–389.

Marks, M. (1957) Stuttering as learned behavior: Theoretical and therapeutic implications. *Journal of South African Logopedic Society, 4,* 10–15.

Marks, M. (1969) Stuttering viewed as a sequence of responses. In B. Gray and G. England, eds., *Stuttering and the conditioning therapies.* Monterey, Calif.: Monterey Institute for Speech and Hearing.

Marland, P. M. (1957) Shadowing: A contribution to the treatment of stammering, *Folia Phoniatrica, 9,* 242–245.

Martin, E. W. (1963) Client-centered therapy as a theoretical orientation for speech therapy. *Asha, 5,* 576–578.

Martin, E. W., Ward, L. M., and Johnson, T. E. (1965) The self as a central concept in speech therapy for the person who stutters. In D. A. Barbara, ed., *New directions in stuttering: Theory and practice.* Springfield, Ill.: Charles C Thomas.

Martin, R. (1962) Stuttering and perseveration in children. *Journal of Speech and Hearing Research, 5,* 332–339.

Martin, R. R., and Siegel, G. M. (1966) The effects of response contingent shock on stuttering. *Journal of Speech and Hearing Research, 9,* 340–352.

Martin, R. R., and Siegel, G. M. (1966) The effects of simultaneously punishing stuttering and rewarding fluency. *Journal of Speech and Hearing Research, 9,* 466–475.

Martin, R. R., and Siegel, G. M. (1969) The effects of a neutral stimulus (Buzzer) on motor responses and disfluencies in normal speakers, *Journal of Speech and Hearing Research, 12,* 179–184.

Martyn, M. M., and Sheehan, J. G. (1968) Onset of stuttering and recovery. *Behaviour Research and Therapy, 6,* 295–307.

Martyn, M. M., Sheehan, J. G., and Slutz, K. (1969) Incidence of stuttering and other speech disorders among the retarded. *American Journal of Mental Deficiency, 74,* 206–211.

Masandilova, I. I. (1968) Preodolenie zaikaniya na materiale uchebnoi programmy 11 klassa v usloviyakh shkol'nogo logopedicheskogo punkta. (Overcoming stuttering utilizing the materials of the instructional program for the 2nd grade under the conditions of the logopedic center servicing the regular school.) *Spetsial'naya Shkola, 1,* 23–27. (Russian)

Massengill, R., Jr. (1965) Phobias present in three stuttering cases. *Perceptual and Motor Skills, 20,* 579–580.

Mast, V. R. (1952) Level of aspiration as a method of studying the personality of adult stutterers. *Speech Monographs, 19,* 196.

Mattmuller-Frick, F. (1959) Wandlungen in der stottererbehandlung auf grund veranderter auslegung des neurosebegriffes. (Changes in the treatment of stuttering on the basis of differences in interpretation of the concept of neurosis.) *Praxis der Kinderpsychologie und Kinderpsychiatrie, 8,* 223–230.

Maxwell, R. D., and Paterson, J. W. (April 12, 1958) Meprobromate in the treatment of stuttering. *British Medical Journal,* pp. 873–874.

May, A. E., and Hackwood, A. (1968) Some effects of masking and eliminating low frequency feedback on the speech of stammerers. *Behaviour Research and Therapy, 6,* 219–223.

Mazars, G., and Mazars, Y. (1957) Intermediatre epileptique dans certains types de begaiement. *Revue Neurologique, 96,* 59–62.

Meyer, V., and Conley, J. (1969) A preliminary report of the treatment of stammer by the use of rhythmic stimulation. In B. Gray and G. England, eds., *Stuttering and the conditioning therapies.* Monterey, Calif.: Monterey Institute for Speech and Hearing.

Meyer, V., and Mair, J. M. M. (1963) A new technique to control stammering: a preliminary report. *Behaviour Research and Therapy. 1,* 251–254.

Miller, C. H. (1962) Psychotherapy in action: A case report. In D. A. Barbara, ed., *The Psychotherapy of Stuttering.* Springfield, Ill.: Charles C Thomas.

Minifie, F. D., and Cooker, H. S. (1964) A disfluency index. *Journal of Speech and Hearing Disorders, 29,* 189–192.

Mironova, S. A. (1967) Ustranenie zaikaniya v usloviyakh detskogo sada. (Elimination of stuttering in kindergarten.) *Spetsial'naya Shkola, 6,* 126–130.

Mogilevskaya, S. N. (1968) Organizatsiya zanyatii po predoleniyu zaikaniya v detskom sadu. (Organization of activities in overcoming stuttering in the kindergarten.) *Spetsial'naya Shkola, 4,* 84–88. (Russian)

Moller, H. (1960) Stuttering, predelinquent, and adjusted boys: A comparative analysis of personality characteristics as measured by the Wise and the Rorschach test. Doctoral dissertation, Boston University School of Education, Boston, Mass.

Moncur, J. P. (1951) Environmental factors differentiating stuttering children from non-stuttering children. *Speech Monographs, 18,* 312–325.

Moncur, J. P. (1952) Parental domination in stuttering. *Journal of Speech and Hearing Disorders, 17,* 155–165.

Moncur, J. P. (1955) Symptoms of maladjustment differentiating young stutterers from non-stutterers. *Child Development, 26,* 91–96.

Moore, G. (February 1954) I've got a secret. *American Magazine,* pp. 32–35.

Moore, M. V. (November 1966) How to help the stutterer. *Sunday School Builder,* pp. 12–14.

Moore, W. E. (1954) Relations of stuttering in spontaneous speech to speech content and to adaptation. *Journal of Speech and Hearing Disorders, 19,* 208–216.

Moore, W. E. (1959) A study of the blood chemistry of stutterers under two hypnotic conditions. *Speech Monographs, 26,* 64–68.

Moore, W. E., Soderberg, G., and Powell, D. (1952) Relations of stuttering in spontaneous speech to speech content and verbal output. *Journal of Speech and Hearing Disorders, 17,* 371–376.

Moravek, M., and Langova, A. (1962) Some electrophysiological findings among stutterers and clutterers. *Folia Phoniatrica, 14,* 305–316.

Moravek, M., and Langova, J. (May 1963) Effect of delayed acoustic afferentation on the speech of stutterers and clutterers. *Activitas Nervosa Superior, 5,* 130–133. (Czech)

Morgenstern, J. J. (1956) Socioeconomic factors in stuttering. *Journal of Speech and Hearing Disorders, 21,* 25–33.

Moser, H. M., Dreher, J., and Adler, S. (1955) Two-digit number transmission by voluntary stuttering. *Journal of Speech and Hearing Disorders, 20,* 388–392.

Mowrer, O. H. (1967) Stuttering as simultaneous admission and denial. *Journal of Communication Disorders, 1,* 46–50.

Mowrer, O. H. (1968) A resume of basic principles of learning. In H. H. Gregory, ed., *Learning theory and stuttering therapy.* Evanston, Ill.: Northwestern University Press.

Mowrer, O. H. (1968) Stuttering as simultaneous admission and denial; or, what is the stutterer "saying"? In H. H. Gregory, ed., *Learning theory and stuttering therapy.* Evanston, Ill.: Northwestern University Press.

Mucchielli, R. (1968) Contribution à une phénoménologie du bégaiement. *Rééduc. orthophon., 34,* 87–91.

Muirden, R. (1968) *Stammering and its correction through the re-education of the speech function.* Springfield, Ill.: Charles C Thomas.

Mulder, R. L. (1961) Student of stuttering as a stutterer. *Journal of Speech and Hearing Disorders, 26,* 178–179.

Muller, A. (1963) Attitude of the physician in relation to a child with speech disorders and current opinions on stuttering. *Confinia Neurologica, 23,* 137–142. (French)

Murphy, A. T. (1953) An electroencephalographic study of frustration in stutterers. *Speech Monographs, 20,* 148. Abstract of doctoral dissertation, University of Southern California, 1952.

Murphy, A. T., and Fitzsimons, R. M. (1960) *Stuttering and Personality Dynamics.* New York: Ronald Press.

Murray, E. (1957) The C. S. Bluemel collection on stuttering. *Journal of Speech Disorders, 22,* 761–763.

Murray, E. (1968) Social learning, personality change, and psychotherapy. In H. H. Gregory, ed., *Learning theory*

389

and stuttering therapy. Evanston, Ill.: Northwestern University Press.

Murray, F. P. (1958) Observations on therapy for stuttering in Japan. *Journal of Speech Disorders, 23,* 243–249.

Mussafia, M. (October 3, 1959) Current views on the problem of stuttering. *Scalpel, 112,* 971–976. (French)

Mussafia, M. (March 19, 1960) Current views on the problem of stammering. *Scalpel, 113,* 231–236. (French)

Mussafia, M. (1964) The role of heredity in language disorders. *Folia Phoniatrica, 16,* 228–238.

Mysak, E. D. (1959) Diagnosis of stuttering as made by adolescent boys and girls. *Journal of Speech and Hearing Disorders, 24,* 29–33.

Mysak, E. D. (1960) Servo theory and stuttering. *Journal of Speech and Hearing Disorders, 25,* 188–195.

Naylor, R. V. (1953) A comparative study of methods of estimating the severity of stuttering. *Journal of Speech and Hearing Disorders, 18,* 30–37.

Naylor, R. V. (1956) A study of the effect of voluntary nonfluency upon frequency and rated severity of audible characteristics of stuttering. *Dissertation Abstracts, 16,* 597–598.

Naylor, R. V. (1960) Helping the stutterer. *Journal of the National Education Association, 49,* 35–36.

Neal, W. R., and White, W. F. (1965) Attitudes of selected employers toward the employment of stutterers. *Southern Speech Journal, 31,* 28–33.

Neely, K. K. (1951) The effect of oral practice in the presence of different conditions of side-tone upon the rate and sound pressure level of the speech of a group of stutterers. Doctoral dissertation, Ohio State University, Columbus.

Neelley, J. N. (1961) A study of the speech behavior of stutterers and non-stutterers under normal and delayed auditory feedback. *Journal of Speech and Hearing Disorders,* Monograph Supplement No. 7, pp. 63–82.

Nekrasova, L. B. (August 1962) Speech rehabilitation in stuttering preschool children. *Voprosy Okhrany Materinstva i Detstva, 7,* 85–86. (Russian)

Newman, P. W. (1954) A study of adaptation and recovery of the stuttering response in self-formulated speech. *Journal of Speech and Hearing Disorders, 19,* 312–321.

Newman, P. W. (1963) Adaptation performances of individual stutterers: Implications for research. *Journal of Speech and Hearing Research, 6*, 293–294.

Neymark, E. J. (1955) Therapy of stuttering on the basis of physiologic treatment of its mechanism. *Zhurnal Nevropatologii i Psikhiatrii, 50*, 518–519. (Russian)

Nuttall, E. C., and Scheidel, T. M. (1965) Stutterers' estimates of normal apprehensiveness toward speaking. *Speech Monographs, 32*, 455–457.

Ockel, H. H. (1959) Concerning the problem of stuttering: Review of literature and personal investigations. *Praxis der Kinderpsychologie und Kinderpsychiatrie, 8*, 213–223.

Ohnsorge, K. (1954) Role of family doctor and parents in therapy of stuttering. *Munchener Medizinische Wochenschrift, 96*, 257–258. (German)

Omel'Chenko, N. A. (October 1961) Stammering in childhood. *Zdravookhanenis Belorussii, 7*, 28–31. (Russian)

Onge, K. St. (1963) The stuttering syndrome. *Journal of Speech and Hearing Research, 6*, 195–197.

Onge, K. St., et al. (1964) Stuttering theory and research. *Journal of Clinical Psychology, 20*, 408–409.

Orchinik, C. W. (1958) On tickling and stuttering. *Psychoanalysis and Psychoanalytic Review, 44*, 25–39.

Oxtoby, E. T. (1955) Frequency of stuttering in relation to induced modifications following expectations of stuttering. In W. Johnson and R. Leutenegger, eds., *Stuttering in children and adults*. Minneapolis: University of Minnesota Press.

Palasek, J. R., and Curtis, W. S. (1960) Sugar placebos and stuttering. *Journal of Speech and Hearing Research, 3*, 223–226.

Parker, C. S., and Christopherson, F. (1963) Electronic aid in the treatment of stammer. *Medical Electronics and Biological Engineering, 1*, 121–125.

Parker, W. (1951) *Pathology of speech*. Englewood Cliffs, N. J.: Prentice-Hall.

Patterson, S. A. (1958) The stammering child. *The Practitioner, 180*, 428–433.

Peins, M. (1961a) Adaptation effect and spontaneous recovery in stuttering expectancy. *Journal of Speech and Hearing Research, 4*, 91–99.

Peins, M. (1961b) Consistency effect in stuttering expectancy. *Journal of Speech and Hearing Research, 4,* 397–398.

Pellman, C. (1962) The relationship between speech therapy and psychotherapy. In D. A. Barbara, ed., *The psychotherapy of stuttering.* Springfield, Ill.: Charles C Thomas.

Pennington, R. C. (1967) *The stuttering child: In the school and in the home.* Danville, Ill.: Interstate.

Penson, E. M. (1952) An exploratory study of the effect of thiamin hydrochloride on adults who stutter. *Speech Monographs, 19,* 197.

Perkins, W. H. (1953) Stuttering as approach-avoidance behavior: A preliminary investigation. *Speech Monographs, 20,* 149. Abstract of doctoral dissertation, University of Missouri, 1952.

Perkins, W. H. (1965) Stuttering: Some common denominators. In D. A. Barbara, ed., *New directions in stuttering: Theory and practice.* Springfield, Ill.: Charles C Thomas.

Perkins, W. H. (1969) Stuttering and discriminative awareness (SRS Research Grant RD-2275-S, Final Report). Washington, D.C.: Dir. of Research and Demonstration Grants, Social and Rehabilitation Service, Dept. of Health, Education and Welfare, 94 pp.

Perkins, W. H., and Curlee, R. F. (1969) Clinical impressions of portable masking unit effects in stuttering. *Journal of Speech and Hearing Disorders, 34,* 360–362.

Peters, R. W., and Simonson, W. E. (1960) Generalization of stuttering behavior through associative learning. *Journal of Speech and Hearing Research, 3,* 9–14.

Peters, T. (1968) Oral language skills of children who stutter. *Dissertation Abstracts, 28,* 5228–5229.

Peterson, H. A. (1969) Affective meaning of words as rated by stuttering and nonstuttering readers, *Journal of Speech and Hearing Research, 12,* 337–343.

Peterson, H. A., Rieck, M. B., and Hoff, R. K. (1969) A test of satiation as a function of adaptation in stuttering. *Journal of Speech and Hearing Research, 12(1),* 110–117.

Petkov, D., and Iosifov, I. (1960) Our experiment with the treatment of stuttering in a treatment-logopedic camp. *Zhurnal Nevropatologii i Psikhiatrii meni S. S. Korsakova, 60,* 903–904.

Phillips, J. (1955) The relation between speech therapy and psychotherapy. *Journal of South African Logopedic Society, 3,* 13–14.

Pierce, C. N., and Lipcon, H.   (1959)   Stuttering: Clinical and electroencephalographic findings. *Military Medicine, 12,* No. 7, 511–519.

Plätzer, O.   (1954)   Das biodrama, eine form der spieltherapie. (Biodrama, a form of play therapy.) *Zeitschrift für Psychotherapie und Medizinische Psychologie, 4,* 297–304.

Pollaczek, P. P., and Homefield, H. D.   (1954)   The use of masks as an adjunct to role playing. *Mental Hygiene* (New York), *38,* 299–304.

Pollitt, J.   (1951)   A review of cases of stammering. *Speech* (London), *15,* 33–41.

Powell, Harold.   (1967)   Child rearing practices reported for young male Negro stutterers and non-stutterers in two South Carolina school districts. *Dissertation Abstracts, 28*(3-A), 1149–1150.

Pringust, G., *et al.*   (1964)   Clinical trial of relaxation in children. *Revue de Neuropsychiatrie Infantile et d'Hygiene Mentale de l'Enfance, 12,* 457–462. (French)

Quarrington, B.   (1953)   The performance of stutterers on the Rosenzweig picture-frustration test. *Journal of Clinical Psychology, 9,* 189–192.

Quarrington, B.   (1956)   Cyclical variations in stuttering frequency and some related forms of variation. *Canadian Journal of Psychology, 10,* 179–184.

Quarrington, B.   (1959)   Measures of stuttering adaptation. *Journal of Speech and Hearing Research, 2,* 105–112.

Quarrington, B., Conway, J., and Siegel, N.   (1962)   An experimental study of some properties of stuttered words. *Journal of Speech and Hearing Research, 5,* 387–394.

Quarrington, B., and Douglass, E.   (November 1960)   Audibility avoidance in nonvocalized stutterers. *Journal of Speech and Hearing Disorders, 25,* 358–365.

Quarrington, B., Seligman, J., and Kosower, E.   (1969)   Goal setting behavior of parents of beginning stutterers and parents of nonstuttering children. *Journal of Speech and Hearing Research, 12,* 435–442.

Quist, R. W., and Martin, R. R.   (1967)   The effect of response contingent verbal punishment of stuttering. *Journal of Speech and Hearing Research, 10,* 795–800.

Razdol'skiy, V. A.   (1965)   On the speech of stutterers when alone. *Zhurnal Nevropatologii i Psikhiatrii, 65,* 1717–1720.

Reichel, C. W. (1964) *Stop stammering and stuttering.* New York: Vantage Press.

Reifenberg, E. (1954) Contributions to the therapy of speech impairment. *Psychiatrie, Neurologie and Medizinische Psychologie,* Leipzig, *6,* 109–112.

Rendi, L. (December 1963) Our experiences with trioxazin and andaxin in phoniatric practice. *Ful-Orr-Gegegy-gyasyat, 9,* 157–160. (Hungarian)

Renen, S. B. V. (1950) Tongue troubles. *Journals Logopaedics, 1,* 16–19.

Renfrew, C. E. (1952) A questionnaire for stammerers. *Speech* (London), *16,* 21–24.

Rethi, A. (1965) Cure of stuttering and of spastic dysphonia by means of inspiratory-expiratory voice production. *Monatsscchrift für Ohrenheilkunde, 99,* 240–246.

Richardson, S. O. (1964) Pediatric evaluation of speech and hearing disorders. *Clinical Pediatrics, 3,* 150–152.

Richenberg, E. (June 1956) Diadochkinesis in stutterers and non-stutterers. *Journal of the Medical Society of New Jersey, 53,* 324–326.

Richter, E. (1965) Physiopathology of stuttering. *Logopedia, 6,* 20–37. (Polish)

Rickard, H. C., and Mundy, M. B. (1964) Direct manipulation of stuttering behavior: An experimental-clinical approach. In L. P. Ullmann and L. Krasner, eds., *Case studies in behavior modification.* New York: Holt, Rinehart and Winston.

Rieber, R. W. (1963) Stuttering and self concept. *Journal of Psychology, 55,* 307–311.

Rieber, R. W. (1965) Word magic, self-alienation and stutterers and non-stutterers. *Journal of Speech and Hearing Research, 9,* 289–296.

Ringel, R. L., and Minifie, F. D. (1966) Protensity estimates of stutterers and non-stutterers. *Journal of Speech and Hearing Research, 9,* 289–296.

Robbins, S. D. (May 1964) 1000 stutterers: A personal report of clinical experiences and research recommendations for therapy. *Journal of Speech and Hearing Disorders, 29,* 178–186.

Robbins, S. D. (1965) Relation between insecurity and onset of stuttering. *Cerebral Palsy Review, 26,* 7–14.

Robinson, F. B. (1951) Effects of changes in the relationship between the speech and the external side-tone level on the oral reading rate of stutterers and non-stutterers.

Doctoral dissertation, Ohio State University, Columbus.

Robinson, F. B. (1962) Nature and treatment of stuttering children. In N. Levin and N. Switzer, eds., *Voice and speech disorders: Medical aspects*. Springfield, Ill.: Charles C Thomas.

Robinson, F. B. (1964) *An introduction to stuttering*. Englewood Cliffs, N. J.: Prentice-Hall.

Robinson, F. B. (1966) What parents and teachers should know about children who stutter. I. *Hearing and Speech News, 34,* 8–10.

Roggemann, W. (1959) Ueber das stottern: Versuch einer diskussion und interpretation der vorliegenden ergebnisse. (Concerning stuttering: An attempt at discussion and interpretation of available findings.) *Praxis der Kinderpsychologie und Kinderpsychiatrie, 8,* 199–213.

Rosenberg, S., and Curtiss, J. (1954) The effects of stuttering on the behavior of the listener. *Journal of Abnormal and Social Psychology, 49,* 355–361.

Rosenthal, T. L. (1968) Severe stuttering and maladjustment treated by desensitization and social influence. *Behaviour Research and Therapy, 6,* 125–130.

Ross, F. L. (1955) A comparative study of stutterers and non-stutterers on a psychomotor discrimination test. In W. Johnson and R. Leutenegger, eds., *Stuttering in children and adults*. Minneapolis: University of Minnesota Press.

Ross, M. M. (1950) Stuttering and the preschool child. *Smith College Studies in Social Work, 21,* 23–54.

Ross, S., and Kohrs, R. (1953) Talking cure for stutterers. *Science Digest, 34,* 55–57.

Rosso, L. J., and Adams, M. R. (1969) A study of the relationship between the latency and consistency of stuttering. *Journal of Speech and Hearing Research, 12,* 389–383.

Rotter, J. B. (1955) A study of the motor integration of stutterers and non-stutterers. In W. Johnson and R. Leutenegger, eds., *Stuttering in children and adults*. Minneapolis: University of Minnesota Press.

Rousey, C. L. (1955) The relationship of prolonged periods of spontaneous speech to severity of stuttering. *Dissertation Abstracts, 15,* 2344.

Rousey, C. L. (1958) Stuttering severity during prolonged spontaneous speech. *Journal of Speech and Hearing Research, 1,* 40–47.

Rousey, C., Goetzinger, C. P., and Dirks, D. (1959) Localization ability of normal, stuttering, neurotic, and hemiplegic subjects. *Archives of General Psychiatry, 1,* 640–645.

Rozental, A. (1968) Logorythmique comme un des moyens d' autopsycholotherapie chez les enfants gegues. (Logorhythmics as one of the methods of autopsychotherapy with stuttering children.) *Journal Francais ORL, 17,* 205–207.

Rozhdestvenskaya, V. I., and Pavlova, A. I. (1967) *Podvizhnye igry dlya zaikayushchegosya doshkil'nika.* (Outdoor games for the stuttering preschool-child.) Moscow: Proveshchenie, 64 pp. (Russian)

Rubenstein, B. C. (1959) Some comments about stuttering for teachers. *Educational Administration and Supervision, 45,* 162–168.

Rumsey, H. S. (1957) *Why stammer?* London: Faber.

Rumsey, H. St. J. (1956) Speech therapy. *British Medical Journal, 2,* 768–769.

Ryle, A. (1961) Stammering and its treatment: A review. *Medical World* (London), *94,* 116–120.

Sadoff, R. L., and Collins, D. J. (1968) Passive dependency in stutterers. *American Journal of Psychiatry, 124,* 1126–1127.

Sadoff, R. L., and Siegel, J. R. (1965) Group psychotherapy for stutterers. *International Journal of Group Psychotherapy, 15,* 72–80.

Samuels, P. R. (1950) A new theory on the relationship of stuttering and handedness. *Journal of Logopaedics* (South Africa), *1,* 26–31.

Sander, E. K. (1959) Counseling parents of stuttering children. *Journal of Speech and Hearing Disorders, 24,* 262–271.

Sander, E. K. (1961) Reliability of the Iowa speech disfluency test. *Journal of Speech and Hearing Disorders,* Monograph Supplement, 7, 21–30.

Sander, E. K. (1963) Frequency of syllable repetition and stutter judgments. *Journal of Speech and Hearing Research, 6,* 19–30.

Sander, E. K. (1965) Comments on investigating listener response to speech disfluency. *Journal of Speech and Hearing Disorders, 30,* 159–165.

Sander, E. K. (1968) Interrelations among the responses of

mothers to a child's disfluencies. *Speech Monographs,* *35,* 187–195.

Santostefano, S. (1960) Anxiety and hostility in stuttering. *Journal of Speech and Hearing Research, 3,* 337–347.

Schacter, M. (1951) Neurotic stammering as a symptom of latent agressiveness: Use of protective psychology technique. *Rivista di Clinica Pediatrica, 49,* 461–469.

Schacter, M. (1967) Aphemia, followed by stuttering, due to psychological trauma in a 4 year old girl. *Acta Paedopsychiatrica, 34,* 13–17.

Schaef, R. A. (1954) An investigation of generalization of stuttering adaptation. *Dissertation Abstracts, 14,* 2404–2405. Abstract of doctoral dissertation, University of Pittsburgh, 1954.

Schaef, R. A. (1955) Use of questions to elicit stuttering adaptation. *Journal of Speech and Hearing Disorders, 20,* 262–265.

Schaef, R. A., and Matthews, J. (1954) A first step in the evaluation of stuttering therapy. *Journal of Speech and Hearing Disorders, 19,* 467–473.

Schilling, A. (1959) Electronystamographic findings as indication of central coordination defect in stutterers. *Archiv fur ohren-nasen-and kehlkopfheikunde vereinigt mit zeitschrift fur hals-nasen-und ohrenheilkunde, 175,* 457–461. (German)

Schilling, A. (1960) Diaphragmatic radiokymograms in stutterers. *Folia Phoniatrica, 12,* 145–153. (German)

Schilling, A. (1963) Adjuvant drugs in therapy of stuttering. *HNO: Wegweiser fur die fachaerztliche praxis, 11,* 300–304. (German)

Schilling, A. (1965) Die behandlung des stotterns. *Folia Phoniatrica, 17,* 365–458.

Schilling, A., and Goeler, D. von (1961) On the question of the analysis of monotony in stutterers. *Folia Phoniatrica, 13,* 202–218. (German)

Schilling, A., and Weiss, H. (March 9, 1962) Determination of relations between intelligence and concentration ability in stuttering children. *Casopis Lekaru Ceskych, 101,* 309–312. (Russian)

Schilling, R., and Schilling, A. (1960) On the diagnosis of early childhood brain injuries in stutterers. *Aktuelle Probleme der Phoniatrie und Logopaedie; Supplementa ad Folia Phoniatrica, 1,* 134–140. (German)

Schlange, H. (1961) Clinical examination findings in stammering and stuttering children. *Monatsschrift fur Kinder-heilkunde, 109,* 493–497. (German)

Schlesinger, I. M., Forte, M., Fried, B. and Melkman, R.   (1965) Stuttering, information lead, and response strength. *Journal of Speech and Hearing Disorders, 30,* 32–36.

Schlesinger, I. M., Melkman, R. and Levy, R.   (1966)   Word length and frequency as determinants of stuttering. *Psychonomic Science, 6,* 255–256.

Schmeer, G.   (1966)   Case history of a child cured of stutter-ing. *Praxis der Kinderpsychologie und Kinderpsychia-trie, 15,* 45–50.

Schmeer, H. I., and Hewlett, I. W.   (1958)   A family ap-proach to stuttering with group therapy techniques. *International Journal of Group Psychotherapy, 8,* 329–341.

Schneider, E.   (1953)   Uber das stottern; ursache, entstehung, verlauf, und heilung. (Stuttering: Its cause, development, course, and treatment.) *Beihefte zur Schweizerischen Zeitschrift für Psychologie und ihre Anwendungen,* No. 22.

Schröder, D.   (1964)   The stuttering child and his treatment. *Neue Blatter für Taubstummenbildung, 18,* 257–263, 336–345.

Sedlacek, C.   (1947–1948)   Reactions of the autonomic nerv-ous system in attacks of stuttering. *Folia Phoniatrica, 1,* 283–284.

Seebandt, G.   (1965)   Ambulant treatment of patients with speech disorders. *Offentliche Gesundheitsdienst, 27,* 343–350. (German)

Seeman, M.   (1951)   Pathogenesis of stuttering. *La Presse Med-icale,* 159.

Senn, M. J. E.   (April 1958)   Lisping, stuttering, baby talk. *McCalls,* p. 75.

Senn, M.   (February 1963)   Child care in Russia: Better than ours? *McCalls,* p. 156.

Seth, G.   (1958)   Psychomotor control in stammering and normal subjects: An experimental study. *British Journal of Psychology, 49,* 139–143.

Shames, G. H.   (1953)   A utilization of adaptation phenomena in therapy for stuttering. *Journal of Speech and Hearing Disorders, 18,* 256–257.

Shames, G. H.   (1957)   An investigation of prognosis and evaluation in speech therapy. *Journal of Speech and Hearing Disorders, 17,* 386–392.

Shames, G. (1969) Operant conditioning and stuttering. In B. Gray and G. England, eds., *Stuttering and the conditioning therapies*. Monterey, Calif.: Monterey Institute for Speech and Hearing.

Shames, G. (1969) Verbal reinforcement during therapy interviews with stutterers. In B. Gray and G. England, eds., *Stuttering and the conditioning therapies*. Monterey, Calif.: Monterey Institute for Speech and Hearing.

Shames, G. H., and Beams, H. L. (1956) Incidence of stuttering in older age groups. *Journal of Speech Disorders, 21,* 313–316.

Shames, G., Egolf, D. B., and Rhodes, R. C. (1969) Experimental programs in stuttering therapy. *Journal of Speech and Hearing Disorders, 34,* 30–47.

Shames, G. H., and Sherrick, E. C. (1965) A discussion of nonfluency and stuttering as operant behavior. In D. A. Barbara, ed., *New directions in stuttering: Theory and practice,* Springfield, Ill.: Charles C Thomas.

Shane, M. L. (1955) Effect on stuttering of alternation in auditory feedback. In W. Johnson and R. Leutenegger, eds., *Stuttering in children and adults*. Minneapolis: University of Minnesota Press.

Shapoff, I. (1954) A stutterer writes to a former teacher. *National Educational Association Journal, 43,* 348–349.

Shearer, W. M. (1961) A theoretical consideration of the self-concept and body image in stuttering therapy. *Asha, 3,* 115.

Shearer, W. M. (1966) Speech: Behavior of the middle ear muscle during stuttering. *Science, 152,* 1280.

Shearer, W. M., and Simmons, F. B. (1965) Middle ear activity during speech in normal speakers and stutterers. *Journal of Speech and Hearing Research, 8,* 203–207.

Shearer, W. M., and Williams, J. D. (1965) Self-recovery from stuttering. *Journal of Speech and Hearing Disorders, 30,* 288–290.

Sheehan, J. G. (1951) Modification of stuttering through nonreinforcement. *Journal of Abnormal and Social Psychology, 46,* 51–63.

Sheehan, J. G. (1953) Theory and treatment of stuttering as an approach-avoidance conflict. *Journal of Psychology, 36,* 27–49.

Sheehan, J. G. (1954a) An integration of psychotherapy and speech therapy through a conflict theory of stuttering. *Journal of Speech and Hearing Disorders, 19,* 474–482.

Sheehan, J. G. (1954b) Rorschach prognosis in psychotherapy and speech therapy. *Journal of Speech and Hearing Disorders, 19,* 217–219.

Sheehan, J. G. (1956) Stuttering in terms of conflict and reinforcement. In E. F. Hahn, ed., *Stuttering: Significant theories and therapies,* 2nd ed. Stanford, Calif.: Stanford University Press.

Sheehan, J. G. (1958a) Conflict theory of stuttering. In J. Eisenson, ed., *Stuttering: A symposium.* New York: Harper & Row.

Sheehan, J. G. (1958b) Projective studies of stuttering. *Journal of Speech and Hearing Disorders, 23,* 18–25.

Sheehan, J. G. (1965) Speech therapy and recovery from stuttering. *The Voice, 15,* 3–6.

Sheehan, J. G. (1968) Stuttering as a self-role conflict. In H. H. Gregory, ed., *Learning theory and stuttering therapy.* Evanston, Ill.: Northwestern University Press.

Sheehan, J. G. (1969a) Cyclic variation in stuttering: Comment on Taylor and Taylor's "Test of predictions from the conflict hypothesis of stuttering." *Journal of Abnormal Psychology, 74,* 452–453.

Sheehan, J. G. (1969b) The role of role in stuttering. In B. Gray and G. England, eds., *Stuttering and the conditioning therapies.* Monterey, Calif.: Monterey Institute for Speech and Hearing.

Sheehan, J. G., Cortese, P. A., and Hadley, R. G. (1962) Guilt, shame, and tension in graphic projections of stuttering. *Journal of Speech and Hearing Disorders, 27,* 129–139.

Sheehan, J. G., Frederick, C. J., Rosevear, W. H., and Spiegelman, M. (1954) A validity study of the Rorschach prognostic rating scale. *Journal of Projective Techniques, 18,* 233–239.

Sheehan, J. G., Hadley, R. G., and Gould, E. (1967) Impact of authority on stuttering. *Journal of Abnormal Psychology, 72,* 290–293.

Sheehan, J. G., and Martyn, M. M. (1966) Spontaneous recovery from stuttering. *Journal of Speech and Hearing Research, 9,* 121–135.

Sheehan, J. G., and Martyn, M. M. (1967) Methodology in studies of recovery from stuttering. *Journal of Speech and Hearing Research, 10,* 396–400.

Sheehan, J. G., Martyn, M. M., and Kilburn, K. L. (1968) Speech disorders in retardation. *American Journal of Mental Deficiency, 73,* 251–256.

Sheehan, J. G., and Voas, R. B. (1954) Tension patterns during stuttering in relation to conflict, anxiety-binding, and reinforcement. *Speech Monographs, 21,* 272–279.

Sheehan, J. G., and Voas, R. B. (1957) Stuttering as conflict: A comparison of therapy techniques involving approach and avoidance. *Journal of Speech and Hearing Disorders, 22,* 714–723.

Sheehan, J. G., and Zelen, S. L. (1955) Level of aspiration in stutterers and non-stutterers. *Journal of Abnormal and Social Psychology, 51,* 83–86.

Sherman, D. (1952) Clinical and experimental use of Iowa scale of severity of stuttering. *Journal of Speech and Hearing Disorders, 17,* 316–320.

Sherman, D. (1955) Reliability and utility of individual ratings of severity of audible characteristics of stuttering. *Journal of Speech and Hearing Disorders, 20,* 11–16.

Sherman, D., and McDermott, R. (1958) Individual ratings of severity of moments of stuttering. *Journal of Speech and Hearing Research, 1,* 61–67.

Sherman, D., and Trotter, W. D. (1956) Correlation between two measures of the severity of stuttering. *Journal of Speech and Hearing Disorders, 21,* 426–429.

Sherman, D., Young, M. A., Gough, K. (1958) Comparison of three measures of stuttering severity. *Proceedings of the Iowa Academy of Science, 65,* 381–384.

Shoemaker, D., and Brutten, E. J. (1969) A two-factor approach to the modification of stuttering. In B. Gray and G. England, eds., *Stuttering and the conditioning therapies.* Monterey, Calif.: Monterey Institute for Speech and Hearing.

Shrum, William F. (1967) A study of the speaking behavior of stutterers and nonstutterers by means of multichannel electromyography. *Dissertation Abstracts, 28*(2-A), 825.

Shtremel, A. K. (1963) Stuttering in left parietal lobe syndrome. *Zhurnal Nevropatologii i Psikhiatrii imeni S. S. Korsakova, 63,* 828–832. (Russian)

Shulman, E. (1955) Factors influencing the variability of stuttering. In W. Johnson and R. Leutenegger, eds., *Stuttering in children and adults.* Minneapolis: University of Minnesota Press.

Shumak, C. (1955) A speech situation rating sheet for stutterers. In W. Johnson and R. Leutenegger, eds., *Stuttering in children and adults.* Minneapolis: University of Minnesota Press.

Sichel, J. P., Renoux, M., and de Bousingen, M. R. (1967) Apport du training autogène au traitement du bégaiement chez l'enfant. *Annales Medico-Psychologiques,* 2(5), 814.

Siegel, G. (1969) Experimental modification of speech dysfluency. In B. Gray and G. England, eds., *Stuttering and the conditioning therapies.* Monterey, Calif.: Monterey Institute for Speech and Hearing.

Siegel, G. M., and Haugen, D. (1964) Audience size and variations in stuttering behavior. *Journal of Speech and Hearing Research, 7,* 383–388.

Siegel, G. M., and Martin, R. R. (1965a) Experimental modification of disfluency in normal speakers. *Journal of Speech and Hearing Research, 8,* 235–244.

Siegel, G. M., and Martin, R. R. (1965b) Verbal punishment of disfluencies in normal speakers. *Journal of Speech and Hearing Research, 8,* 245–251.

Siegel, G. M., and Martin, R. R. (1966) Punishment of disfluencies in normal speakers. *Journal of Speech and Hearing Research, 9,* 208–218.

Siegel, G. M., and Martin, R. R. (1967a) Interpersonal approaches to the study of communication disorders. *Journal of Speech and Hearing Disorders, 32,* 112–120.

Siegel, G. M., and Martin, R. R. (1967b) Verbal punishment of disfluencies during spontaneous speech. *Language and Speech, 10*(4), 244–251.

Siegenthaler, B. M., and VanHattum, R. J. (1959) Characteristics of adult patients enrolled in an intensive speech and hearing therapy program. *Speech Monographs, 26,* 295–299.

Silverman, E. M., and Williams, D. E. (1967) A comparison of stuttering and nonstuttering children in terms of five measures of oral language development. *Journal of Communication Disorders, 14*(4), 305–309.

Silverman, F. H., and Williams, D. E. (1967) Loci of disfluencies in the speech of nonstutterers during oral reading. *Journal of Speech and Hearing Research, 10,* 790–794.

Silverman, F. H., and Williams, D. E. (1968) A proportional measure of stuttering adaptation. *Journal of Speech and Hearing Research, 11*(2), 444–448.

Simpson, B. C. (1966) *Stuttering therapy: A guide for the speech clinician.* Danville, Ill.: Interstate.

Sittig, E. (1952) Symptomatology of stuttering. *International*

Record of Medicine and General Practice Clinics, 165, 567–570.

Skalbeck, O. M. (1956) The relationship of expectancy of stuttering to certain other designated variables associated with stuttering. *Dissertation Abstracts, 16,* 1738.

Sklar, B. (1969) A feedback model of the stuttering problem —an engineer's view. *Journal of Speech and Hearing Disorders, 34,* 226–230.

Smith, A. M. (1953) Treatment of stutterers (on basis of psychoneurotic personality) with carbon dioxide. *Diseases of the Nervous System, 14,* 243–244.

Smith, D. R. (September 1954) They call themselves block busters. *American Mercury,* pp. 79–81.

Smith, L. W. (1967) Stuttering therapy then and now. *Today's Speech, 15,* 15–17.

Snidecor, J. C. (1955) Tension and facial appearance in stuttering. In W. Johnson and R. Leutenegger, eds., *Stuttering in children and adults.* Minneapolis: University of Minnesota Press.

Snyder, M. A. (1957) Counseling for parents of stuttering children. *Psychiatric Quarterly,* Supplement, *31,* 102–111.

Snyder, M. A. (1958) Stuttering and coordination. *Logos, 1,* 36–43.

Snyder, M. A. (1962) Evaluating in personality of the stutterer. In D. A. Barbara, ed., *The psychotherapy of stuttering.* Springfield, Ill.: Charles C Thomas.

Snyder, M. A., Henderson, D., Murphy, M., and O'Brien, R. (1958) The personality structure of stutterers as compared to that of parents of stutterers. *Logos, 2,* 97–105.

Soderberg, G. A. (1959) A study of the effects of delayed side-tone on four aspects of stutterers' speech during oral reading and spontaneous speech. Doctoral dissertation, Ohio State University, Columbus.

Soderberg, G. A. (1962a) Phonetic influence upon stuttering. *Journal of Speech and Hearing Research, 5,* 315–320.

Soderberg, G. A. (1962b) What is average stuttering? *Journal of Speech and Hearing Disorders, 27,* 85–86.

Soderberg, G. A. (1966) The relations of stuttering to word length and word frequency. *Journal of Speech and Hearing Research, 9,* 584–589.

Soderberg, G. A. (1967) Linguistic factors in stuttering. *Journal of Speech and Hearing Research, 10,* 801–810.

403

Soderberg, G. A. (1968) Delayed auditory feedback and stuttering. *Journal of Speech and Hearing Disorders, 33,* 260–267.

Soderberg, G. A. (1969) Delayed auditory feedback and the speech of stutterers: A review of studies. *Journal of Speech and Hearing Disorders, 34,* 20–29.

Solomon, N. D. (1952) A comparison of rigidity of behavior manifested by a group of stutterers compared with "fluent" speakers in oral and other performances as measured by the Einstellung-effect. *Speech Monographs, 19,* 198.

Sortini, A. J. (1955) Twenty years of stuttering research. *Exceptional Children, 25,* 181–183, 196.

Soufi, A. (1960) One-month stutterer. *Journal of Speech and Hearing Disorders, 25,* 411.

Speech Foundation of America (1960) *On stuttering and its treatment.* Memphis, Tenn.: M. Fraser.

Speech Foundation of America (1962) *Stuttering: Its prevention.* Memphis, Tenn.: M. Fraser.

Speech Foundation of America (1963) *Stuttering words.* Memphis, Tenn.: M. Fraser.

Speech Foundation of America (1964) *Stuttering: Treatment of the young stutterer in the schools.* Memphis, Tenn.: M. Fraser.

Speech Foundation of America (1966) *Stuttering: Training the therapist.* Memphis, Tenn.: M. Fraser.

Speech Foundation of America (1968) *Stuttering: Successes and failures in therapy.* Memphis, Tenn.: M. Fraser.

Speidel, L. M. (1963) A Rorschach experiment with stutterers and a control group. *Praxis der Kinderpsychologie und Kinderpsychiatrie, 12,* 241–245. (German)

Spielberger, C. D. (1954) The effects of stuttering behavior and response set upon tachistoscopic visual recognition thresholds. *Dissertation Abstracts, 14,* 2397–2398. Abstracts of doctoral dissertation, State University of Iowa.

Spielberger, C. D. (1956) The effects of stuttering behavior and response set on recognition thresholds. *Journal of Personality, 24,* 33–45.

Spriestersbach, D. C. (1951) Objective approach to investigation of social adjustment of male stutterers. I. *Journal of Speech and Hearing Disorders, 16,* 250–257.

Staats, L. C. (1955) Sense of humor in stutterers and non-stutterers. In W. Johnson and R. Leutenegger, eds., *Stut-*

tering in children and adults. Minneapolis: University of Minnesota Press.

Stammering cured when speech not heard. (November 19, 1955) *Science Newsletter,* p. 323.

Starbuck, H. B. (1952) The adaptation effect in stuttering behavior and its relation to breathing. *Speech Monographs, 19,* 198–199.

Starbuck, H. B. (1954) Determination of severity of stuttering and construction of an audio-visual scale. *Dissertation Abstracts, 14,* 2158. Abstract of doctoral dissertation, Purdue University.

Starbuck, H. B., and Steer, M. D. (1953) Adaptation effect in stuttering speech behavior and normal speech behavior. *Journal of Speech and Hearing Disorders, 18,* 252–255.

Starbuck, H. B., and Steer, M. D. (1954) The adaptation effect in stuttering and its relation to thoracic and abdominal breathing. *Journal of Speech and Hearing Disorders, 19,* 440–449.

Stein, L. (1949) Emotional background of stammering. *British Journal of Medical Psychology, 22,* 189–193.

Stein, L. (1951) The psychological structure of stammering. *Quarterly Bulletin of the British Psychological Society, 2,* 32.

Stein, L. (1954) Stammering as psychosomatic disorder. *Folia Phoniatrica, 6,* 12–46.

Stennet, N. E. (1964) *A workbook for stutterers.* Chicago: King.

Stern, E. (1955) Speech recording in stuttering therapy. *Journal of the South African Logopedic Society, 3,* 7–9.

Steven, M. (1963) The language of stuttering. *Journal of Indiana Speech and Hearing Association, 22,* 55–64.

Stewart, J. L. (April 1959) Problem of stuttering in certain North American Indian Societies. *Journal of Speech and Hearing Disorders,* Supplement, *6,* 1–87.

Strean, H. S. (1967) A note on the treatment of a stutterer in a group. *Journal of the Long Island Consultation Center, 5,* 41–44.

Streifler, M., and Gumpertz, F. (1955) Cerebral potentials in stuttering and cluttering. *Confinia Neurologica, 15,* 344–359.

Stromsta, C. P. (1956) A methodology related to the determination of the phase angle of bone-conducted speech sound energy of stutterers and nonstutterers. *Dissertation Abstracts, 16,* 1738–1739.

Stromsta, C. P. (1959) Experimental blockage of phonation by distorted sidetone. *Journal of Speech and Hearing Research, 2,* 286–301.

Stromsta, C. P. (1965) A procedure using group consensus in stuttering therapy. *Journal of Speech and Hearing Disorders, 30,* 277–279.

Stroobant, R. I. (1952) A psychological study of some stammering children. *New Zealand Speech Therapists Journal, 7,* 7–12.

Stunden, A. A. (1965) The effects of time pressure as a variable in the verbal behavior of stutterers. *Dissertation Abstracts, 26,* 1784–1785

Stuttering: Causes and treatment. (February 1963) *Good Housekeeping,* p. 152.

Stuttering clue to how Indians treated young. (February 21, 1953) *Science Newsletter,* p. 114.

Stuttering studies. (April 14, 1952) *Newsweek,* p. 64.

Sutton, S., and Chase, R. A. (1961) White noise and stuttering. *Journal of Speech and Hearing Research, 4,* 72.

Sutu, A., Mironescu, D., Cocinschi, R., Tirziu, O. and Miscoiu, M. (1964) Clinical and electroencephalographic contributions to a study of the pathogenesis of stammering. *Pediatrica, 8,* 39–49.

Swartout, J. M., and Benson, W. F. (April 1952) When stuttering is normal. *Today's Health, 30,* 38–40.

Szalka, V. (1965) The pathogenesis of stuttering and its pharmaceutical therapy. *Fül-orr-gégegyógyószat, 11,* 26–31.

Tabata, O. An analytic study of self-consciousness and interpersonal feeling in stuttering children. *Kyoto Daigaku Kyoikugakubu Kiyo, 12,* 46–60. (Japanese)

Tanberg, M. C. (1955) A study of the role of inhibition in the moment of stuttering. In W. Johnson and R. Leutenegger, eds., *Stuttering in children and adults.* Minneapolis: University of Minnesota Press.

Tate, M. W., and Cullinan, W. L. (1962) Measurement of consistency of stuttering. *Journal of Speech and Hearing Research, 5,* 272–283.

Tate, M. W., Cullinan, W. L., and Ahlstrand, A. (1961) Measurement of adaptation in stuttering. *Journal of Speech and Hearing Research, 4,* 321–329.

Tawadros, S. M. (1957) An experiment in the group psychotherapy of stutterers. *International Journal of Sociometry, 1,* 181–189.

Taylor, A. (1968) The effect of affect-laden words on perceptual thresholds of stutterers. *Dissertation Abstracts, 29,* 763–764.

Taylor, I. K. (1966a) The properties of stuttered words. *Journal of Verbal Learning and Verbal Behavior, 5,* 112–118.

Taylor, I. K. (1966b) What words are stuttered? *Psychological Bulletin, 65,* 233–242.

Taylor, I. K., and Taylor, M. M. (1967) Test of predictions from the conflict hypothesis of stuttering. *Journal of Abnormal and Social Psychology, 72,* 431–433.

Thile, Edmund L. (1967) An investigation of attitude differences in parents of stutterers and nonstutterers. *Dissertation Abstracts, 28*(5-B), 2174–2175.

Tomatis, A. (1956) Relations entre l'audition et la phonation, *Extait des Annals des Telecommunications, 2,* 10–19.

Travis, L. E. (1957) The unspeakable feelings of people with special reference to stuttering. In L. E. Travis, ed., *Handbook of speech pathology,* New York: Appleton.

Trojan, F. A. (1965) A new method in the treatment of stuttering: The kinetic discharge therapy. *Folia Phoniatrica, 17,* 195.

Trojan, L., and Weins, H. (1963) Studien zur stottertherapie, *Folia Phoniatrica, 15,* 42–67.

Trombly, T. (1965) Responses of stutterers and normal speakers to a level of aspiration. *Central States Speech Journal, 16,* 179–181.

Trotter, W. D. (1953) A study of the severity of the individual moments of stuttering under the conditions of successive readings of the same material. *Dissertation Abstracts, 13,* 891. Abstract of doctoral dissertation, State University of Iowa.

Trotter, W. D. (1955) The severity of stuttering during successive readings of the same material. *Journal of Speech and Hearing Disorders, 20,* 17–25.

Trotter, W. D. (1956) Relationship between severity of stuttering and word conspicuousness. *Journal of Speech and Hearing Disorders, 21,* 198–201.

Trotter, W. D., and Brown, L. (1958) Speaking time behavior of the stutterer before and after speech therapy. *Journal of Speech Research, 1,* 48–51.

407

Trotter, W. D., and Kools, J. A. (1955) Listener adaptation to the severity of stuttering. *Journal of Speech and Hearing Disorders, 20,* 385–387.

Trotter, W. D., and Lesch, M. M. (1967) Personal experiences with a stutter-aid. *Journal of Speech and Hearing Disorders, 32,* 270–272.

Truhlarova, M. (1962) Results of control examination of the speech of stuttering patients treated at the phoniatry department of Professor Seeman in Prague 7–10 years ago. *Ceskoslovenska Otolaryngologie, 11,* 20–29. (Czech)

Turetskiy, M. Y. (1954) Clinical-physiologic analysis of stammering in young children: Preliminary report. Pediatriyn, no. 3, 51–56. (Russian)

Tuttle, E. (1952) Hyperventilation in a patient who stammered: Methedrine as an adjunct to psychotherapy. *American Journal of Medicine, 13,* 777–779.

Ugulava, T. K. (1968) Nekotorye psikhicheskie osobennosti detei preddoshkol'nogo vozrasta i ikh rol' v razvitii zaikaniya. (Some psychological features of children of prekindergarten age and their role in the development of stuttering.) *Spetsial'naya Shkola, 2,* 89–94. (Russian)

Umeda, K. (1963) *Study and therapy of stuttering.* Tokyo: Seisei Gakwin.

Vandierendonck, R. (1962) Trial and synthesis of the problem of stuttering (evaluation of therapy). *Belgisch Tijdschrift voor Geneeskunde, 18,* 225–244. (Dutch)

Vandierendonck, R., et al. (1964) The laterality test in stutterers. A quantitative and qualitative investigation. *Belgisch Tijdschrift voor Geneeskunde, 20,* 850–857. (Dutch)

Van Riper, C. (1951) Therapy for stutterers. *Speech and Hearing Therapist* (Indiana), 10, 5–12.

Van Riper, C. (1953) The treatment of stuttering. *Speech* (London), 17, 17–20.

Van Riper, C. (1954) Stuttering. Chicago: National Society of Crippled Children and Adults.

Van Riper, C. (1955a) The conquest of stuttering, *Journal of the South African Logopedic Society, 3,* 18–20.

Van Riper, C. (1955b) The role of reassurance in stuttering therapy. *Folia Phoniatrica, 7,* 217–222.

Van Riper, C. (1958a) Adventures in stuttering therapy. In

J. Eisenson, ed., *Stuttering: A symposium.* New York: Harper & Row.

Van Riper, C. (1958b) Stammering. In *Conquering physical handicaps*, Proceedings of the First Pan-Pacific Rehabilitation Conference, Sydney, Australia.

Van Riper, C. (1963a) How stuttering perpetuates itself. *Logopeden*, 9, 4–6. (Norwegian)

Van Riper, C. (1963b) *Speech correction: Principles and methods.* 4th ed. Englewood Cliffs, N. J.: Prentice-Hall.

Van Riper, C. (1968) Prognostic factors in stuttering. *Journal of the South African Logopedic Society*, 15, 7–13.

Van Riper, C., and Gruber, L. (1957) *A casebook in stuttering.* New York: Harper & Row.

Van Riper, C., and Hull, C. J. (1955) The quantitative measurement of the effect of certain situations on stuttering. In W. Johnson and R. Leutenegger, eds., *Stuttering in children and adults.* Minneapolis: University of Minnesota Press.

Van Thal, J. H. (1957) Observations on unusual behavior by stammerers. *Folia Phoniatrica*, 9, 42–44.

Vette, G., and Goven, P. (1966) *A manual for stuttering therapy.* Pittsburgh: Stanwix House.

Villarreal, J. J. (1950) Two aspects of stuttering therapy. *Journal of Speech and Hearing Disorders*, 15, 215–220.

Villarreal, J. J. (1962) The role of the speech pathologist in psychotherapy. In D. A. Barbara, ed., *The psychotherapy of stuttering.* Springfield, Ill.: Charles C Thomas.

Villarreal, J. J., and Blackwell, T. (1951) Projective tests in planning therapy for stutterers. *Southern Speech Journal*, 16, 251–259.

Vlasova, N. A. (1962) Prevention and treatment of stuttering in children in the U.S.S.R. *Ceskoslovenska Otolaryngologie*, 11, 30–32. (Czech)

Vlasova, N. A. (1963) Value of the complex method of treatment of stuttering in children. *Folia Phoniatrica*, 16, 39–43. (French)

Volterra, V., et al. (1964) EEG contribution to the study of Pavor Nocturnus. *Rivista di Neurologia*, 34, 88–100. (Italian)

von Staabs, G. (February 1952) Treatment of stuttering by repetition of single child growth phases in experience with the Sceno test play therapy. *Psyché*, pp. 688–706.

409

Wallen, V. (1959) A Q-technique study of the self-concepts of adolescent stutterers and non-stutterers. Doctoral dissertation, Boston University School of Education, Boston, Mass.

Wallen, V. (1961a) Stutterer with a low I.Q. *Journal of Speech and Hearing Disorders, 26,* 89.

Wallen, V. (1961b) Primary stuttering in a twenty-eight-year-old adult. *Journal of Speech and Hearing Disorders, 26,* 394.

Walnut, F. (1954) A personality inventory item analysis of individuals who have other handicaps. *Journal of Speech and Hearing Disorders, 19,* 220–227.

Walton, D. (1958) Learning theory, personality, drug-action and the treatment of stammering. *Bulletin of the British Psychological Society, 36,* 37–38. Abstract.

Walton, D., and Black, D. A. (1958) The application of learning theory to the treatment of stammering. *Journal of Psychosomatic Research, 3,* 170–179.

Walton, D., *et al.* (1963) The relevance of generalization techniques to the treatment of stammering and phobic symptoms. *Behaviour Research and Therapy, 1,* 121–125.

Weinberg, B. (August 1964) Stuttering among blind and partially sighted children. *Journal of Speech and Hearing Disorders, 29,* 322–326.

Weinstock, J. J. (1968) A child psychiatrist's view of therapy for stuttering. *Journal of Speech and Hearing Disorders, 33*(1), 15–20.

Weiss, D. A. (1950) The relation between cluttering and stuttering: A preliminary investigation of the problem of stuttering. *Folia Phoniatrica, 2,* 252–262. (German)

Weiss, D. A. (1960) Therapy for cluttering. *Folia Phoniatrica, 12,* 216–228.

Weiss, D. A., and Beebe, H. (1950) *The chewing approach in speech and voice therapy.* White Plains, N.Y.: S. Karger, 19–38.

Weissova, B., and Handzel, L. (1962) The problem of familial stuttering on the basis of parathyroid gland insufficiency. *Ceskoslovenska Otolaryngologie, 11,* 57–60. (Czech)

Welch, I. L. (1960) An investigation of the listening proficiency of stutterers. Doctoral dissertation, University of Missouri, Columbia.

Wendahl, R. W., and Cole, J. (1961) Identification of stuttering during relatively fluent speech. *Journal of Speech and Hearing Research, 4,* 281–286.

Wertheim, E. X. (1967) The family as a psychosomatic unit: A case study. *Australian Psychologist, 2*(1), 167 (abstract).

West, R. (1958) An agnostic's speculation about stuttering. In J. Eisenson, ed., *Stuttering: A symposium.* New York: Harper & Row.

West, R. (1964) The land of silence. *Voice, 13,* 15–18.

West, R., and Ansberry, M. (1968) *The rehabilitation of speech.* 4th ed. New York: Harper & Row.

Weuffen, M. (1961) A study on word finding by normal and stuttering children and adolescents from 8–16 years of age. *Folia Phoniatrica, 13,* 255–268.

Wiesenhütter, E. (1955) Anthropological interpretation of stuttering. *Zeitschrift für Psychotherapie und Medizinische Psychologie, 5,* 64–75.

Wilhelm, W. (1958) Subjective speech tempo. *Psychologische Rundschau, 9,* 53–57.

Williams, D. E. (1953) An evaluation of masseter muscle action potentials in stuttered and non-stuttered speech. *Speech Monographs, 20,* 190. Abstract of doctoral dissertation, State University of Iowa, 1952.

Williams, D. E. (1955a) Intensive clinical case studies of stuttering therapy. In W. Johnson and R. Leutenegger, eds., *Stuttering in children and adults.* Minneapolis: University of Minnesota Press.

Williams, D. E. (1955b) Masseter muscle action potentials in stuttered and nonstuttered speech. *Journal of Speech and Hearing Disorders, 20,* 242–261.

Williams, D. E. (1957) A point of view about stuttering. *Journal of Speech and Hearing Disorders, 22,* 390–397.

Williams, D. E. (1959) Effects of meprobamate on stuttering. *American Practitioner and Digest of Treatment, 10,* 1734–1736.

Williams, D. E. (1968) Stuttering therapy: an overview. In H. H. Gregory, ed., *Learning theory and stuttering therapy.* Evanston, Ill.: Northwestern University Press.

Williams, D. E., and Kent, L. R. (1958) Listener's evaluations of speech interruptions. *Journal of Speech and Hearing Research, 1,* 124–136.

Williams, D. E., and Roe, A. M. (1960) Teachers, parents and stutterers. *Education, 80,* 471–475.

Williams, D. E., and Silverman, F. H. (1968) Note concerning

411

articulation of school-age stutterers. *Perceptual and Motor Skills, 27,* 713–714.

Williams, D. E., Silverman, F. H., and Kools, J. A. (1969) Disfluency behavior of elementary school stutterers and nonstutterers: the consistency effect. *Journal of Speech and Hearing Research, 12,* 30–38.

Williams, D. E., Silverman, F. H., and Kools, J. A. (1969) Disfluency behavior of elementary-school stutterers and nonstutterers: loci of instances of disfluency. *Journal of Speech and Hearing Research, 12,* 308–318.

Williams, J. D. (1954) A study of stuttering adaptation under assumed minimization of anxiety motivation. *Dissertation Abstracts, 14,* 2343–2344. Abstract of doctoral dissertation, State University of Iowa, 1954.

Willmore, L. (1960) The adult stammerer. *Practitioner, 184,* 621–625.

Wilson, A. W. (1964) Inability to open the mouth: An unusual psychosomatic symptom. *Comprehensive Psychiatry, 5,* 271–278.

Wilson, D. M. (1951) A study of the personalities of stuttering children and their parents as revealed through projection tests. *Speech Monographs, 18,* 133.

Wilson, R. G. (1950) A study of expressive movements in three groups of adolescent boys, stutterers, non-stutterers maladjusted and normals, by means of three measures of personality, Mira's Myokinetic Psychodiagnosis, the Bender-Gestalt, and figure drawing. Doctoral dissertation, Western Reserve University, Cleveland.

Wilton, G. (1950) *How to overcome stammering.* New York: Harper & Row.

Wingate, M. E. (1956) An experimental investigation of the effect produced by calling attention to stuttering. *Dissertation Abstracts, 16,* 1722.

Wingate, M. E. (1959) Calling attention to stuttering. *Journal of Speech and Hearing Research, 2,* 326–335.

Wingate, M. E. (1962a) Evaluation and stuttering. *Journal of Speech and Hearing Research, 27,* 106–115, 244–257, 368–377.

Wingate, M. E. (1962b) Personality needs of stutterers. *Logos: Bulletin of the National Hospital for Speech Disorders* (New York), *5,* 35–38.

Wingate, M. E. (1964) Recovery from stuttering. *Journal of Speech and Hearing Disorders, 29,* 312–321.

Wingate, M. E. (1964) A standard definition of stuttering. *Journal of Speech and Hearing Disorders, 29,* 484–489.

Wingate, M. E. (1966a) Prosody in stuttering adaptation. *Journal of Speech and Hearing Research, 9,* 550–556.

Wingate, M. E. (1966b) Behavioral rigidity in stutterers. *Journal of Speech and Hearing Research, 9,* 626–629.

Wingate, M. E. (1966c) Stuttering adaptation and learning. I. The relevance of adaptation studies to stuttering as learned behavior. *Journal of Speech and Hearing Disorders, 31,* 148–156.

Wingate, M. E. (1966d) Stuttering adaptation and learning. II. The adequacy of learning principles in the interpretation of stuttering. *Journal of Speech and Hearing Disorders, 31,* 211–218.

Wingate, M. E. (1967) Slurvian skill of stutterers. *Journal of Speech and Hearing Research, 10,* 844–848.

Wischner, G. J. (1950) Stuttering behavior and learning: Preliminary theoretic formulation. *Journal of Speech and Hearing Disorders, 15,* 324–335.

Wischner, G. J. (1952a) Anxiety-reduction as reinforcement in maladaptive behavior: Evidence in stutterers' representations of the moment of difficulty. *Journal of Abnormal Psychology, 47,* 566–571.

Wischner, G. J. (1952b) Experimental approach to expectancy and anxiety in stuttering behavior. *Journal of Speech and Hearing Disorders, 17,* 139–154.

Wischner, G. J. (1969) Stuttering behavior, learning theory and behavior therapy: problems, issues and progress. In B. Gray and G. England, eds., *Stuttering and the conditioning therapies.* Monterey, Calif.: Monterey Institute for Speech and Hearing.

Wischner, G. J., and Goss, A. E. (1960) Pictorial representations of situations involving threat. Illustration. *Journal of Clinical Psychology, 16,* 196–200.

Wohl, M. T. (1955) The sequellae of stammer. *Speech* (London), *9,* 68–70.

Wolpe, J. (1969) Behavior therapy of stuttering: Deconditioning the emotional factor. In B. Gray and G. England, eds., *Stuttering and the conditioning therapies.* Monterey, Calif.: Monterey Institute for Speech and Hearing.

Wolski, W. (1967) Speech and language disorders in children. *Clinical Pediatrics, 6,* 599–601.

Woody, D. J. (1968) The effects of certain operant conditioning techniques in the control of stuttering. *Journal* of Speech and Hearing Association of Virginia, 9, 14–20.

Worster-Drought, C. (1968) Speech disorders in children. *Developmental Medicine and Child Neurology, 10,* 427–440.

Wulffert, N. F. (1964) Recent work in Bulgaria on the treatment of logoneuroses. *Review of Soviet Medical Sciences, 1,* 57–61.

Wyatt, G. L. (1958) Developmental crisis theory of stuttering. *Language and Speech, 1,* 250–264.

Wyatt, G. L. (1958) Mother-child relationship and stuttering in children. *Dissertation Abstracts, 19,* 881–882.

Wyatt, G. L., and Herzan, H. M. (1962) Therapy with stuttering children and their mothers. *American Journal of Orthopsychiatry, 32,* 645–649.

Yastrebova, A. V. (1962) Osobennoste Ustnoi e Pis-Mennoi Rechi u Zackyushchelhsya Uchashchekhsya, *(Peculiarities in the oral and written speech of stuttering pupils.)* Moscow: Institute of Defectology.

Yastrebova, A. V. (1968) Iz opyta raboty s zaikayushchimisya uchashchimisya. (From the experience of working with stuttering pupils.) *Spetsial'naya Shkola, 3,* 124–133. Russian)

Yates, A. (1969) The relationship between theory and therapy in the clinical treatment of stuttering. In B. Gray and G. England, eds., *Stuttering and the conditioning therapies.* Monterey, Calif.: Monterey Institute for Speech and Hearing.

Yates, A. J. (August 1963) Recent empirical and theoretical approaches to the experimental manipulation of speech in normal subjects and stammerers. *Behaviour Research and Therapy, 1,* 95–119.

Young, E. H. (1958) A personal experience with speech. *Journal of Speech and Hearing Disorders, 23,* 136–142.

Young, E. H. (1965) The motokinesthetic approach to the prevention of speech disorders, including stuttering. *Journal of Speech and Hearing Disorders, 30,* 269–273.

Young, M. A. (1960) Predicting severity of stuttering. Doctoral dissertation, State University of Iowa, Iowa City, Iowa.

Young, M. A. (1964) Identification of stutterers from recorded samples of their "fluent speech." *Journal of Speech and Hearing Research, 7,* 302–303.

Young, M. A. (1965) Audience size, perceived situational difficulty, and stuttering frequency. *Journal of Speech and Hearing Research, 8,* 401–407.

Young, M. A. (1969) Observer agreement: Cumulative effects of rating many samples. *Journal of Speech and Hearing Research, 12,* 135–143.

Young, M. A. (1969) Observer agreement: Cumulative effects of repeated ratings of the same samples and of knowledge of group results. *Journal of Speech and Hearing Research, 12,* 144–155.

Young, M. A., and Prather, E. (1962) Measuring severity of stuttering using short segments of speech. *Journal of Speech and Hearing Research, 5,* 256–262.

Zaliouk, A. (1954) Une méthode de traitement de la dysphémia (begaiement) chez enfants et adultes. (A method of treatment of sysphemia (stuttering) in children and adults.) *Encéphale, 43,* 337–346.

Zaluek, D. (1961–1962) Hagimgum: Avhana vedarkhey ripuy. (Stammering: Its diagnosis and healing.) *Hahinukh, 34,* 39–42.

Zelen, S. L., Sheehan, J. G., and Bugental, J. F. T. (1954) Self-perception in stuttering. *Journal of Clinical Psychology, 10,* 70–72.

Zerneri, L. (1966) Attempts to use delayed speech feedback in stuttering therapy. *Journal Francais d' Oto-Rhino-Laryngologie et Chirurgie Maxillo-Faciale, 15,* 415–418. (French)

Zürneck, E. (1964) On appropriate aid for stuttering children. *Ceffentliche Gesundheitsdienst, 26,* 17–21. (German)

INDEX

Designed by Michel Craig   70 71 72 73 7 6 5 4 3 2 1